T0073064

Principles and Practice of Health Promotion and Public Health

Principles and Practice of Health Promotion and Public Health brings together the disciplines and fields of study that inform the work of promoting health into one book and provides many examples of practice.

It starts with understanding ourselves and our health and continues with chapters on working in health promotion and public health; epidemiology; research methods and evidence-based practice; health psychology; communicating health; health education; health promotion; public health; health protection; arts and health; tackling tobacco, alcohol and drugs; tackling overweight; promoting health in workplaces and promoting health within the National Health Service. Together these communicate the core principles of how to prevent disease and promote health when working with individuals, communities and populations in any country across the world. The book focusses on adults' health and includes international and UK examples. *Principles and Practice of Health Promotion and Public Health* complements *Priorities for Health Promotion and Public Health*, published in 2021. Both are core texts for those studying health promotion or public health and supplementary texts for students of healthcare and social care. They are ideal for public health practitioners and members of the wider public health workforce.

Sally Robinson is a Visiting Reader in Health Promotion and Public Health at Canterbury Christ Church University.

Principles and Practice of Health Promotion and Public Health

Edited by Sally Robinson

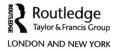

Routledge
Taylor & Francis Group

LONDON AND NEW YORK

Designed cover image: © Getty Images

First published 2023
by Routledge
4 Park Square, Milton Park, Abingdon, Oxon OX14 4RN

and by Routledge
605 Third Avenue, New York, NY 10158

Routledge is an imprint of the Taylor & Francis Group, an informa business

British Library Cataloguing-in-Publication Data
A catalogue record for this book is available from the British Library

Library of Congress Cataloging-in-Publication Data
Names: Robinson, Sally, editor.
Title: Principles and practice of health promotion and public health /
edited by Sally Robinson.
Description: Third edition. | Abingdon, Oxon ; New York, NY : Routledge,
2023. | Series: Canterbury public health series | Includes
bibliographical references and index. |
Identifiers: LCCN 2022032745 (print) | LCCN 2022032746 (ebook) | ISBN
9781032411248 (hbk) | ISBN 9780367423445 (pbk) | ISBN 9780367823696 (ebk)
Subjects: LCSH: Health promotion--United Kingdom. | Public health--United
Kingdom. | Medicine, Preventive--United Kingdom.
Classification: LCC RA427.8 .P7534 2023 (print) | LCC RA427.8 (ebook) |
DDC 362.10941--dc23/eng/20220729
LC record available at https://lccn.loc.gov/2022032745
LC ebook record available at https://lccn.loc.gov/2022032746

ISBN: 978-1-032-41124-8 (hbk)
ISBN: 978-0-367-42344-5 (pbk)
ISBN: 978-0-367-82369-6 (ebk)

DOI: 10.4324/9780367823696

Typeset in Times New Roman
by KnowledgeWorks Global Ltd.

Contents

List of figures   vii
List of tables   x
List of boxes   xii
List of contributors   xiv
Preface   xvii
Acknowledgements   xviii

PART I
Fundamentals of health promotion and public health practice   1

1 Understanding ourselves and our health   3
   SALLY ROBINSON

2 Working in health promotion and public health   28
   LOUISE HOLDEN, EM RAHMAN, BRANWEN THOMAS AND SALLY ROBINSON

PART II
Disciplines and fields of study   61

3 Epidemiology   63
   RAJEEB KUMAR SAH AND GAIL SHEPPARD

4 Research methods and evidence-based practice   89
   ELISABETTA CORVO, JOANNE CAIRNS AND SALLY ROBINSON

5 Health psychology   113
   MURRAY ALLEN

6 Communicating health   133
   SALLY ROBINSON

7 Health education   157
SALLY ROBINSON

8 Health promotion   194
SALLY ROBINSON

9 Public health   225
RAJEEB KUMAR SAH, DEVENDRA RAJ SINGH, LALITA KUMARI SAH
AND SALLY ROBINSON

10 Health protection   249
MERADIN PEACHEY

11 Arts and health   275
TRISH (PATRICIA) VELLA-BURROWS AND CHRISTINA DAVIES

PART III
Tackling priorities for health promotion and public health   295

12 Tackling tobacco, alcohol and drugs   297
SALLY ROBINSON

13 Tackling overweight   323
SALLY ROBINSON

PART IV
Promoting health within settings   353

14 Promoting health in workplaces   355
SALLY ROBINSON

15 Promoting health in the National Health Service   382
SALLY ROBINSON

Index   409

Figures

1.1   Neurons   4
1.2   The bioecological model of human development   6
1.3   Cultural messages influence the ideal self, self-concept and self-esteem   8
1.4   Maslow's hierarchy of needs   10
1.5   The biopsychosocial model   14
1.6   Sustainable development goals   21
1.7   Interdependent healthy people in a healthy society and healthy planet   22
2.1   Public health domains and functions   29
2.2   The public health workforce   31
2.3   UK Public Health Skills and Knowledge Framework   43
2.4   WHO-ASPHER Competency Framework   45
2.5   The CompHP core competencies for health promotion   49
3.1   Life expectancy for males and females in the UK between 1980 to 1984
      and 2018 to 2020   64
3.2   UK population pyramid, 2020 ($n = 67,886,004$)   65
3.3   A bill of mortality February 21st to 28th 1664   70
3.4   John Graunt's data based on the bills of mortality 1647 to 1659   71
3.5   Number of male deaths in the UK by the leading causes, 2001 to 2018   73
3.6   Observational studies   77
3.7   Age-specific incidence rates of cancer in the UK, 2016 to 2018   78
3.8   Teenage pregnancies in Scotland by age at conception, 1994 to 2019   79
3.9   Cohort study design   81
3.10 Case-control study design   82
3.11 Experimental studies   83
5.1   The health belief model   117
5.2   The theory of reasoned action   118
5.3   The theory of planned behaviour   119
5.4   The transtheoretical model   121
5.5   The common-sense model   124
6.1   The communications continuum: moving audiences towards
      health action   148
7.1   The General Board of Health, 1846   160
7.2   Broadsheet: cholera and water, 1866   161
7.3   Hygiene demonstration cabinet, 1895   162
7.4   A School for Mothers, 1907   163
7.5   Protests against COVID-19 coronavirus regulations in London   165

7.6	The health continuum	168
7.7	A sticker illustrates the preventive model/medical approach, dated between 1950 and 1970	173
7.8	A poster illustrates the preventive model/behaviour change approach, 1988	175
7.9	A leaflet demonstrates a holistic approach to health and self-help	178
7.10	A poster illustrates a resource to support self-empowerment	187
8.1	Health promotion comprises four models	195
8.2	Ottawa Charter for Health Promotion	198
8.3	From community disempowerment to empowerment	211
8.4	Priorities for the European Healthy Cities Network 2019 to 2024	214
9.1	Sir Edwin Chadwick	226
9.2	Three domains of public health practice	230
9.3	Healthcare need, supply and demand	235
9.4	Five steps of a health needs assessment	236
9.5	Five stages of a health impact assessment	243
10.1	The disease triangle	250
10.2	Transmission cycle of malaria	250
10.3	Global disease burden by cause, 1990 to 2019, measured as disability-adjusted-life years per year	251
10.4	Campylobacter gastroenteritis poisoning from restaurant pâté, Scotland 2006 ($n = 47$ diners)	253
10.5	Control measures may be introduced at any step of managing an outbreak	254
10.6	The body produces a specific antibody for every new antigen	257
10.7	Confirmed cases of measles in Wales from 1996 to 2020	258
10.8	Fatal injuries to employees and the self-employed by the most common kinds of accidents, 2016/17 to 2020/21	266
10.9	Non-fatal injuries to employees by the most common kinds of accidents, 2020 to 2021	267
10.10	Percentage uptake of cervical screening among women (25 to 64 years), Scotland 2020 to 2021	271
11.1	Five art forms with examples	276
11.2	Arts engagement across primary, secondary and tertiary prevention	281
12.1	The UK national needle exchange symbol	300
12.2	Example of health warnings on a packet of cigarettes	312
12.3	Stoptober 2021	313
13.1	Energy balance	324
13.2	Gastrointestinal tract	325
13.3	Energy imbalance and gaining body fat	327
13.4	Energy imbalance and losing body fat	328
13.5	Eatwell Guide	336
13.6	Yo-yo dieting	337
13.7	Ice cream consumption in dieters and non-dieters	338
13.8	Liquid lunches	341
13.9	The microbiome, health and body fat	344
14.1	Quality of work by socio-economic classification, 2020	360
14.2	Nine hazard pictograms to indicate a hazardous chemical	363

14.3   How the psychosocial work environment influences workers' health   364
14.4   Demand/control model   365
14.5   Effort/reward imbalance at work   366
14.6   Work-related psychosocial experiences of workers in England
       aged 50 to 69 years, 2018   367
14.7   CIPD wellbeing model   376
14.8   WHO Healthy workplace model   377
15.1   The health system should draw attention to the social and
       environmental determinants of health   389
15.2   'Falling Leaves' by Sian Tucker at Chelsea and Westminster Hospital,
       London   390
15.3   'Jos' by Jonathan Delafield Cook at Chelsea and Westminster Hospital,
       London   391
15.4   'Assembly450' by Joy Gerrard at Chelsea and Westminster Hospital,
       London   391
15.5   'Radiance' by Adam Nathaniel Furman at Chelsea and Westminster
       Hospital, London   392
15.6   Zola's river   395
15.7   Navigating Antonovsky's river of life between ease and dis-ease   398
15.8   The salutogenic umbrella   399

Tables

1.1	Human values	5
1.2	Examples of disciplines, fields of study, sectors and agencies which contribute to health	25
2.1	Examples of job roles within the UK public health workforce	34
2.2	Using PHSKF competencies to support a social prescriber's work objectives	44
2.3	WHO-ASPHER competencies relating to collaboration and partnerships	46
2.4	A personal development plan referencing WHO-ASPHER competencies	47
2.5	WHO-ASPHER competencies for working in health promotion and addressing health inequity (EPHO 4)	48
2.6	Examples of career routes	57
3.1	Most common causes of female deaths in the UK, 1915 to 1975	74
3.2	Validity of a screening test	85
4.1	Glossary of research terms	91
4.2	Useful databases for searching for health promotion and public health evidence	93
4.3	A critical appraisal tool	95
4.4	Philosophy, methodology, methods and question types	98
4.5	Types of questions	99
4.6	Advantages and disadvantages of online qualitative research	103
6.1	Verbal and non-verbal communication in therapeutic, person-centred, one-to-one communication	140
7.1	Disease prevention versus health education	169
7.2	Preventive, educational and empowerment models	170
7.3	The preventive model	172
7.4	Methods to meet learning objectives	180
8.1	Models of health promotion	196
8.2	Global conferences on health promotion	200
8.3	Political ideologies	202
8.4	Comparing health promotion with public health	221
9.1	A summary of the five waves of public health	228
9.2	Examples of health indicators for England	233
10.1	Worldwide distribution, infections and deaths in recent pandemics	254
10.2	Preventing food poisoning from fruit and vegetables	260

10.3 UK mass screening programmes offered through the National Health Service 269

11.1 Examples of pivotal works in the arts and health field, 1996 to 2021 279

11.2 Healthy arts framework 282

12.1 UK drug penalties 298

12.2 Health promotion interventions to reduce substance-related harm 309

12.3 Health warnings on cigarette packets across the world, 2021 311

12.4 Health warnings and alcohol across the world, 2016 312

13.1 Estimated average requirements for energy 327

13.2 Comparison of calorie expenditure between sedentary behaviour and moderate activity 329

13.3 UK Physical Activity Guidelines 330

13.4 Carbohydrates 330

13.5 Examples of recommended portion sizes 332

13.6 Factors which encourage and discourage excess body fat 346

14.1 Death rates by occupation in England and Wales, 2001 to 2011 359

14.2 Examples of causes of injuries, illness and death at work by British industries 362

14.3 Current UK smokers by occupation, 2019 372

14.4 Heavy alcohol consumption among UK workers aged 40 to 46 years, by occupation, 2006 to 2010 ($n = 100,817$) 372

14.5 UK average sitting times by occupation, 2019 ($n = 1,200$ workers; 10 worksites) 373

15.1 Comparison of the NHS in the 1950s to a modern health system 386

Boxes

1.1	Health	11
1.2	1944	13
1.3	Stanley	16
1.4	Constitution of the World Health Organization	19
1.5	The social work setting	20
1.6	Health promotion in Nazi Germany	23
2.1	Health improvement lead for mental health	32
2.2	Registered principal public health practitioner	52
2.3	Registered psychologist and registered public health specialist	54
3.1	From outbreak to pandemic: COVID-19 coronavirus	66
3.2	Some epidemiological calculations	73
4.1	From researcher to student	93
4.2	Example of a questionnaire	100
4.3	Example of an interview guide	104
6.1	Assessing readability	135
6.2	Writing to express the experience of cancer	138
6.3	Mass communication and COVID-19 coronavirus in the UK	143
6.4	UK COVID-19 coronavirus media campaign	144
7.1	Power	158
7.2	Kitty Wilkinson, the 'saint of the slums'	161
7.3	Fresh air	162
7.4	Salutogenesis	169
7.5	Be Clear on Cancer	173
7.6	Five Ways to Wellbeing	181
7.7	Becoming a good listener	182
7.8	Learning to recognise we have choices	185
7.9	Being a self-empowered person	186
8.1	How health promotion models work together	197
8.2	Ethical health promotion practice	204
8.3	Singing to improve community cohesion in Italy during the COVID-19 pandemic, Spring 2020	208
8.4	Threats to community cohesion in the UK during the COVID-19 pandemic, January 2021	208
8.5	A community-based initiative using educational and empowerment models of health promotion	210
8.6	Healthy living centres	211

8.7	Examples of community action using an empowerment model of health promotion	212
8.8	Belfast Healthy City	214
8.9	A Healthy New Town: Bicester, Oxfordshire	216
9.1	Techniques for prioritising needs	237
10.1	Bhopal: the world's worst industrial disaster, 1984	262
10.2	Chernobyl: the world's worst nuclear disaster, 1986	263
10.3	Emergency response to Novichok poisoning in Salisbury, 2018	263
11.1	BBC Music Day, 2019	283
11.2	Singing for breathing	284
11.3	*Promesas y Traiciones* (Promises and betrayals)	286
11.4	The Creative Arts Pilot Project	288
12.1	Biopsychosocial: drug, set and setting model	300
12.2	Historical overview of tackling alcohol, drug and tobacco use in the United States of America and the United Kingdom	303
12.3	Weekly drinking guidelines	314
12.4	Cocaine Anonymous	317
13.1	Counting calories in crunchy nut peanut butter	333
13.2	Emotional eating as compulsive eating	334
13.3	The 2-Day Diet	343
14.1	Supporting a migrant workforce	369
14.2	Building workers' resilience	371
14.3	Work Ready	375
15.1	The creation of the NHS as separate from public health (the public's health)	385
15.2	#Hello my name is	393
15.3	Social prescribing	397
15.4	Hospice ward manager	400

Contributors

Murray Allen was a clinical exercise physiologist in cardiac rehabilitation and morbid obesity programmes for the National Health Service and a British Association of Sport and Exercise Sciences accredited sport scientist. Murray delivered behaviour change training for health professionals and applied his expertise to promote health behaviour changes for patients with complex comorbidities. In 2018, he joined the public health team at Canterbury Christ Church University. His teaching includes physical activity and health, psychology and health, health promotion, and major health and lifestyle issues.

Joanne Cairns is undertaking a research fellowship, funded by Yorkshire Cancer Research at Hull York Medical School (HYMS), on inequalities and cancer screening uptake. Before moving to HYMS, Jo was a lecturer in health promotion and public health at Canterbury Christ Church University (2017–2019). Previously, Jo worked for Alcohol Research UK as a senior research and policy officer (2016–2017). She also worked as a post-doctoral research associate and teaching fellow at Durham University (2012–2016) upon successful completion of her PhD in health geography. Jo's research and teaching experience are interdisciplinary spanning across social sciences, public health and medicine.

Elisabetta Corvo earned a degree in Jurisprudence before moving into public health and health promotion. Her PhD explored the effectiveness and transferability of an English model of health promotion to Italy. Afterwards she worked as a research fellow for the Department of Public Health and Infectious Disease at Sapienza University, Rome. She is course director of the MSc Global Public Health at Canterbury Christ Church University and leads the Public Health and Wellbeing Observatory. Her current research is focussed on health literacy, social capital and arts and health. Her teaching includes research methods and social aspects of health.

Christina Davies is a senior research fellow at the University of Western Australia. Her multi-award-winning research focusses on the areas of arts-health, health promotion and mental wellbeing. For the past 20 years, Christina has worked in academic, government and market research settings. Locally, nationally and internationally, she has successfully translated her arts-health research into policy and practice, with a number of her publications ranked by Altmetric in the top 1% of articles by attention internationally, e.g. *The art of being mentally healthy* and *The art of being healthy*.

Louise Holden is a visiting lecturer at Canterbury Christ Church University and has held numerous senior roles in the NHS, local government and Civil Service shaping national and local workforce strategies and building the evidence for effective interventions. She is currently responsible for establishing a workforce programme to improve the health of Londoners. As a registered public health practitioner, Louise contributes to UKPHR's quality assurance processes as a trained moderator. Her interests include standards setting, curriculum design and quality improvement.

Meradin Peachey has worked in healthcare and public health for 40 years, recently as director of public health for Kent and Berkshire West. Her career began as a nurse and she became one of the first non-medical public health consultants in England. She served as vice president of the Faculty of Public Health. Her health protection work has included enhancing immunisation programmes, protection from tuberculosis, leading emergency planning and the COVID-19 coronavirus response in Berkshire. With Master's degrees in Health Management and Global Public Health, Meradin now works as an independent consultant supporting sustainability across the world.

Em Rahman leads public health workforce development for Health Education England in South East England. His career has included developing behaviour change services, capacity building, workforce development, sexual health and community development; at local, regional and national levels. Em leads the Wessex UKPHR public health practitioner scheme. As a registered health promotion practitioner with IUHPE, Em is committed to supporting individuals and workforces through training and education, to recognise the role they have in addressing health inequalities.

Sally Robinson led the public health team at Canterbury Christ Church University from 2003 to 2018 and is now a visiting reader. She has developed, led and taught a wide range of courses for undergraduates, postgraduates and professionals working in public health, healthcare and education. She is an experienced supervisor of PhDs and external examiner to other universities. Her research and scholarship have centred on public health nutrition, health promotion and children's health and wellbeing.

Lalita Kumari Sah is a postgraduate researcher at Canterbury Christ Church University. She completed her BSc Medicine and Bachelor of Surgery (MBBS) at Zhengzhou University in China, followed by an MSc Public Health at London Metropolitan University, UK. She has worked to promote the health and wellbeing of diverse communities as a medical doctor in Nepal and within the UK National Health Service. Her publications span mental health and wellbeing, maternal and child health and global health inequalities.

Rajeeb Kumar Sah is a senior lecturer in public health at the University of Huddersfield. Previously, he was the course director for MSc Global Public Health at Canterbury Christ Church University. He has extensive experience in teaching public health to diverse groups of undergraduate and postgraduate students. He trained as a medical doctor and is an interdisciplinary researcher with a particular interest in international aspects of health and education. His research and publications include global public health, health inequalities, sexual and reproductive health/rights and mental health.

Gail Sheppard worked as an exercise physiologist in NHS cardiac rehabilitation prior to joining the public health team at Canterbury Christ Church University. Gail has led the academic team since 2018 and is a senior fellow of Advance HE. Her PhD research focusses on sedentary behaviour at work. Gail has been a member of the British Association of Cardiovascular Prevention and Rehabilitation (BACPR) since 2009, acting as Scientific Officer from 2011 to 2015. She is co-editor of BACPR's second edition of *Cardiovascular Prevention and Rehabilitation in Practice* guidelines (2020).

Devendra Raj Singh is a postgraduate researcher at the University of Huddersfield. He completed an MSc Health Promotion and Public Health at Canterbury Christ Church University. He has more than ten years' experience teaching and working in global and public health. His work has spanned health needs assessments, maternal and child health, sexual and reproductive health/rights and adolescent health. He has worked for various national and international organisations, including United Nations agencies. He has taught and supervised public health, nursing and pharmacy students and published extensively in international peer-reviewed journals.

Branwen Thomas works for Health Education England as a public health workforce lead for South East England. Her experience includes assuring the quality of educational programmes across the private sector, third sector, NHS and Civil Service, and leading the refreshed public health practitioner programme across the Thames Valley. More recently, she has supported the training of practitioners in response to the COVID-19 coronavirus pandemic. She has a keen interest in mentoring, developing networks for shared learning, social mobility and inclusion.

Trish (Patricia) Vella-Burrows is a visiting principal research fellow at the Sidney De Haan Research Centre for Arts and Health and a visiting lecturer in arts and health at Canterbury Christ Church University. As director of research for the Canterbury Cantata Trust, she is researching the impact of music on people living with degenerative neurological conditions. Trish is also director of Music4Wellbeing, a community interest company. Trish is interested in developing integrated models of care for people with dementia that equally address the holistic needs of family carers, care staff and those for whom they care.

Preface

In 2021, we published *Priorities for Health Promotion and Public Health* to support learning about 'what' health concerns have the most damaging effects on many people's lives and need to be prioritised, particularly in the UK. *Principles and Practice of Health Promotion and Public Health* is designed to explain 'how' we protect and promote people's health. These disciplines and fields of study inform practice within all countries and can be applied to any public health concern. Both books focus on working with adults and are designed to support those students and practitioners who want to understand more about improving everyone's health.

Acknowledgements

With thanks to Noah Silver for graphic design and Peter Main for his reading and comments.

Part I

Fundamentals of health promotion and public health practice

1 Understanding ourselves and our health

Sally Robinson

Key points

- Introduction
- What is a person?
- Vision of a healthy society
- A concept of health
- Summary

Introduction

This chapter argues that understanding people is central to understanding their health. It discusses a person as an evolving human being shaped by interactions between their biology, psychology and socio-cultural context. A person's life, their values and aspirations are unavoidably entwined with what health means for them. People live within societies where those with influence, and their vision of a healthy society, can powerfully shape how people's health is perceived and managed. We consider the influence of the medical model, the biopsychosocial model and the World Health Organization. Contemporary discussions suggest that health may be a person-centred, time-dependent, positive and holistic concept, but these ideas continue to be debated.

What is a person?

There may be as many answers to the question, "What is a person?" as there are people who have lived. It depends on perspective. In the 17th century, the philosopher Descartes famously argued that a person was the union of a physical body and a separate thinking mind. For many, metaphysical aspects such as the mind, soul or spirit are essential components of personhood and may continue after the body has died. Various scholars have distinguished a person from a 'non-person' by arguing a person is conscious, self-aware, intelligent, able to reason, engage in moral judgements and can be held accountable by other persons for their actions (White, 2013). Here, we explore a person as a continuously evolving human being shaped by the interrelationships between their biology, psychology and their social context.

A person may be described in terms of their nature, that is their genes; the water, fat, protein and minerals that make up their body, and the brain as its control centre. Nature is never static; it is influenced by the environment. For example, neuroscientists point to the ever-changing patterns of neurons in the brain which grow or wither

DOI: 10.4324/9780367823696-2

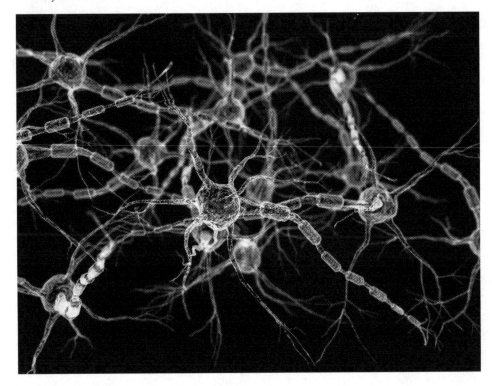

Figure 1.1 Neurons

Source: OlgaReukova/Shutterstock.com

in response to a person's physical, emotional and social experiences (Figure 1.1). The brain's ability to rewire, its plasticity, means we can learn and improve knowledge and skills because with each repetition the exact neuronal pathway is reinforced. The brain stores memories, some we can consciously recall, some we cannot. The oldest 'memories' relate to the instincts to 'fight, flight or freeze' in response to danger, seated in the neurons at the base of the brain, inherited from humans' reptile ancestors. The brain contains the emotional memories of interpersonal experiences that help a person to recognise and read faces and tune into the internal states of another person (Cozolino, 2006). These affect how a person reacts to events, situations and other people. For example, negative experiences encourage the neurons of the brain to record certain social interactions, perhaps certain people, as potentially threatening. When these reappear, the brain sends alert signals throughout the body to be physically ready to defend or attack. It simultaneously suppresses the functioning of the upper parts of the brain that allow a person to think clearly and rationally. In turn, this can have a negative impact on a person's communication, such as 'being lost for words' and their behaviour, such as aggression. Positive social experiences enable the brain to develop in a way that helps a person to trust and to engage in thinking, problem-solving and empathy so a person can communicate, learn and thrive.

Social psychologists also describe the human brain as being essentially social. They argue that by living and working together, people improve their chances of fulfilling their most basic needs: to survive and reproduce. It is people's abilities to think and

Table 1.1 Human values

Values	Essential motivations within the value
Self-direction	Freedom, independent thinking and actions, choosing, creating
Stimulation	Excitement, challenge, novelty, daring
Hedonism	Pleasure or sensuous gratification for oneself
Achievement	Personal success, demonstrating competence and meeting cultural standards
Power	Prestige and social status, control over people and resources
Security	Harmony, safety, stability within the self and with, and among, others
Conformity	Restraint of actions and impulses which may harm or upset others or violate social norms
Tradition	Commitment, respect, acceptance of customs and ideas within one's culture
Benevolence	Preserving and enhancing the welfare of others
Universalism	Understanding, tolerance, appreciation and protection of the welfare of people and nature

Source: Schwartz (2012).

feel that enable them to interact with people and the world. More than being social animals, Baumeister and Bushman (2014) argue people are cultural animals. Culture represents a dynamic social system of shared ideas, beliefs and values, which include those around food, language, customs and a shared sense of history. Where people's 'natural' instincts and drives such as thirst, hunger, aggression, sex or avoiding pain – to meet the primary needs of survival or reproduction – are activated, it is culture that might apply the brakes through rules of restraint. Cultural rules include laws, religious guidance, manners, codes of conduct and so forth. 'Society' refers to the people who share the culture. At times, a person will experience internal conflict between their impulses to fulfil personal values versus their need to adhere to the cultural values of the society in which they live (Table 1.1). To avoid punishment, they apply self-discipline, apply the cultural rules and control their own 'selfish'/natural impulses. For example, despite feeling hungry, we may avoid eating an apple because we know the sound of crunching will disturb others. It would be culturally unacceptable. The benefits of people living within a culture are that it enables people to be social, to live together, to share and to accumulate the knowledge and wisdom to help them to live well for longer.

Thinking point:

> Consider which one of the human values in Table 1.1 resonates most strongly with your own personality and goals. How important is the fulfilment of this value to your own health? Consider which values may conflict with one another. Which are most evident among your family or friends?

Bioecological model

Bronfenbrenner, a developmental psychologist, described a person, like all living things, as being at the heart of their own ecosystem. His bioecological model (Bronfenbrenner and Ceci, 1994; Bronfenbrenner and Morris, 1998; Tudge *et al.*, 2009) was one of the first examples of a social-ecological model. He suggested that a person

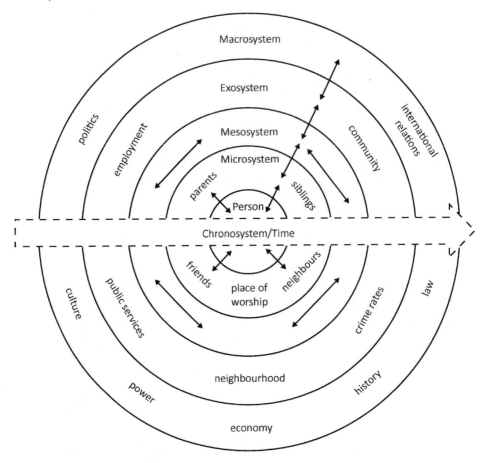

Figure 1.2 The bioecological model of human development

develops through the synergistic interconnections between their personal characteristics, their immediate socio-cultural context, their interactions and across time
(Figure 1.2).

- Person – an active biopsychosocial human organism comprising, for example, genes,
  age, sex, gender, physical characteristics, personality, temperament, cognitive and
  emotional intelligence, skills and personal resources such as their education
- Context – four interconnected systems of rules, norms, routines and the social
  roles people play:
  - microsystem, the immediate environment where the individual spends much
    time, e.g. family, peers, people in the local neighbourhood
  - mesosystem, how those in the microsystem interact with each other
  - exosystem, indirect influences from the wider community, e.g. a peaceful or
    violent neighbourhood, local employment levels and workplaces
  - macrosystem, the broad culture with its shared values and beliefs, social
    norms, political and socio-economic factors

- Processes (proximal processes) – regular, reciprocal, enduring and increasingly complex interactions between the person and people, objects and symbols in their environment. The word 'proximal' implies interactions with elements close to the person but, in the context of today's world, this is questioned (Griffore and Phenice, 2016). For example, we can be closely interacting via the Internet. The young Swedish environmental activist Greta Thunberg directly interacted with her microsystem, mesosystem and macrosystem. She went from discussions with her family to being invited to address the World Economic Forum in January 2020
- Time/chronosystem – interactions alter both the developing person and their environment over time. Thunberg changed others and was also changed herself (Hook, 2021). Time includes the time that interactions take and their repetition; the frequency and patterns of interactions over weeks or years; the influence of broader historical or cultural time periods such as living in the digital age; interactions and transitions over a person's lifespan and through generations

The self

Some psychologists look at the same process of a person's development from the inside by focussing on the person's self. Baumeister and Bushman (2014) write,

> "The self comes into being at the interface between the inner biological processes of the human body and the socio-cultural network to which the person belongs."

(p. 74)

The self is created within a person's interactions with others. It begins with Winnicott's observation that the mother's face, and how it looks to her baby, is the mirror in which the baby first begins to identify 'his own self' (Winnicott, 1971). If the baby sees delight, the baby learns he is a delight. If the baby sees impatience, he learns he is an irritation. The self is created and recreated as we move through life.

- A person's self-concept is how they describe themselves. It is a motivator in that a person usually behaves in ways that fit their own perception of who they are. This includes identity, such as having a gender identity, a work identity, a religious identity and a health identity
- A person's self-concept is made up of their self-image and their ideal self (Figure 1.3)
- A person's self-image is initially guided by the views and feedback of others. If a person is repeatedly told that they are frail, they develop an image of themselves as a frail person
- A person's ideal self is what they aspire to becoming and this is often influenced by what is desirable and valuable in their culture. For example, social pressures to be fit and strong
- A person's self-esteem is the difference between their self-image and their ideal self. It is about how much a person values their self. Someone who has a self-image of being frail and whose ideal self is to be fit and strong may have low self-esteem. People have a strong need to be liked and feel valued to maintain or improve their self-esteem, and this is dependent on their relationships with others

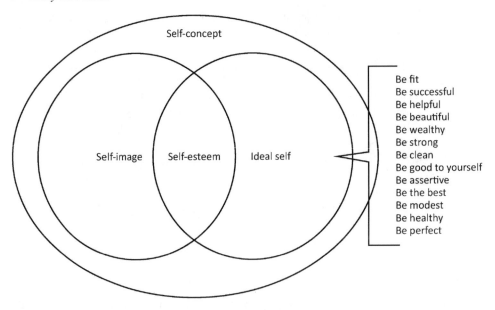

Figure 1.3 Cultural messages influence the ideal self, self-concept and self-esteem

Not only is a person's self-concept influenced by society and its culture, but so is their body. The sociologist Erving Goffman wrote about the body's significance to non-verbal communication (Jacobson and Kristiansen, 2015). Its expressions, gestures, clothing and behaviours allow others to label and classify a person, to accept or to alienate. The body is not only intrinsic to a person's self-identity but also to their social identity. A person is embodied because the body is both something that one 'has' and something one 'is'. Fox (2018) writes,

> "The lived body is a rich source of meaning for people, in sickness and in health; people make sense of their lives by reflecting on their bodily experience."
>
> (p. 266)

He proposed that the body is both biological and social.
    The biological body is

- about anatomical and physiological systems and processes such as circulation and sensation
- a repository where cultural values of fitness, health, beauty and performance are demonstrated
- a consumer of products
- a resource to support living life and engaging with the world

The social body

- is what we sense and experience every day
- is a repository of meaning shaped by others

- is full of cultural symbolism, e.g. the heart as love; or the body as a tomb which houses a soul which is freed at death or a temple through which we communicate our inner worth
- presents a social identity, e.g. eco-warrior, police officer or rapper
- is a focus for self-observation, discipline and control, e.g. grooming or exercise
- is the object through which the powerful control, some might say 'civilise' others, e.g. subjecting bodies to work routines governed by a clock, or to mass observation by closed-circuit television (CCTV)

Thinking point:

Think about your body and the way you present it to others. Consider how it looks and how it behaves. How has this been shaped by the culture in which you live and what does it tell others about you?

Therefore, the material body

- is always both biological and social
- is about what it can do and what it can produce, e.g. move an obstacle or produce a solution
- comprises relations, which means the way things are connected
- has relations with that which is non-human, e.g. gravity, the air we breathe, chemicals and time which deteriorates the body
- has relations to that which is human. It engages with human culture and products, e.g. social institutions such as universities, economic and political systems, people such as friends or a nation, social roles, the arts, clothes and historical artefacts
- is a combination of its physical, psychological and social relations
- has capacities which may be called upon in different contexts at different times. These capacities are dependent on the body's physical, psychological and social relations

Carl Rogers (1961), a humanistic psychologist and the founder of person-centred counselling, writes that a person,

"... discovers that he exists only in response to the demands of others, that he seems to have no self of his own, that he is only trying to think, feel and behave in a way that others believe he ought to think, feel and behave."

(p. 110)

Rogers argues that everyone, knowingly or not, is striving to become their true self, the person they truly are. It is a life-long process of bringing together their self-image with their ideal self. Maslow (1943) explains the process as a hierarchy comprising five goals which are often, but not always, addressed in the same order (Figure 1.4). He argues a person first needs to address their physiological needs, that is the food, air and water we need to keep the biology of the body functioning. Then they become preoccupied with addressing their need for safety. Once this is satisfied, they are restless to

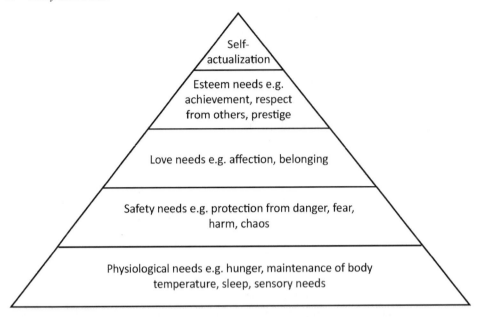

Figure 1.4 Maslow's hierarchy of needs

fulfil their need for love and a sense of belonging with other people, and then they turn to needing confidence, self-respect, self-esteem and the esteem of others. When these four goals are met, Maslow suggests a person becomes restless again to reach their potential. They are motivated to do what they are meant to do. He writes,

> "A musician must make music, an artist must paint, a poet must write, if he is to be ultimately happy. What a man can be, he must be. This need we may call self-actualization."
>
> (Maslow, 1943, p. 382)

> *A person may be understood as a continuously evolving human being who develops over time, is shaped by interactions between their biology, psychology and their socio-cultural context, and is striving towards their true self.*

A person's health

The true, self-actualised self, impelled by the whole human organism, is associated with notions of optimal health for both Rogers and Maslow. Their work influenced the work of Rosemarie Parse, a nursing theorist. Where Rogers wrote about 'becoming a person', Parse wrote about 'human becoming', and she defined health as each person's own experience of valuing that can be known only to them. She proposed,

> "Health is lived experience … one's quality of life … because the person alone knows what his or her own life is like, what is important, and what the possibilities are … Quality of life can only be described by the person … living the life …"
>
> (Pilkington, 1999, p. 22)

Box 1.1 Health

"By health I mean the power to live a full, adult, living, breathing life in close contact with what I love – the earth and the wonders thereof – the sea – the sun. All that we mean when we speak of the external world. I want to enter into it, to be part of it, to live in it, to learn from it, to lose all that is superficial and acquired in me and to become a conscious direct human being. I want, by understanding myself, to understand others. I want to be all that I am capable of becoming so that I may be (and here I have stopped and waited and waited and it's no good – there's only one phrase that will do) *a child of the sun*. About helping others, about carrying a light and so on, it seems false to say a single word. Let it be at that. *A child of the sun*.

Then I want to work. At what? I want so to live that I work with my hands and my feeling and my brain. I want a garden, a small house, grass, animals, books, pictures, music ... warm, eager, living life – to be rooted in life – to learn, to desire to know, to feel, to think, to act. That is what I want. And nothing less."

(Source: Mansfield, 2006, pp. 250, 251, written in 1922)

A person's view of what health means to them is unavoidably entwined with their experience of being a living, and some would add 'doing' person and how they see themselves biologically, psychologically and socially. It is shaped over their lifetime by others, by the real and perceived power of others, and how the person thinks they are seen by others. It is judged against their own values and against the values of others. Peter Baelz, a professor of morals and theology, summarises,

"Physical and mental health have a social dimension, social and political well-being have a value dimension, and values are rooted and grounded in some kind of a vision of a healthy society."

(Baelz, 1987, p. 27)

Thinking point:

Who decides the vision of a healthy society, community, group or family?

A person's view of what health means to them is entwined with their experiences as a fully living person, biologically, psychologically and socially. It is shaped, and changed, over time by personal and social values.

Vision of a healthy society

Those with influence shape the vision of a healthy society. Socially sanctioned health-related systems and interventions are underpinned by beliefs about what health means and how it is best achieved. In the last 150 years, important influences have included the medical model, the biopsychosocial model and the World Health Organization.

Medical model

During the 20th century in Western societies, the guardians of the vision of a healthy society were largely members of the medical scientific community who defined health as an absence of disease. Influenced by the philosophy of Descartes, scientific methods had been used for over four centuries to understand the physical body of a person, leaving the Church to focus on their mind and soul (Moon, 1995). Biomedical scientists, doctors and professions allied to medicine developed, and continue to develop, expertise in physical malfunctions which cause physical and mental disease. The central tenets of the medical model of health and illness are that disease

- arises within the physical body, which is viewed as a machine
- is a malfunction of the body
- is a deviation from a norm or a standard that is agreed by the medical scientific community
- includes the presence of a germ or a physical malfunction such as a blockage, sprain or irregular blood chemistry
- can be prevented, diagnosed, treated and cured using the rules and rigour of science
- can be understood by a reductionist approach which means studying the body's systems, organs and tissues at a microscopic level. Understanding the parts will bring about an understanding of the whole
- can be explained with reference to physiology, the functioning of the body; and to biochemistry, the chemicals within the body
- comprises observable physiological and biochemical measurements, which are much more important than the person's account of their experience, e.g. sociologists who observed antenatal clinics recorded,

"OBSTETRICIAN: [reading case notes] Ah, I see you've got a boy and a girl
PATIENT: No, two girls.
OBSTETRICIAN: Really. Are you sure? I thought it said … [checks in notes] oh no, you're quite right, two girls."

(Graham and Oakley, 1991, p. 111)
(Robinson, 2021)

The process of detection, measurement, understanding and treatment of one malfunction/disease in one human is likely to be transferable to many humans, at best, it is a 'one size fits all' universal approach with benefits for humankind. Similarly, epidemiologists observe and measure disease in populations, identify common causes or risk factors such as being sedentary or consuming alcohol, and encourage universal changes to health-related behaviour to prevent disease in a population. Clean water, reductions in smoking-related diseases, vaccinations, antibiotics, physiotherapy and routine surgical procedures represent some of the great successes of using this science-based medical model. It has saved, and continues to save, very many lives from disease and death.

Box 1.2 1944

"He shivered in the sand with the shock and loss of blood. Hours went by. He remembered lying semi-conscious on the famous Mulberry harbour, waiting to be evacuated – planes and bombs and bullets whizzing by. Then he woke in Leicester Infirmary in England. He was in a ward full of D-Day casualties. He was alive.

How had the filthy shrapnel wounds not poisoned him? He looked for his precious binoculars beside his bed but they were gone. Damn. Someone had pinched them. Yet he'd been given a gift far more rare and valuable. Every few hours a nurse was injecting him with a new drug. Fleming's miracle, fresh from Brooklyn. Penicillin. In the ward, amazed servicemen gathered around each other's beds to show off their rapidly healing wounds. Their generation had never seen its like before. A medical wonder. An antibiotic. They were the first warriors in history to have their wounded bodies cleansed of internal infection by this new medicine. He never forgot the gift. He'd later scoff at the complacency of his children, who'd pop antibiotics for every tiny cough or cut. 'You don't know you're born,' he'd say. He was right. Dad was born in an age when a cut from a rose thorn could grow septic and kill – or when a simple streptococcal infection could silently eat the heart. Now physical trauma had a new foe ..."

(Source: McGann, 2017, p. 140)

The aim of the medical model is to achieve an absence of disease.

Bio-psychosocial model

During the 1970s, feminists (Phillips and Rakusen, 1978), theologians (Illich, 1977), policymakers (Lalonde, 1981), disability rights campaigners (Finkelstein, 1980), the World Health Organization (1978) and many 'ordinary' people expressed concerns about the limitations of the disease-centred medical model. They recognised its strengths, but from all sides came arguments that the vision of a healthy society needed to reflect contemporary understandings of a person as a whole being in relation to others and encompass more than an absence of disease within the body.

Within the medical community, one contributor to the debate was George Engel, an American psychiatrist with an interest in changing medical practice. In 1977, Engel defined illness as being the human experience of a disease. He argued the most important skill of a doctor is to listen and then analyse a person's subjective account of their illness; it is essential to making the diagnosis and providing appropriate treatment and care. He also recognised that the person's experience is strongly influenced by the social context of their lives. For example, a person will only believe themselves to be ill if their experience fits with their personal perception of what an illness is, and this is likely to be informed by mainstream beliefs about illness in their family and culture. People who live within a society that has a strong adherence to a traditional model of health and illness may attribute their cough to a spirit or a sin; those who live in a society that has a strong adherence to a social model of health and illness may attribute the same cough to living in cold, damp housing; those within a society that values the medical model of health and illness may attribute the cough to a germ (Robinson, 2021). At a macro level, organisations and policies designed to protect and support the public's health are created and maintained according to what a society values at that moment and in that place. A society that believes illness is the result of spiritual distress may build a health system around spiritual resources such as temples or churches; one that believes illness is the result of poverty will invest in actions such as rectifying poor housing; one that believes illness is something to be detected by science may invest in laboratories and technology; one that believes illness is the result of unhealthy personal behaviours may invest in counselling, education or social marketing. It is not about which is right or wrong, it is about recognising how personal and social values shape each person's perceptions of their own experience. Engel recognised that a person's experience of a physical or mental illness cannot be limited to bodily measurements, it is a blend of the anatomical, physiological, biochemical, psychological, cultural and social. The strict boundaries of the medical model do not allow this. He wrote,

> "The boundaries between health and disease, between well and sick, are far from clear and never will be clear, for they are diffused by cultural, social and psychological considerations."

> (Engel, 1977, p. 132)

Engel proposed his biopsychosocial model (Figure 1.5) as a way for medical practitioners to bring together the patient's experience and the measurements that indicated malfunction/disease. He hoped it would act as a blueprint for medical research, teaching and care. Today we see it described as a model of clinical care, health, health and illness, stress, disability, pain and so forth (Bolton and Gillett, 2019; Borrell-Carrió *et al.*, 2004; Karunamuni *et al.*, 2020; Miaskowski *et al.*, 2019; WHO, 2002) and it

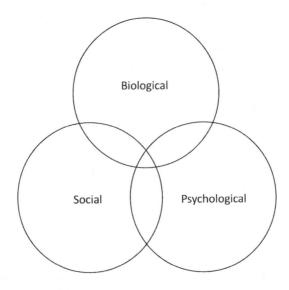

Figure 1.5 The biopsychosocial model

has become central to the work of some healthcare professions such as occupational therapy. In contrast to the disease-centredness of the medical model, the biopsychosocial model communicates the importance of a holistic and person-centred approach to these matters; a blending of the psychological experience, human biology and the social context in which people live.

In 2020, Karunamuni and colleagues published their investigation into whether the biopsychosocial model can be supported by evidence. Their review of a large body of research concluded that there is substantial evidence to demonstrate the relationships between a person's biology, psychology, social context and their subjective wellbeing.

- Biological factors include a person's body including its organs and cells
- Psychological factors include a person's lived/subjective experiences, feelings, mental states, goals, attitudes, intentions and behaviour
- Social factors include a person's interpersonal experiences, life events, social policies, culture and social circumstances

The authors found evidence for the six pathways:

- B-P Biological factors influence psychological factors, e.g. physical health conditions and pain affect life satisfaction. Having access to shelter, water and good nutrition protect the body and a person's subjective wellbeing
- P-B Psychological factors influence biological factors, e.g. negative feelings, such as stress, affect the nervous and immune systems, which can lead to low-grade chronic inflammation in the body. Low-grade inflammation is associated with the development of cardiovascular disease, some cancers and autoimmune diseases. Repeatedly dwelling on a stressor, rumination, intensifies the effects on the body. The 'placebo effect' refers to the way a person's expectations of a 'dummy' treatment can lead to physical, measurable changes in the body
- P-S Psychological factors influence social factors, e.g. positive feelings are more likely to lead to social relationships and negative feelings to social conflict
- S-P Social factors influence psychological factors, e.g. abuse, unemployment and social exclusion negatively affect a person's subjective wellbeing; whereas social belonging and social support are protective. Living in places where the rule of law, human rights and political freedoms are protected are associated with higher levels of subjective wellbeing
- S-B Social factors influence biological factors. This is usually mediated by psychological factors such as people's thoughts, feelings and attitudes, e.g. early childhood experiences predict vulnerability to a range of physical and mental health issues in later life. Persistent loneliness has negative biological consequences leading to adverse health outcomes. A change in the law, such as the compulsory wearing of seatbelts, can have a large impact on accident prevention
- B-S Biological factors influence social factors. The impact of biological factors on social factors is also usually mediated by psychological factors, e.g. a painful injury or disease can reduce a person's energy and motivation to join social events and to exert social influence. A person's body may conform or deviate from perceptions of social norms and elicit social stigma or social praise, thus closing or opening social opportunities for subjective wellbeing

Box 1.3 Stanley

Stanley arrived in the UK with his mother on HMT Empire Windrush in 1948 from Jamaica. It is 2017 and Stanley, now 72 years old, lives on a housing estate in Glasgow. He has not worked in full-time employment since 1985 when he lost his job at the coal mine. He is a heavy smoker and has a chronic cough. He hasn't been seen for a couple of weeks.

Biological – Stanley's lungs are fragile, irritated and inflamed. He has chronic bronchitis, which is likely to have been caused by tobacco smoke and coal dust. He is addicted to nicotine.

Psychological – In 1975, Stanley experienced a major loss. His friend died of pneumoconiosis, which he later found out was caused by inhaling coal dust. Since then, he has worried about his own cough. Stanley knows that smoking tobacco is harmful to health, but he feels twitchy and irritable if he doesn't smoke and he says that smoking helps him to have a really good cough which temporarily clears his chest. Smoking represents a shared behaviour with his ex-miner mates. Their friendship is very important to him, it's where he most feels a sense of belonging and remembers 'the good days' with pride. Although he sometimes feels a bit low, he puts on a big smile and keeps going. Recently he hasn't the motivation to get out of bed. He smokes in bed, and his chest hurts. He feels his life is worthless.

Social – Stanley spent his early life in the UK living in poverty. He was often cold, hungry and insecure. He found it difficult to make friends due to wide-spread racial discrimination. At school, he was bullied and often felt isolated. He found that smoking was a way to fit in with some of the other lads and he would imagine himself as the film star Sidney Poitier lighting a cigarette. He left school to work in the local coal mine. Among the mining community, he made good friends. He had a stable weekly wage, a decent home and three square meals a day. He joined the miners' trade union and took a leading role, initially fighting for better health and safety and later during the miners' strikes. They lost, and the mine was closed in 1985. The resulting high unemployment meant the whole community became poorer financially, spiritually and socially. He has heard rumours that he might be deported back to Jamaica because he doesn't have the required documents to prove he is a UK citizen.

B-P Being cold and hungry contributed to Stanley's feelings of insecurity as a child; having a really good cough, from inhaling tobacco smoke, makes Stanley feel temporarily better; his painful chest is contributing to his current lack of motivation.

P-B Stanley's feelings of isolation encouraged him to start smoking which contributed to bronchitis; a lack of motivation encourages him to stay in bed and smoke which inflames his lungs.

P-S Stanley's need for acceptance encouraged his friendship with smokers at school; motivated by bereavement he joined with other miners to fight for better health and safety standards; anxieties about deportation evoke memories of feeling excluded as a child and have led him to socially isolate himself in bed.

S-P Racial discrimination and bullying made Stanley feel isolated; poor health and safety standards in the mines led to his bereavement; social inclusion by mining friends encouraged his self-esteem and confidence to lead the miners; unemployment and potential deportation has led to a loss of motivation.

S-B Smoking in films and social isolation encouraged Stanley's uptake of smoking; poor health and safety standards in the mines led to respiratory illnesses and his friend's death.

B-S Stanley's friend's death led to a social movement to improve miners' health; his bronchitis and painful chest encourages him to stay in bed and avoid social engagement.

The aim of the holistic and person-centred biopsychosocial model is to understand a person's experience of health or illness in the context of the interconnections between their biology, psychology and social context.

World Health Organization

During the 20th century, another vision of a healthy society emerged from the World Health Organization whose primary role is to coordinate health across the world. It was also seeking something more holistic and person-centred than the absence of disease. The World Health Organization has argued health is,

"... not merely the absence of disease or infirmity ..."

(WHO, 1946, p. 1)

It is a,

"... positive concept emphasizing social and personal resources, as well as physical capacities."

(WHO, 1986, p. 1)

Health is,

"... a resource for everyday life, not the objective of living,"

(WHO, 1986, p. 1)

and it includes,

"... physical, mental and social wellbeing,"

(WHO, 1946, p. 1; 1986, p. 1)

where 'wellbeing' is defined as a positive, subjective state. This is associated with a person's quality of life which comprises six domains: physical, psychological, level of independence, spiritual beliefs, social relations and the environment. Quality of life is,

"An individual's perception of their position in life in the context of the culture and value systems in which they live and in relation to their goals, expectations, standards and concerns. It is a broad ranging concept affected in a complex way by the person's physical health, psychological state, personal beliefs, social relationships and their relationship to salient features of their environment ... [this] subjective evaluation ... is embedded in a cultural, social and environmental context."

(WHO, 1998, p. 3)

Health is person-centred and linked to personal values. To achieve health,

> "An individual or group must be able to identify and realize aspirations, to satisfy needs,"
>
> (WHO, 1986, p. 1)

rather like moving up Maslow's hierarchy. It requires skills to be able to achieve it. People need the ability,

> "… to change of cope with the environment,"
>
> (WHO, 1986, p. 1)

which recognises people do not live in a bubble but within a culture, a society and a physical environment which can be enabling or constraining. Health is,

> "… a complete state of physical, mental and social wellbeing."
>
> (WHO, 1946, p. 1; WHO, 1986, p. 1)

The words 'complete state' have been criticised by many authors for making health into an unattainable and idealistic concept. Perhaps no one would achieve health, it is too illusive. However, in the context of understanding health as including a person's subjective wellbeing, being a person-centred aspiration, about achieving one's true self, being self-actualised, being what a person feels they were meant to be, and then being able to use this health as a resource to support their lives, it makes more sense. For the World Health Organization, health is less a definitive, objective, universal, measurable outcome and more about the *processes and conditions of enablement* which will allow each person to achieve whatever 'a complete state of physical, mental and social wellbeing' means for them. Enablement is associated with individual autonomy, democracy, equality and human rights (WHO, 1946; 1986; 1998; 2009).

Health for all

In 1981, the World Health Organization launched its *Global Strategy for Health for All by the Year 2000*, which declared the international community would work towards all people across the world being healthy by 2000. This meant people being able to work productively; participate in their communities; be free from avoidable disease and disability; growing up, living and dying with grace; enjoying a fair distribution of the resources that support health and having the power to shape their own lives. The year 2000 has passed, but the 'health for all' movement continues at the centre of the World Health Organization's approach to health promotion.

Health as a human right

Today, the World Health Organization's vision of a healthy society clearly states that health is a universal human right (WHO, 2017). The right to health means that a person has the right to control their own health. For example, they have sexual and reproductive rights and they have the right to protect their health, including their body, from being violated, such as from non-consensual medical treatment, forced institutionalisation and torture. A person also has the right to enjoy optimum health through opportunities

Box 1.4 Constitution of the World Health Organization

"… the following principles are basic to the happiness, harmonious relations and security of all peoples:

Health is a state of complete physical, mental and social wellbeing and not merely the absence of disease or infirmity.

The enjoyment of the highest attainable standard of health is one of the fundamental rights of every human being without distinction of race, religion, political belief, economic or social condition.

The health of all peoples is fundamental to the attainment of peace and security and is dependent upon the fullest cooperation of individuals and [member] States.

The achievement of any [member] State in the promotion and protection of health is of value to all.

Unequal development in different countries in the promotion of health and control of disease, especially communicable disease, is a common danger.

Healthy development of the child is of basic importance; the ability to live harmoniously in a changing total environment is essential to such development.

The extensions of all peoples of the benefits of medical, psychological and related knowledge are essential to the fullest attainment in health.

Informed opinion and active cooperation on the part of the public are of the utmost importance in the improvement of the health of the people.

Governments have a responsibility for the health of their peoples which can be fulfilled only by the provision of adequate health and social measures."

(Source: WHO, 2020a, p. 1. This is the 1946 version with subsequent amendments included. Reproduced with permission from the World Health Organization)

that are available equally to all other persons. Achieving health equity, fairness across a society, means prioritising the needs of those who are the most disadvantaged and ensuring health is not subject to discrimination on the grounds of race, age, ethnicity, sexuality, disability and so forth. It means targeting discriminatory practices and abuses of power as well as having policies and legal systems to ensure rights are respected. The right to health is indivisible from other human rights, such as the right to food, sanitation, housing, clean and accessible water, clean air and education. A human rights approach is person-centred, which includes enabling people to gain the knowledge and skills they need to fully participate in matters that affect their health. More widely, a region, state, nation or country must enable a range of key agencies, stakeholders and sectors beyond government to participate in developing, planning and evaluating the work needed to achieve a healthy society for all. This is summed up in the title of the World Health Organization's 2019 global action plan *Stronger Collaboration, Better Health* (WHO, 2019).

Healthy settings

The World Health Organization has been drawing attention to the physical and social quality of the settings in which people live, learn, play and work for almost 40 years. These include cities, villages, workplaces, homes, islands, hospitals, universities and prisons (WHO, 2022) (see Chapters 8 and 15). Settings are places, or social contexts, where we see physical, social, organisational or environmental factors influencing people's health (Box 1.5). For example, in a workplace, the 'settings approach' draws attention to buildings, facilities, culture and the degree to which employees can influence their quality of life at work.

During the 21st century, the World Health Organization, as part of the United Nations, committed to the *2030 Agenda for Sustainable Development* which aims to address the global challenges of climate change, environmental degradation, poverty, inequality, peace and justice (UN, 2015) (Figure 1.6). There is a symbiotic relationship between health and development because people's health is shaped by personal, social and environmental factors over time, across their life course, and because the ultimate healthy setting is a healthy planet. A healthy society is only possible within a healthy planet, and both create and depend upon healthy people. The means

---

Box 1.5 The social work setting

Jermaine Ravalier was aware of a high level of sickness absence across the UK social care sector and the reputation for social work being a very stressful occupation. He carried out research with 1,333 social workers to understand their working conditions. He found low job satisfaction and presenteeism, which means working when unwell. Many social workers were thinking of leaving their job. The causes of their significant stress and related outcomes included experiencing

- high workload, e.g. having a high number of cases, many of which were complex cases; having too few social workers to deal with the demand and excessive administration
- poor managerial support, e.g. managers who did not fully understand the role of the social worker and managers who set unrealistic time scales alongside unrealistic expectations
- lack of regular supervision from experienced colleagues
- a culture of blame which included a lack of respect for their work from politicians and the public and a poor understanding of the difficulties of the job
- 'hot desking,' not having a permanent desk and computer
- lack of opportunities for flexible working and, for some, inadequate pay

At the heart of the social workers' stress was the combination of highly demanding work, feeling they had little control and poor managerial support.

(Source: Ravalier, 2019)

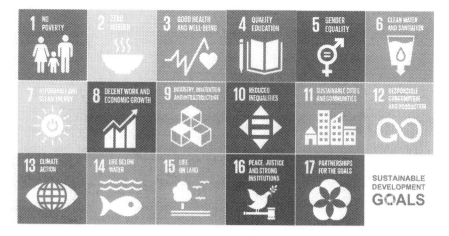

Figure 1.6 Sustainable development goals

Source: ALX1618/Shutterstock.com

to achieving a healthy society is through people working in partnership with one another.

> "Health and wellbeing are shaped by the conditions in which people are born, grow, work and age, and these are in turn shaped by social, economic and environmental factors. The reverse is also true. Health and well-being drive broader sustainable development including reductions in poverty and inequality, better educational outcomes, and inclusive economic growth. Health and well-being promote resilience, sustainability, equity and human security."
>
> (WHO, 2019, p. 65. Reproduced with permission from the World Health Organization)

The World Health Organization views health as a human right. People have the right to control their health based on their own values, it is person-centred. Health is a resource for living not the reason for life. It is a holistic concept, comprising absence of disease and quality of life. It is more achievable when people are fully enabled within a healthy setting.

A concept of health

A concept of health may be

- person-centred – a human right which reflects each person's life and their values
- time dependent – health changes over the life course, across generations and eras
- positive – health is being able to achieve aspirations and meet needs; subjective wellbeing and a good quality of life
- holistic – health is created through interactions between the biological, psychological and social. These may be further broken down into physical, mental, emotional, sexual, social and spiritual dimensions, which are discussed in Chapter 7. In turn, these are influenced by a person's interactions with their wider social and physical environment. This may be represented as a social-ecological model (Figure 1.7)

These ideas provide a useful start, but they also present challenges.

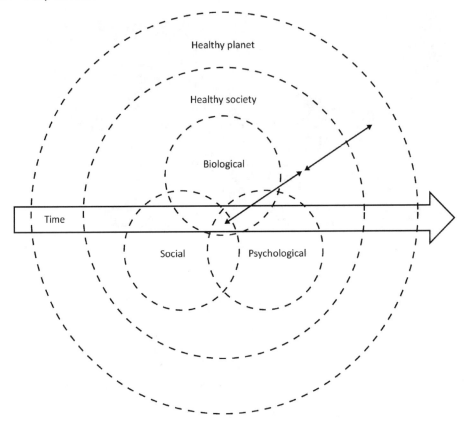

Figure 1.7 Interdependent healthy people in a healthy society and healthy planet

Person-centred

- A person-centred approach to health means we must first understand people, their beliefs, self-concept, values, needs, aspirations and the context in which their lives have been and are being lived. Listening, learning and responding appropriately takes time, skills and other resources which may not be available or which people choose not to make available
- A person-centred approach may lead to tensions when one person's actions to protect or promote their own health impacts negatively on others
- Health is often determined by power. For example, the power of governments, professional bodies or commercial businesses who promote, deliver or enforce their own circumscribed vision of a healthy society versus the power of the individual to know and assert their own wishes in accordance with their own values

Thinking point:

> Thinking about current advertising and the messages they convey, what does health mean to a pharmaceutical company, to a company selling holidays, a business selling a diet product and a fitness guru on social media? See Box 1.6 and consider what health meant to the Nazi party in the early 1940s.

Box 1.6 Health promotion in Nazi Germany

Dr Leonard Conti, the leader of health within the Third Reich, became aware of German research which indicated smoking was related to lung cancer. Antismoking propaganda was disseminated by the Hitler Youth and the League of German Girls, soldiers were forbidden to smoke on the streets, and smoking was banned in schools and, by 1943, in public places for anyone under 18 years. By 1944 it was banned on trains and buses and in workplaces, public buildings, care homes and hospitals. There were discussions about whether those with self-inflicted smoking-related illnesses should be given medical care. Along with smoking, the German healthy lifestyle campaigns also discouraged the drinking of alcohol. Adolf Hitler was vehemently against smoking and did not drink alcohol.

The promotion of a healthy lifestyle was part of the racial hygiene movement. It was believed that tobacco and alcohol would poison genes and damage the purity of the German people, the Aryan 'master race'. Other racial hygiene activities included persecuting Jews, homosexuals and those with learning disabilities; 'preventive death sentences' for those identified as potential murderers and euthanasia programmes which murdered 70,000 people deemed to be 'mentally or physically defective.' The message from Hitler was that every German was responsible for all Germans and they did not have the right to damage their body with drugs.

(Source: Smith, 2004; Smith *et al.*, 1994)

- A person-centred approach means enabling people with the knowledge, skills and resources to reach their personal goals for health. However, person-centredness may be interpreted as health being a personal matter and divorced from health as a social concept. For example, disability can be understood as a personal attribute or a socially constructed one. Many argue it is how society is organised that is 'dis-abling', not any individual within it. A social concept of health can complement and facilitate person-centredness

Time

- Health is dependent on time. The urgency to attend to the health emergencies of today may conflict with attending to the health emergencies of tomorrow. The former is often high value, visible, known and immediate; the latter is often low value, not yet fully known, invisible and arguably can be delayed. It is difficult to win a political election by promising to prevent health problems that have not yet arrived
- Personal concepts of health change over lifetimes, generations, eras and sometimes daily. Health-related decisions and actions need to be understood in their contemporary context

Positive

- Working with a negative definition of health, meaning health is defined as only the 'absence of disease', has advantages compared to working with a more complex, positive definition of health. Researching malfunctions in the body using highly valued, rigorous and respected scientific methods which produce data that can be generalised to every human is very different to researching the more contested concept of health. The latter necessitates the use of quantitative and qualitative social scientific research methods such as questionnaires, interviews, case studies and social observations. Historically, these have been perceived as lower status than scientific research, partly because they do not always produce findings that can be generalised to others. This has had implications for funding and acceptance. However, awareness of the limitations of scientific research and of the potential insights to be gained from social scientific research are increasingly recognised as vital for working with a positive definition of health

- Treating disease or injury is often given higher priority by society than disease prevention; and preventing disease and injury is often given higher priority than the social and educational actions that will enable people to achieve their aspirations for wellbeing and a good quality of life. It is difficult to measure disease that has been prevented, but it is even harder to measure and demonstrate the health benefits of a long-term investment in people's lives

- Working with a positive definition of health means allowing it into mainstream, socially inclusive thinking. A positive concept of health includes the individual who reports being healthy, feeling fulfilled, achieving their aspirations and living as their true self in the *presence* of an identified disease or infirmity, which they have successfully learnt to live with. There are many people; some with disabilities, some with a chronic or terminal illness, and some with neither; for whom health 'as a positive concept' is a much more meaningful way to think about health and how we can achieve it, but this is more rarely represented in culture, for example in films, television drama and documentaries, than the fight against disease

Holistic

- If health is as broad as life, there are no experts. The health of a society becomes everyone's business and no practitioner, professional, agency or government can claim unquestioning expertise or authority over people's health. Yet practitioners, professionals, agencies and governments are often given this authority

- A holistic approach can be interpreted as pertaining to the 'whole person', as if they lived in a bubble, without recognising the wider context in which a person lives and dies. By focussing only on one person at a time, we fail to see that poor health, illness, disease and early death are not random but often predictable and, to some extent, preventable

- A holistic approach requires a broad understanding of all the factors that influence health, it is inherently an interdisciplinary field of study like education. Yet, historically, single disciplines have enjoyed a higher status in UK research and wider academia

- A holistic approach to an individual's health may involve interprofessional working among, for example, a nurse, social worker, occupational therapist and a hospital chaplain. While each brings their knowledge and experience, they also bring their own professional visions of health associated with the professional bodies which guide their professional education and allow them to practise. Successful interprofessional working takes skill, mutual respect, time and patience

- A holistic approach to a population's health requires multi-disciplinary, multi-agency, multi-sectoral and international partnerships to understand people's health and to work towards improvements, but such a broad remit may permit unwelcome encroachments into every aspect of everyone's lives

Table 1.2 Examples of disciplines, fields of study, sectors and agencies which contribute to health

Disciplines/fields of study	Sectors	UK national/regional agencies	International agencies
Arts and health	Business	Cancer Research UK	Bill & Melinda Gates
Biomedical science	Criminal justice	Department for the	Foundation
Education	Education	Environment, Food &	Befrienders Worldwide
Environmental	Health and care	Rural Affairs	Centers for Disease
science	Hospitality	Department of Health	Control and
Epidemiology	Housing	(NI)	Prevention (USA)
Geography and	Local government	Department of Health	Center for Reproductive
health	Sport and leisure	and Social Care (UK)	Rights
Health economics	Voluntary	Food Standards Agency	Elton John AIDS
Health promotion		Health Protection	Foundation
Philosophy		Scotland	European Commission
Politics		Local authorities	Food and Agriculture
Psychology		Local health boards	Organization
Social anthropology		Mind	International Monetary
Social policy		NHS Wales	Fund
		Public health	Oxfam
		observatories	Water Aid
		The Health Foundation	World Bank
			World Health
			Organization

There is no definitive definition of health. Contemporary thinking suggests it may be person-centred, time-dependent, positive and holistic. We need to recognise and respect individuals' values and their lives, and to work in partnership with them and others, if we are to support and improve people's health.

Summary

This chapter has

- explored a person as a biological, psychological and social being who changes over time and in relation with their own ecosystem
- suggested that a person's view of what health means to them is tied up with their experience of living in a society with its culture, and by their personal needs, values and aspirations
- provided examples of how people with influence and their vision of a healthy society can shape how individuals and populations understand and resource their health
- explored some contemporary ideas about health as a person-centred, time-dependent, holistic and positive concept

Further reading

Buchanan, D.R. (2020) *A humanistic approach to health promotion.* Newcastle upon Tyne: Cambridge Scholars

Duncan, P. (2006) *Critical perspectives on health.* London: Macmillan

Nettleton, S. (2020) *The sociology of health and illness.* 4th edn. Cambridge: Polity Press

Useful website

World Health Organization. Available at: www.who.int

References

Baelz, P.R. (1987) 'Philosophy of health education', in Sutherland, I. (ed) *Health education: perspectives and choices*. Cambridge: National Extension College Trust Ltd, pp. 20–38

Baumeister, R.F. and Bushman, B.J. (2014) *Social psychology and human nature*. 3rd edn. Belmont: Wadsworth, Cengage Learning

Bolton, D. and Gillett, G. (2019) 'Biopsychosocial conditions of health and disease', in Bolton, D. and Gillett, G. (eds) *The biopsychosocial model of health and disease: new philosophical and scientific developments*. London: Palgrave/Macmillan, pp. 109–145

Borrell-Carrió, F., Suchman, A.L. and Epstein, R.M. (2004) 'The biopsychosocial model 25 years later: principles, practice and scientific enquiry', *Annals of Family Medicine*, 2(6), pp. 576–582

Bronfenbrenner, U. and Ceci, S.J. (1994) 'Nature-nurture reconceptualized in developmental perspective: a bioecological model', *Psychological Review*, 101(4), pp. 568–586

Bronfenbrenner, U. and Morris, P.A. (1998) 'The ecology of developmental processes', in Damon, W. and Lerner, R.M. (eds) *Handbook of child psychology: theoretical models of human development*. 5th edn. New York: John Wiley and Sons, pp. 993–1028

Cozolino, L.J. (2006) *The neuroscience of human relationships*. London: W.W. Norton and Co.

Engel, G.L. (1977) 'The need for a new medical model: a challenge for biomedicine', *Science*, 196(4286), pp. 129–136

Finkelstein, V. (1980) *Attitudes and disabled people: issues for discussion*. New York: World Rehabilitation Fund. Available at: https://disability-studies.leeds.ac.uk/wp-content/uploads/sites/40/library/finkelstein-attitudes.pdf (Accessed 21st June 2022)

Fox, N.J. (2018) 'Reconceptualising bodies', in Scambler, G. (ed) *Sociology as applied to health and medicine*. London: Macmillan/Palgrave, pp. 263–276

Graham, H. and Oakley, A. (1991) 'Competing ideologies of reproduction: medical and maternal perspectives on pregnancy', in Currer, C. and Stacey, M. (eds) *Concepts of health, illness and disease. A comparative perspective*. Oxford: Berg, pp. 97–115

Griffore, R.J. and Phenice, L.A. (2016) 'Proximal processes and causality in human development', *European Journal of Educational and Development Psychology*, 4(1), pp. 10–16

Hook, L. (2021) 'FT Magazine. Greta Thunberg: "It just spiralled out of control."' *Financial Times*, March 31st. Available at: https://www.ft.com/content/6ee4bb03-3039-446a-997f-91a7aef5f137 (Accessed 21st June 2022)

Illich, I. (1977) *Limits to medicine: medical nemesis: the expropriation of health and medicine*. 2nd edn. Harmondsworth: Penguin

Jacobson, M.H. and Kristiansen, S. (2015) *The social thought of Erving Goffman*, London: Sage

Karunamuni, N., Imayama, I. and Goonetilleke (2020) 'Pathways to well-being; untangling the causal relationships among biopsychosocial variables', *Social Science and Medicine*, 112846 doi: 10.1016/j.socscimed.2020.112846

Lalonde, M. (1981) *A new perspective on the health of Canadians*. Ottawa: Government of Canada

Mansfield, K. (2006) *Journal of Katherine Mansfield*. London: Persephone Books

Maslow, A. (1943) 'A theory of human motivation', *Psychological Review*, 50(4), pp. 370–396.

McGann, S. (2017) *Flesh and blood. A history of my family in seven sicknesses*. London: Simon and Shuster

Miaskowski, C., Blyth, F., Nicosia, F., Haan, M., Keefe, F., Smith, A. and Ritchie, C. (2019) 'A biopsychosocial model of chronic pain for older adults', *Pain Medicine*, 21(9), pp. 1793–1805

Moon, G. (1995) 'Health care and society', in Moon, G. and Gillespie, R. (eds) *Society and health. An introduction to social science for health professionals.* London: Routledge, pp. 49–64

Phillips, A. and Rakusen, J. (1978) *Our bodies ourselves. A health book by and for women.* London: Viking

Pilkington, F.B. (1999) 'An ethical framework for nursing practice: Parse's human becoming theory', *Nursing Science Quarterly*, 12(1), pp. 21–25

Ravalier, J.M. (2019) 'Psycho-social working conditions and stress in UK social workers', *British Journal of Social Work*, 49(9), pp. 371–390

Robinson, S. (2021) 'Social context of health and illness' in Robinson, S. (ed) *Priorities for health promotion and public health. Explaining the evidence for disease prevention and health promotion.* London: Routledge, pp. 3–33

Rogers, C. (1961) *On becoming a person. A therapist's view of psychotherapy.* London: Constable and Co.

Schwartz, S.H. (2012) 'An overview of the Schwartz theory of basic values', *Online Readings in Psychology and Culture*, 2(1) doi:10.9707/2307-0919.1116

Smith, D.G. (2004) 'Lifestyle, health and health promotion in Nazi Germany', *BMJ (Clinical Research Edn.)*, 329(7480), pp. 1424–1425

Smith., D.G., Ströbele, S.A. and Egger, M. (1994) 'Smoking and health promotion in Nazi Germany', *Journal of Epidemiology and Community Health*, 48(3), pp. 220–223

Tudge, J.R.H., Payir, A., Merçon-Vargas, E., Cao, H., Liang, Y., Li, J. and O'Brian, L. (2009) 'Still misused after all these years? A reevaluation of the uses of Bronfenbrenner's bioecological theory of human development', *Journal of Family Theory and Review*, 8(4), pp. 427–445

United Nations (2015) *Transforming our world: the 2030 agenda for sustainable development.* Available at: https://sustainabledevelopment.un.org/content/documents/21252030%20Agenda%20for%20Sustainable%20Development%20web.pdf (Accessed 21st June 2022)

White, F.J. (2013) 'Personhood: an essential characteristic of the human species', *The Linacre Quarterly*, 80(1), pp. 74–97

Winnicott, D. (1971) *Playing and reality.* London: Routledge

World Health Organization (1946) *Constitution.* Geneva: World Health Organization

World Health Organization (1978) *Declaration of Alma-Ata. International conference on primary health care, Alma-Ata, USSR, 6–12 September 1978.* Available at: https://www.euro.who.int/__data/assets/pdf_file/0009/113877/E93944.pdf (Accessed 21st June 2022)

World Health Organization (1981) *Global strategy for health for all by the year 2000.* Geneva: World Health Organization

World Health Organization (1986) *Ottawa charter for health promotion.* Available at: https://www.canada.ca/content/dam/phac-aspc/documents/services/health-promotion/population-health/ottawa-charter-health-promotion-international-conference-on-health-promotion/charter.pdf (Accessed 21st June 2022)

World Health Organization (1998) *WHOQOL user manual.* Available at: https://www.who.int/publications/i/item/WHO-HIS-HSI-Rev.2012.03 (Accessed 21st June 2022)

World Health Organization (2002) *Towards a common language for functioning, disability and health.* Geneva: World Health Organization

World Health Organization (2009) *Milestones in health promotion. Statements from global conferences.* Geneva: World Health Organization

World Health Organization (2017) *Human rights and health.* Available at: https://www.who.int/news-room/fact-sheets/detail/human-rights-and-health (Accessed 21st June 2022)

World Health Organization (2019) *Stronger collaboration, better health. Global action plan for healthy lives and well-being for all.* Geneva: World Health Organization

World Health Organization (2020) *Basic documents.* 49th edn. Geneva: World Health Organization

World Health Organization (2022) *Healthy settings.* Available at: https://www.who.int/teams/health-promotion/enhanced-wellbeing/healthy-settings (Accessed 21st June 2022)

2 Working in health promotion and public health

Louise Holden, Em Rahman, Branwen Thomas and Sally Robinson

Key points

- Introduction
- The UK public health workforce
- Competencies for working in health promotion and public health
- Registration of health promotion and public health professionals
- Examples of career routes
- Summary

Introduction

This chapter describes the structure and breadth of the UK public health workforce and provides examples of different job roles. Competencies are the knowledge, skills and behaviours needed to do a job effectively, and the chapter outlines four competency frameworks that set professional standards and support the public health workforce to progress their careers. The chapter explains the importance of professional registration and continuous professional development. It provides several examples to illustrate the varied ways that people enter and progress through their public health and health promotion careers.

The UK public health workforce

In the UK, we describe those who work to improve health and reduce health inequalities as the 'public health workforce'. As everyone has the potential to make a positive contribution to the health of others, the workforce is very broad, comprising people with different skills, knowledge and backgrounds. Their work supports the health of people across the life course, that is from birth to the final stages of life, and takes place in a range of work settings. For example, individuals may work in a laboratory, office, community venue, hospital, clinic, in outdoor spaces or across combinations of these (DH, 2012). By working in partnership, the workforce aims to address the determinants of health, as illustrated in Figure 2.1. Public health work is described in terms of domains and functions.

DOI: 10.4324/9780367823696-3

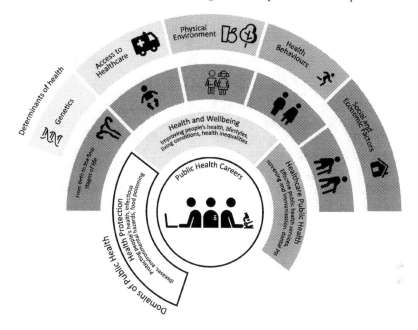

Figure 2.1 Public health domains and functions

Source: YHPHN, 2021. Reproduced with permission from YHPHN

Domains

The UK public health workforce needs to cover three inter-related domains of work: health improvement, health protection and healthcare public health (FPH, 2020; UK Public Health, 2020).

- Health and wellbeing, also known as health improvement, concerns health promotion and includes reducing health inequalities, e.g. health needs assessment, partnership working, community development, advocacy and building resources to support the population's health
- Health protection incorporates preventing and controlling infectious diseases, emergency planning, risk management and protecting people from environmental health hazards, e.g. in the air, water or food, or from dangerous chemical incidents
- Healthcare public health refers to planning integrated health and care services which are equitably distributed, meet the population's needs, are regularly evaluated, safe and effective

For example, in the UK during the COVID-19 coronavirus pandemic, the need for 'test, trace and isolate' (health protection) met public vulnerabilities such as health inequalities (health improvement) and limitations in the National Health Service (healthcare public health). These challenges needed,

> "… a workforce of adequate size … appropriately trained and developed, skilled in the three [domains] and supported by the necessary science, research, data and intelligence."

> (UK Public Health, 2020, p. 2)

Functions

All three domains include three underlying functions: public health intelligence, academic public health and workforce development (FPH, 2020).

- Public health intelligence involves gathering knowledge about the health and health needs of a population and then using this knowledge to inform a plan of action. It includes collecting, generating, analysing and interpreting data, and then communicating the evidence to others. Examples of data include births and deaths, hospital admissions, smoking prevalence, obesity rates, teenage conception rates, vaccine uptake, income and educational attainment
- Academic public health comprises research, the application of public health evidence, evaluating public health interventions, being advocates for evidence-based public health and teaching
- Workforce development involves working with partners to agree the standards for an effective, safe and resilient public health system. This includes setting standards for the workforce who deliver public health programmes and interventions. Workforce development may include mapping and counting the workforce; identifying where there are recruitment gaps in key roles, now or in the future; designing and commissioning (purchasing) training or education to fill the gaps; and creating opportunities for the workforce to develop strong peer networks where mutual learning can take place

Thinking point:

> Which of these three public health domains and three underlying functions best reflect your interests?

Workforce categories

The public health workforce comprises three broad categories: public health specialists, public health practitioners and the wider public health workforce (DH, 2012) (Figure 2.2). Specialists and practitioners are defined as the core public health workforce.

Public health specialists

Public health specialists are educated in all three public health domains but may specialise in one or more domains during their career. The specialist public health workforce encompasses professionals from diverse and varied backgrounds who have higher qualifications in public health. These individuals occupy senior positions and exclusively, or substantially, focus on population health. Specialists work at local, regional and national level in the National Health Service, local and central government and higher education.

Public health practitioners

Public health practitioners may work within one preferred domain or they may choose jobs, across their career, which span all three domains. Many public health

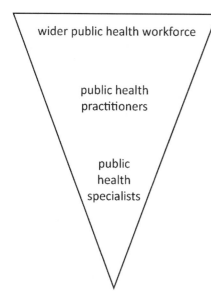

The wider public health workforce makes a contribution to public health e.g. teachers, local business leaders, local councillors, social workers, transport engineers, housing officers, care assistants and clinicians such as radiographers, nurses, paramedics, dietitians, therapists and doctors

Public health practitioners spend all their time in public health practice e.g. health improvement practitioners, smoking cessation advisors, social prescribers, health visitors, environmental health officers, community development workers, oral health promoters, school nurses, public health nutritionists, public health analysts and public health scientists. Senior/principal practitioners lead areas of work

Public health specialists are strategic leaders, senior managers and senior scientists e.g. public health specialists in screening, health protection, children and young people, mental health, epidemiology etc.; directors of public health; public health consultants and professors in public health.

Figure 2.2 The public health workforce

practitioners begin their careers studying a discipline such as social science or a profession such as teaching or nursing. Some, such as environmental health officers or graduates in public health, hold a public health qualification. Examples of public health practitioner roles include health visitors, school nurses, health promotion/ improvement practitioners, smoking cessation advisors and environmental health officers. Practitioners spend all their time improving the health of populations, communities, groups or individuals. They can be found in front-line roles or in middle or senior management. They usually work in the health sector, local and central government, the independent sector and voluntary sector.

Wider public health workforce

The wider public health workforce is the most diverse of the three workforce categories and includes anyone whose work makes a positive impact on people's health and wellbeing. It comprises paid and unpaid workers across many sectors including education, science, retail, leisure and hospitality (CfWI, 2015). Individuals can be found working at any level of an organisation, from the front-line to chief executive. This wider public health workforce comprises three types of job roles:

- people who have direct contact with individuals or communities, e.g. general practitioners, registered nurses and midwives, dentists, opticians, pharmacists, social care workers, teachers, housing officers and fitness professionals
- leaders and advocates, e.g. local councillors, chief executives, board members, headteachers, police chief constables and faith leaders
- influencers of the social determinants of health, e.g. people employed in town planning and licensing or those working in public transport

(PHE, 2019)

Some jobs can include more than one type of role. The key distinction between the public health practitioner workforce and the wider public health workforce is how much of their job comprises public health. Practitioners usually spend their whole time involved in one or more of the three public health domains and functions, and would describe their job to others as 'working in public health'. Those within the wider public health workforce would not describe the main purpose of their job as 'public health', but would recognise that their work influences people's health. If we invest in training, motivating and empowering this wider public health workforce, it offers huge potential for improving the population's health and wellbeing (CfWI, 2015; UK Public Health, 2020).

Job roles

The public health workforce includes an array of different job roles which affect, and can potentially improve, the health and wellbeing of populations. They work across a range of sectors and organisations, and across the three domains of public health. Examples are shown in Box 2.1 and Table 2.1.

Box 2.1 Health improvement lead for mental health

Tell us about your route into public health.

"My route into public health was unconventional. I left school with no qualifications aged 16 and went to work as a sewing machinist in a bra factory. I married at age 17 and had four children. When I was 30, I went to an open learning college where I studied Maths and English. I did well and managed to get a place at the University of Glasgow to study Social Sciences, as I had a keen interest in poverty and health inequalities. In my final year of university, I worked as a volunteer for a local community health project over the summer and this paved the way for my career in public health/health improvement. In 1994, at the age of 35, I graduated with a Master of Arts degree in Social Science. This was no mean feat with a nine year old and three other children under the age of four. Then, I got a permanent contract at a community health project to lead the work related to sexual health, addictions, poverty and inequalities. I continued with my education and completed a postgraduate diploma (PGDip) in Community Education as well as a PGDip in Health Promotion and finally a (top up) MSc in Public Health. I then moved jobs and went to work in one of Scotland's national demonstration projects, Have a Heart Paisley, where I was the team leader. This post was high profile and gave me enormous opportunities and exposure to policy and strategy work; it was also my route into the NHS. It allowed me to work in areas of health inequalities and poverty as well as community engagement and empowerment which is a passion of mine. I stayed there for nine years and then moved into my current role as health improvement lead for mental health in Scotland's largest health board, NHS Greater Glasgow and Clyde."

Please describe your current role.

"My current role as health improvement lead for mental health is varied and interesting. I lead a team of senior health improvement practitioners who contribute to the early intervention/prevention agenda, focussing on public mental health across the life course. Our work spans perinatal, infant, child, youth and adult mental health; as well as self-harm, suicide prevention, resource development and training. We work in a variety of settings including community, schools, clinical areas, prisons and the third (voluntary) sector. I contribute to the development of Scotland's national policies and strategies, for example I am the representative for health improvement within a national Managed Clinical Network that seeks to co-ordinate primary, secondary and tertiary care. I am involved in the national mental health work, funded by the Scottish Government, as part of the remobilisation/recovery effort for restarting services that were paused during the COVID-19 pandemic. This has led to exciting opportunities for our third sector partners, across six health and social care partnerships, to create innovative approaches to public mental health. I have also led the development of new ways of working as we adapted to the challenges of the COVID-19 crisis; in particular the adaptation and development of training and support for our staff groups and partners."

"My public health journey has taken me through a wide range of health improvement topics in my work, from sexual health, addictions, poverty and inequality and ultimately to mental health, which underpinned much of my previous work. In addition to my substantive post, I am also a coordinator for the UK Public Health Register (UKPHR) Scottish Practitioner Scheme, and I get the equivalent of one day a week to cover this role. I became involved with the Scheme when it first started in Scotland in 2012 and was registered as a public health practitioner in 2013. I continue to be an assessor for practitioner registration. I am also a workforce champion within my health board where I support workforce development around the *UK Public Health Skills and Knowledge Framework* (PHSKF)."

What advice would you give to someone who is thinking about a career in public health?

- "Public health is a diverse and fascinating discipline. It is wide and varied, and no two days are ever the same
- I would say if a career in public health interests you, then go for it! There is a wide range of exciting roles to choose from and the opportunities are vast. There is a great sense of personal satisfaction in the knowledge that you are making a difference (however small)
- I have been really fortunate in my career in that I get to work in areas that I am passionate about i.e. health inequalities where hopefully I contribute to eradicating the health divide. I am also passionate about lifelong learning and see education as a way out of poverty, and I am living proof of that
- Passion and hard work are key if you want to make a difference
- Public health matters!!"

Heather Sloan
Health improvement lead for mental health, registered public health practitioner and UKPHR assessor
November 2021
Reproduced with permission

Table 2.1 Examples of job roles within the UK public health workforce

Job title/role	Overview of the role	Training and/or education	Salary range per annum (2021)	Domain(s)	Workforce category
Health champion	Health champions are typically voluntary roles. They work with local communities supporting health promotion initiatives and signposting people to services. They also engage in health and wellbeing-related conversations to support behaviour change or behaviour-focused action. Their role can be an adjunct to an existing job role, e.g. pharmacy assistant.	The training for health champions varies, but it normally includes a basic understanding of health, the risk factors for poor health and communication skills. Many learn about health-related behaviour change through the Making Every Contact Count (MECC) e-learning programme.	Voluntary	Health improvement	Wider public health
Smoking cessation advisor	Smoking cessation advisors, sometimes called stop smoking advisors or stop smoking specialists, motivate and support people who want to stop smoking for good. They work with individuals and groups in community centres, GP practices and other settings that are accessible to the public. Over several weeks, they help people to set goals and develop action plans towards quitting, as well as offering nicotine replacement therapy (NRT). They may also be involved in health promotion campaigns with communities such as Stoptober.	Smoking cessation advisors undertake nationally accredited smoking cessation training which includes motivational interviewing techniques and learning about NRT.	£22,000–£31,000	Health improvement	Public health practitioner

(Continued)

Table 2.1 Examples of job roles within the UK public health workforce (*Continued*)

Job title/role	Overview of the role	Training and/or education	Salary range per annum (2021)	Domain(s)	Workforce category
Social prescriber	Social prescribers, also called link workers, work with people who are vulnerable or disadvantaged within healthcare, communities and other settings. They support individuals, their families and carers with issues relating to their health and wellbeing. This includes working with people over many sessions to help them to develop their confidence, a sense of control, the skills to manage and improve their health, and to enable them to live independently. Typically, social prescribers work with GP practices or in the voluntary sector, but their role is evolving and being utilised more widely.	Social prescribers are trained to NVQ Level 3 or equivalent. Their learning includes communication skills, community engagement, emotional resilience, motivational interviewing or coaching skills, partnership working, and evaluation and monitoring.	£24,000–£30,000	Health improvement	Wider public health
Recovery worker	Recovery workers, or support, time and recovery (STR) workers, aim to enable adults and young people with mental health diagnoses or learning disabilities to improve their health and wellbeing. They provide advice and practical support across a range of issues such as homelessness, substance misuse, social exclusion and unemployment. They are employed by the voluntary sector, National Health Service and local government, and are often based in community venues, health centres and GP practices.	There are no set entry requirements for this post, however sometimes employers may ask for a qualification in a health-related field or equivalent experience. In addition to on-the-job learning, some recovery workers may work towards qualifications in mental health or substance misuse.	£19,000–£22,000	Health improvement	Wider public health

(*Continued*)

Table 2.1 Examples of job roles within the UK public health workforce (*Continued*)

Job title/role	Overview of the role	Training and/or education	Salary range per annum (2021)	Domain(s)	Workforce category
Community development worker	Community development workers (CDWs) help communities to bring about social changes which will improve their quality of life. CDWs may work in a geographical area or with a specific population, e.g. as a mental health CDW, or working with black and ethnic minority communities or older people. Their work includes community mapping, service navigation, advocacy, community engagement and one-to-one support. They are usually employed by local authorities or the voluntary sector, and are based in community venues or other settings that are accessible to the public.	Typically, CDWs are graduates or those with equivalent experience. They may have a degree in health promotion or public health, social sciences or community development, and a passion for helping communities. Once in post, they can access on-the-job training, e.g. mental health training or asset-based community mapping.	£21,000–£36,000	Health improvement	Wider public health
Oral health promoter	Oral health promoters (OHPs) provide oral health education for education and healthcare professionals, community groups and individuals such as children or older adults living in care homes. They also collect data to monitor and evaluate oral health outcomes.	Typically, OHPs are graduate dental care practitioners registered with the General Dental Council (GDC), and some have a certificate in oral health promotion/education. They have a good understanding of the determinants of health and oral health inequalities.	£26,000–£32,000	Health improvement	Public health practitioner

(*Continued*)

Table 2.1 Examples of job roles within the UK public health workforce (*Continued*)

Job title/role	Overview of the role	Training and/or education	Salary range per annum (2021)	Domain(s)	Workforce category
Health protection practitioner	Health protection practitioners work within teams that protect the public from infectious diseases and other non-infectious health hazards, e.g. tuberculosis, e-coli, sexually transmitted infections and COVID-19 coronavirus. They collect, monitor, analyse and interpret health-related data (surveillance) and collaborate with multiple agencies to manage and prevent infections and disease. Health protection teams are based within national organisations and local authority public health departments.	Health protection practitioners are graduates such as registered nurses, environmental health officers or public health practitioners. They engage with health protection-related continuous professional development (CPD) to keep up to date with the latest evidence and practice.	£38,000–£63,000	Health protection	Public health practitioner
Environmental health officer	Environmental health officers (EHOs) deal with noise and environmental pollution; food safety and hygiene; workplace health; housing standards and health protection. They work in teams within local authorities.	EHOs undertake a degree, a degree apprenticeship or post-graduate qualification in Environmental Health. Some practitioners attain chartered status with the Chartered Institute of Environmental Health (CIEH). They are expected to undertake continuous professional development.	£23,000–£45,000	Health protection	Public health practitioner

(*Continued*)

Table 2.1 Examples of job roles within the UK public health workforce *(Continued)*

Job title/role	Overview of the role	Training and/or education	Salary range per annum (2021)	Domain(s)	Workforce category
Health visitor	Health visitors (HVs) develop 'early intervention' public health initiatives to support families with children, from birth to five, towards the 'best start in life.' This includes child protection, parental education and visiting homes to carry out the 'mandated checks' which assess each child's health and development. HVs work within local authorities, children's centres and other venues which are accessed by families.	HVs are registered with the Nursing and Midwifery Council (NMC). Nurses and midwives complete post-graduate education to become a specialist community public health nurse (SCPHN) specialising in health visiting. Continuous professional development is mandatory.	£30,000–£38,000	Health improvement	Public health practitioner
Occupational health nurse	Occupational health nurses (OHNs) focus on health and care in the workplace, supporting the prevention of work-related health problems, and promoting healthy living and working conditions. OHNs work for a range of employers including local authorities, National Health Service, the voluntary sector and the private sector.	Nurses complete post-graduate education to become a specialist community public health nurse (SCPHN) specialising in occupational health nursing. (Other SCPHNs include school nurses, health visitors and public health nurses). Continuous professional development is mandatory.	£21,000–£45,000	Health improvement	Public health practitioner
Public health analyst	Public health analysts form part of the public health intelligence workforce. They collect, analyse and interpret health-related data/information which is used to identify a population's health needs and inform the planning of public health initiatives. Typically, they work across the three domains of public health and are employed in local authorities, the National Health Service, national agencies and the civil service.	Those who work within the intelligence workforce are typically graduates in subjects such as epidemiology, geography or data analysis. They receive further on-the-job training around the use of data and information software.	£21,000 starting salary	Health improvement/ Health protection/ Healthcare public health	Public health practitioner/ specialist

(Continued)

Table 2.1 Examples of job roles within the UK public health workforce (*Continued*)

Job title/role	Overview of the role	Training and/or education	Salary range per annum (2021)	Domain(s)	Workforce category
Lecturer in public health	Lecturers in public health are normally employed by universities, and work in one or more of the domains of public health. They develop and lead undergraduate and post-graduate modules and programmes; provide lectures, seminars and tutorials. Many are engaged in research which involves applying for funding and actively contributing to the creation and dissemination of public health evidence. Those with experience lead and manage teams, projects and departments.	Typically, lecturers in public health have a master's degree and/or a PhD in health promotion and/or public health or a closely related field. They have a variety of academic and/or professional backgrounds which can include disciplines such as psychology or nutrition; or professional backgrounds such as cardiac rehabilitation or medicine. Lecturers are expected to work towards fellowship of Advance HE. Continuous professional development is necessary.	£33,000 starting salary	Health improvement/ Health protection/ Healthcare public health	Public health practitioner/ specialist
Health improvement practitioner	Health improvement practitioners typically work in local authority/local health board public health teams where they manage or lead an area of work, e.g. public health mental health, behaviour change, substance misuse, diet, etc. The role varies and may include the commissioning, development and delivery of programmes and services.	Entry routes into this type of role vary. Some practitioners have relevant degrees such as health promotion, public health, nutrition, sport and health or social sciences; some may have professional qualifications such as occupational therapy and others follow three-year apprenticeships to gain a public health degree along with UKPHR practitioner registration. Increasingly, job descriptions are stipulating public health practitioner registration as a requirement.	£22,000–£39,000	Health improvement	Public health practitioner

(*Continued*)

Table 2.1 Examples of job roles within the UK public health workforce (*Continued*)

Job title/role	Overview of the role	Training and/or education	Salary range per annum (2021)	Domain(s)	Workforce category
Public health principal	A public health principal, sometimes called a public health manager or senior public health practitioner, is a role that sits between a public health practitioner and consultant. They are responsible for a portfolio of public health work. They provide specialist knowledge, leadership, strategic direction, policy advice and develop long-term plans for public health priorities. They work collaboratively with others, and are typically based in local authorities.	Typically, principals are registered public health practitioners with a master's degree in public health or equivalent. They may also be registered health professionals. They have received leadership training and are actively engaged with ongoing continuous professional development.	£48,000–£65,000	Health improvement	Public health practitioner
Public health consultant	Public health consultants lead the work to address a population's health needs, based on the evidence. They provide specialist technical advice and help to develop policies and strategies. Their job title reflects the domain of public health in which they specialise, e.g. consultant in healthcare public health. Typically, they work in local authorities/health boards, the National Health Service, national agencies and the civil service.	Consultants complete the 48-month Public Health Speciality Training Programme which comprises a master's degree in public health and the completion of professional exams. Individuals with significant public health experience can submit a retrospective portfolio demonstrating how they meet the public health specialist standards to the UKPHR or GMC. Consultants are registered with either the GMC or UKPHR, and continuous professional development is mandatory.	£71,095–£93,764	Health improvement/ Health protection/ Healthcare public health	Public health specialist

(*Continued*)

Table 2.1 Examples of job roles within the UK public health workforce *(Continued)*

Job title/role	Overview of the role	Training and/or education	Salary range per annum (2021)	Domain(s)	Workforce category
Dental public health consultant	Consultants in dental public health lead the work to improve oral health in their locality. They offer expert input into a range of dental public health programmes and support colleagues to develop dental services and other related services, such as those dealing with food and nutrition. Typically, they work in local authorities/health boards, the National Health Service, other national agencies and the civil service.	Consultants have usually completed an approved four-year minimum training programme in Dental Public Health, a master's degree in dental public health or the equivalent and must be on the General Dental Council specialist list in dental public health.	£71,095–£93,764	Health improvement/ Health protection/ Healthcare public health	Public health specialist
Director of public health	Directors of public health have a strategic leadership role, and statutory responsibilities, to protect and improve the health of their population and to reduce health inequalities. They are responsible for public health budgets which are used to commission services such as weight management, smoking cessation or health visiting. They actively work across the wider/ social determinants of health.	Directors of public health have often worked as public health consultants, have substantive experience, and have both leadership qualifications and experience.	£100K +	Health improvement/ Health protection/ Healthcare public health	Public health specialist

A range of job roles contribute to improving the health and wellbeing of individuals and the population. Individuals work in a range of sectors and organisations, and across the three domains of public health.

Competencies for working in health promotion and public health

A competency describes the knowledge, technical skills and behaviours needed to do a job effectively. For example, a plumber needs many competencies including knowing how plumbing systems work, having the technical skills to replace a sink and behaving in a professional and courteous manner in people's homes. An assessor will decide whether an apprentice plumber is competent to practise by checking the apprentice's practice against an approved list of plumbing competencies. A list of competencies is called a competency framework and there is a plethora of competency frameworks for different job roles.

Competency frameworks

- inform the content of education/training courses and their assessment
- set out the agreed standards against which the quality of people's work is monitored and assessed
- help employers to identify where their workforce may need further education/training
- inform recruitment, selection and employment processes such as the competencies outlined in a job description
- can help individuals to identify what they have learnt, their areas of expertise and what they need to learn as part of their life-long learning across their whole career
- can help individuals to identify what they need to learn, or do, to meet the requirements for professional registration

We will describe four public health competency frameworks, each of which can be used by individuals or organisations. Like the apprentice plumber who may have developed some plumbing competencies when working in a previous job, public health competencies can be developed across a wide range of job roles. While each framework uses different terminology, their common competencies include being able to

- communicate effectively to improve health outcomes and reduce health inequalities
- collaborate with, and lead, others to drive improvements in health
- use public health intelligence, and epidemiological and statistical methods, to understand and address population health and wellbeing, and health inequalities
- Assess and apply evidence to plan the delivery of effective public health interventions or services
- practise professionally, ethically and legally to minimise risk and harm to others

UK Public Health Skills and Knowledge Framework (PHSKF)

The first UK public health competency framework, the *UK Public Health Skills and Knowledge Framework* (PHSKF) (Figure 2.3), was developed in 2008 and updated in 2016 (PHE/PHA/PHW/NHS Scotland, 2016). The framework aims to provide the benchmark, a single point of reference, for public health competencies across the UK.

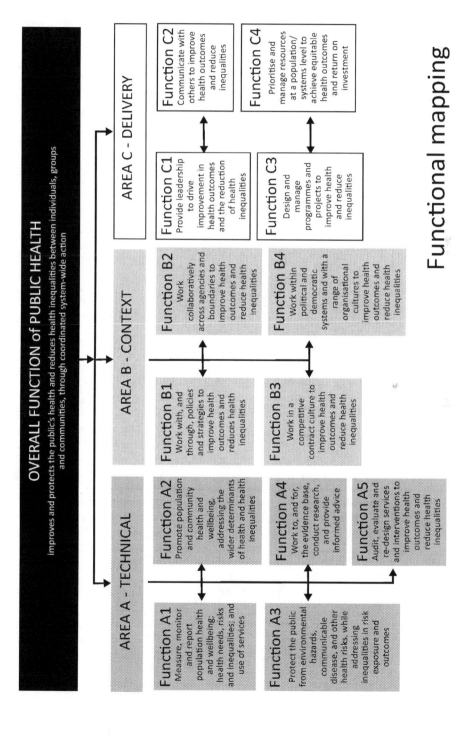

Figure 2.3 UK Public Health Skills and Knowledge Framework

Source: PHE/PHA/PHW/NHS Scotland, 2016, p. 10. Reproduced under the terms of the Open Government Licence v.3.0

This framework is written for the public health specialist, practitioner and the wider public health workforce. It is divided into three Areas of activity:

- A – technical
- B – context
- C – delivery

Each Area includes four or five public health competencies which are called Functions. Each Function is divided into Sub-functions which explain what actions are required to meet the public health competency. Table 2.2 illustrates how a social prescriber

Table 2.2 Using PHSKF competencies to support a social prescriber's work objectives

Public Health Knowledge and Skills Framework			Objectives for the year ahead
Area	*Function (public health competency)*	*Sub-function (action to meet competency)*	
Area A TECHNICAL	**Function A1** Measure, monitor and report population health and wellbeing, health needs, risks and inequalities; and use of services.	**Subfunction A1.1** Identify data needs and obtain, verify and organise that data and information. **Subfunction A1.2** Interpret and present data and information.	Visit the local public health team to understand the local data sets, how to use them and seek advice about how to best present data and information.
	Function A2 Promote population and community health and wellbeing, addressing the wider determinants of health and health inequalities.	**Subfunction A2.6** Facilitate change (behavioural and/or cultural) in organisations, communities and/or individuals.	Attend appropriate training to develop my skills to support behaviour change with an individual.
Area B CONTEXT	**Function B2** Work collaboratively across agencies and boundaries to improve health outcomes and reduce health inequalities.	**Subfunction B2.5** Connect communities, groups and individuals to local resources and services that support their health and wellbeing.	Design and co-develop a website of services available across health, care and voluntary sector in collaboration with local partners.
Area C DELIVERY	**Function C3** Design and manage programmes and projects to improve health and reduce health inequalities.	**Subfunction C3.4** Track and evaluate programme/project progress against schedule(s) and regularly review quality assurance, risks and opportunities to realise benefits and outcomes.	Lead on evaluation of local pilot of strength-based programme for the over 70s to evaluate impact on health and social isolation.

might use the PHSKF to prepare for their annual appraisal/performance review meeting with their line manager. They have identified four public health competencies (Functions A1, A2, B2 and C3). They reflect on their work and identify where they have already acquired expertise, what competencies they need to develop and the specific objectives/tasks for the year ahead which will help to achieve this.

WHO-ASPHER Competency Framework

The *World Health Organization-Association of Schools of Public Health in the European Region's (WHO-ASPHER) Competency Framework for the Public Health Workforce in the European Region* is aimed at the core public health workforce and includes three levels of competence: competent (level 3), proficient (level 2) and expert (level 1). Published in 2020, it was developed to provide a comprehensive and consistent framework for addressing the population's health needs across Europe. Figure 2.4 shows it has three major categories.

- 'Content and context' concentrates on the technical and scientific competencies of public health practice including ethical practice
- 'Relations and interactions' focuses on the ability to effectively communicate technical and scientific knowledge to lead and work in partnership with others to improve the population's health
- 'Performance and achievement' addresses competencies to ensure evidence-based decisions are made through reflective practice

These are divided into 10 sections, each encompassing a total of 84 public health competencies.

The WHO-ASPHER Competency Framework categories are:

Content and context
1. Science and practice
2. Promoting health
3. Law, policies and ethics
4. One Health and health security

Relations and interactions
5. Leadership and systems thinking
6. Collaboration and partnerships
7. Communication, culture and advocacy

Performance and achievement
8. Governance and resource management
9. Professional development and reflective ethical practice
10. Organisational literacy and adaptability

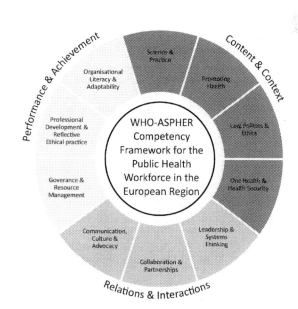

Figure 2.4 WHO-ASPHER Competency Framework

Source: WHO-ASPHER, 2020, p. 12. Reproduced with permission from World Health Organization Europe

To demonstrate how this framework can be used, we will take the example of a public health practitioner whose ambition is to gain further experience, be given more responsibility and apply for a senior position such as a public health principal. The practitioner is working with several organisations within the local community to prevent and tackle substance misuse. Specifically, they decide to focus on their ability to work collaboratively with others and develop their leadership skills. They read the category 'Relations and interactions' and go to 'Section 6 Collaboration and partnerships' which contains two competencies, 6.1 and 6.2 (Table 2.3). The practitioner

Table 2.3 WHO-ASPHER competencies relating to collaboration and partnerships

Relations and interactions

Section 6. Collaboration and partnerships

Effective collaboration; building alliances and partnerships; networking and connecting; working with and building interdisciplinary and intersectoral networks; dealing with and managing stakeholders

Competency	Competent (level 3)	Proficient (level 2)	Expert (level 1)
6.1 Works across sectors in organisational structures at the local, national and international levels.	My competency in public health means that I work with a range of stakeholders from various organisations or sectors who are mainly based within my locality.	My proficiency in public health means that I effectively work with a range of stakeholders from various organisations and sectors across my local area with others across the region or country.	My leadership role requires me to have the necessary expertise to establish and work with partner organisations in various sectors, potentially at local, national or international level.
6.2 Understands the interdependence, integration and competition among healthcare sectors and various actors who have interests in public health issues.	I understand that to be competent in my role, I must work with a wide range of stakeholders. I attempt to understand their priorities and motivations.	I realise that to be proficient in my role and to establish effective partnerships, I must understand the priorities and motivations of a wide range of stakeholders.	Given the importance of collaboration and partnership working within public health, in my leadership role, I analyse the priorities and motivations of individuals and organisations. Based on this analysis and the goals I aim to address, I decide on the approach I will take for future relationships such as accommodation, avoidance, collaboration, competition and compromise.

Source: Adapted from WHO-ASPHER, 2020, p. 46

Table 2.4 A personal development plan referencing WHO-ASPHER competencies

Sections (which relate to the needs identified)	Objectives for the year ahead	Public health competency (to be achieved)	Target date (by which competency will be achieved)
Collaboration and partnerships	Deputise for the principal at the regional Children's & Young People's forum to build networks and develop opportunities to lead regional programmes of work. Lead on the development and uptake of alcohol brief intervention training with GP practices as part of a regional Alcohol Strategy.	6.1 Works across sectors in organisational structures at the local, national and international levels	12 months 8 months
Leadership and systems thinking	Contribute to the Tobacco Control Strategy by leading on the 'smoke free environments' chapter. Undertake a 360-degree review to understand strengths and areas of development for personal effectiveness and leadership.	5.1 Inspires and motivates others to work towards a common vision, programme and/or organisational goals	6 months 3 months

focuses on 6.1, reads the competency and assesses their work as being at level 3 (competent). They learn they would need to lead a programme of work in their local community, a region or even nationally, and work with a wider range of organisations, stakeholders and policymakers, to meet the 6.1 competency at level 2 (proficient). The practitioner considers what they could do over the next year to gain the experience needed to achieve proficiency and they write this on their personal development plan (Table 2.4). They decide not to focus on competency 6.2 this year.

Next, staying within the same category, the practitioner finds 'Section 5 Leadership and systems thinking' which comprises nine competencies. They focus on competency 5.1 'Inspires and motivates others to work towards a common vision, programme and/or organisational goals'. The practitioner assesses their practice to be at level 3 (competent), decides to work towards level 2 (proficient), considers what experience they need and adds this to their personal development plan (Table 2.4). The plan includes a 360-degree review which is a way for individuals to receive constructive feedback from peers, colleagues and stakeholders, on their strengths and areas for development. For example, the feedback may include how well they interact with others and raise awareness about any blind spots. A year later, the practitioner will repeat the process.

The WHO-ASPHER framework helpfully illustrates which competencies are essential for a particular area of work, each of which will include a range of specific job roles. They call these areas of work essential public health operations (EPHOs), rather like the three UK public health domains. The ten EPHOs include the work of disease prevention, including the early detection of illness; the work of health protection including environmental and occupational protection, food safety and so forth; and the work of surveillance and population wellbeing. For example, for those public health professionals whose career is focussed on health promotion and reducing health inequity, there are eight priority competencies to be achieved, eventually to the level of expert. These are shown in Table 2.5.

Table 2.5 WHO-ASPHER competencies for working in health promotion and addressing health inequity (EPHO 4)

EPHO 4: Health promotion including action to address social determinants and health inequity

The purpose of this EPHO is to promote population health and wellbeing by addressing inequalities and the broader social and environmental determinants. Supportive environments need to be created and community assets strengthened to empower individuals and populations to have healthier lifestyles and behaviour across the life course. Multisectoral action is needed to create healthy environments and to reduce inequalities and risk factors in social and environmental determinants of health.

Competencies

2.1 Assesses the focus and scope of initiatives to promote health by assessing the need to achieve positive changes in individual and community health.

2.2 Knows, supports and engages in health promoting and health literacy activities and programmes for implementing good practices to promote health at a population level and specific organisation or institutional level.

2.3 Uses evidence-based methods and strategies, social participation and intersectoral approaches as tools for promoting health and influencing public policies affecting health.

2.4 Evaluates the effectiveness of activities to promote health geared towards producing changes at the community and individual levels and in public or social policy to benefit health and quality of life.

2.5 Fosters citizen empowerment and engagement within the community, developing capabilities that are valuable to actively participate in the development and decision-making of a healthy community.

2.6 When needed, generates or promulgates factual information to counteract industry marketing in relation to nutrition, tobacco cessation, reducing alcohol consumption, etc.

2.8 Understands and addresses the upstream fundamental causes of health inequalities and downstream consequences (such as drug and alcohol abuse and smoking) in ensuring equitable access to health services.

5.8 Catalyses change (behavioural and/or cultural) in the organisation, communities and/or individuals.

7.8 Advocates for healthy public policies and services that promote and protect the health and wellbeing of individuals and communities.

Source: Adapted from WHO-ASPHER, 2020, p. 61

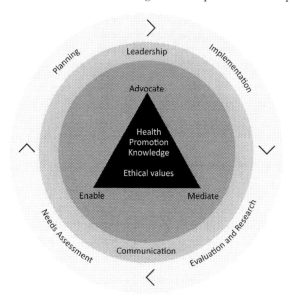

Figure 2.5 The CompHP core competencies for health promotion

Source: Barry *et al.*, 2012. Reproduced with permission from IUHPE

International Union for Health Promotion and Education

The International Union for Health Promotion and Education (IUHPE) is an international network of professionals and institutions dedicated to health promotion. Their competency framework was originally developed as part of the project *Developing Competencies and Professional Standards for Health Promotion Capacity Building in Europe* (CompHP) (Barry *et al.*, 2012). It supports health promotion practice, based on addressing the five principles of the *Ottawa Charter for Health Promotion* discussed in Chapter 8. The framework comprises nine standards across 11 domains of core competency (Figure 2.5). Ethical values and health promotion knowledge are central and underpin all the domains.

UK Public Health Register Practitioner Standards for Registration

The *UK Public Health Register* (UKPHR) Practitioner Standards for Registration were published in April 2011 and updated, after extensive UK-wide consultation, in April 2019 (UKPHR, 2020). This competency framework of 'standards' was developed with reference to the *National Health Service Knowledge and Skills Framework*, the *National Occupational Standards for the Practice of Public Health* (Skills for Health, 2004) and the *UK Public Health Skills and Knowledge Framework* (PHSKF). It sets the minimum standards of knowledge and skills that a public health practitioner needs to be able to deliver safe, effective and evidence-based public health. Examples of the 34 standards (competencies) include

- demonstrate knowledge of existing and emerging legal and ethical issues in own area of practice
- act in ways that acknowledge and recognise people's expressed beliefs and preferences

- act in ways that promote the ability of others to make informed decisions
- apply evidence to improving own area of work
- demonstrate knowledge of the nature of health inequalities and how they might be monitored
- demonstrate the ability to make valid interpretations of the data and/or information and communicate these clearly to a variety of audiences
- demonstrate knowledge of the risks to health and wellbeing relevant to own area of work and of the varying scale of risk
- demonstrate awareness of the effect the media has on public perception
- communicate effectively with a range of different people using different methods

(UKPHR, 2020, pp. 4–7)

Competency frameworks can be used by individuals to understand the competencies they need to work effectively in health promotion and public health. They support reflection, personal and professional development, including career planning.

Thinking point:

Evaluate your own competencies. Which are your strengths and which would you need to develop if working in public health?

Registration of health promotion and public health professionals

The competencies for working in health promotion and public health are also used in the context of registration. Registration refers to a professional register such as those held by the Nursing and Midwifery Council (NMC), General Medical Council (GMC), General Dental Council (GDC) and Health and Care Professions Council (HCPC). Regulation via registration exists to protect the public against the risk of harm when receiving treatment or care. Each name on the register has met both academic and vocational competencies, they adhere to the profession's ethical code and they have kept their practice up to date throughout their career with additional learning, often called continuing professional development. They can call themselves 'registered'. The registers can be accessed by the public, including employers. If a professional fails to meet the profession's standards, they can lose their license to practise and be 'removed from the register'.

In the UK, when developing the current structure of the UK's public health workforce, employers argued that this workforce needed to be registered to ensure safe and ethical practice, and to provide parity with other health and care professions working at a similar level of responsibility. For example, a new graduate with a degree in public health, which is an academic, not a professional qualification, who begins work as a smoking cessation advisor will not be named on any register. While some professionals who initially qualified and registered as clinical professionals may move into a public health role. For example, a midwife who is qualified to practice midwifery care then moves into a public health role such as a community development worker (women's health). The NMC register is mostly concerned with standards of care; a public health register is concerned with the standards of public health work. The UK needed a registration system that could cover the needs of both the smoking cessation advisor and the community development worker.

Thinking point:

> Consider the ways in which the public health workforce could harm the public. Why do we need safe and ethical public health practice?

UK Public Health Register (UKPHR)

Today, all those who are appointed to public health specialist posts are expected to be registered with either the General Medical Council, the General Dental Council or the UK Public Health Register (UKPHR). The UKPHR is a voluntary register, accredited by the Professional Standards Authority, and a national accreditation organisation (PSA, 2021). Many public health specialists with non-medical backgrounds and most public health practitioners, such as smoking cessation advisors, work towards becoming registered with the UKPHR.

- To become registered and use the title 'registered public health specialist,' individuals either complete:

    - the Faculty of Public Health's Public Health Speciality Training Programme

  or

    - those with extensive experience working at specialist level can apply to submit a retrospective portfolio of evidence of their competencies for assessment against the public health specialist curriculum (FPH, 2020)

To use the title 'registered public health practitioner', the individual needs to

    - complete the public health practitioner apprenticeship (degree)

  or

    - submit a retrospective portfolio of evidence of their competencies for assessment against the 34 practitioner standards outlined in the *UKPHR Practitioner Standards for Registration* (UKPHR, 2020).

If successful, the individual is added to the UK Public Health Register (Box 2.2). Support for those wishing to work towards registration is provided by regional or local public health departments across the UK. Once registered, like all registered professionals, they are expected to follow a professional code of conduct. The UKPHR's code states registrants must:

- make the health and protection of the public their prime concern
- be honest and trustworthy
- protect confidentiality
- maintain high standards of professional and personal conduct
- know the limits of their competence and act within them
- respect the dignity of individuals and treat everyone fairly
- cooperate with the teams with which they work and interact

(UKPHR, 2014)

Box 2.2 Registered principal public health practitioner

Tell us about your route into public health.

"I completed my MSc in Health and Social Care Leadership in 2013. I have worked in the NHS for 27 years. During this time, I worked as health partnership lead for one of the North Wales local health boards. I was jointly responsible for drafting, consulting with others and then implementing the Health, Social Care and Wellbeing Strategy (2008–2011) for the county. This required a whole systems approach to ensure inclusive public engagement and community involvement. The experience provided an opportunity to further strengthen the collaboration between, and integration of, all partners with the aim to significantly improve the health and wellbeing of the local population. On reflection, this was the start of my route into public health.

"In 2016, I joined the local public health team as a senior public health practitioner and in 2017, completed two modules of the master's degree in Public Health: Health Economics and Epidemiology. To demonstrate my experience and commitment to public health, I also worked to become registered as a UK public health practitioner on the UK Public Health Register (UKPHR). In 2018, as part of my continuing professional development, and because I have a passion for supporting others, I qualified as an ILM7 executive coach and mentor awarded by the Institute of Leadership and Management.

"I now have over five years' experience in the local public health team, and have worked as a principal public health practitioner for almost three years now. I am committed to supporting others and have recently undertaken the UKPHR public health practitioner registration assessor training and assessed my first portfolio. I recently participated in the Healthcare Leadership Model led by the NHS Leadership Academy. Some of the 360 degree feedback I received included,

'Jackie is a positive role model and supports the development of others in her team, the wider organisation and across the PH system in Wales and UK. She is an advocate 'champion' for professional recognition of the PH workforce.'"

Please describe your current role.

"Since March 2020, the priority for our team has been to support the COVID-19 response, and as such, roles and responsibilities had to change accordingly. The team embraced and adapted as necessary. Each, and every one of us, rose to the challenges of working in such a fluid environment, working from home and undertaking new roles with limited lead-in time or training. As a UKPHR registered public health practitioner, I continue to contribute to the Test, Trace, Protect (TTP) strategy demonstrating my practice across the UKPHR standards.

"In addition, I am the principal early years lead for the team and I seize opportunities to influence the public health improvement agenda, engaging at a strategic level with diverse partners. I am particularly proud to have led all of the team's achievements in the 'early years space' over the last 18 months. We have:

- provided women and families with the Solihull online resources (to support parenting) at a time when it was probably most needed
- provided Solihull Parenting Training for our partners/colleagues
- established a quality improvement programme to support infant feeding

and

- commissioned and driven the work to gain deeper insight into healthy weight in pregnancy, which will inform our future plans for tackling maternal obesity across our region

"I actively contribute to the senior leadership team and principal group for peer support and challenge. I currently line manage five team members providing support and advice to meet objectives and to promote health and wellbeing.

"The current climate of the NHS and Public Health is one of constant change, I use my planning and organisational skills to support the unpredictable nature of the principal practitioner role to respond to competing demands. I do this by making judgements based on risks, reprioritising and adapting mine and others' work where necessary. I thrive in this fluid environment."

What advice would you give to someone who is thinking about a career in public health?

"Go for it, public health needs people who want to make a difference to population health!

As a starting point, I would advise you to:

- take a look at the four nation's public health websites and their respective strategic plans
- visit the Faculty of Public Health website
- take a look at the UKPHR standards to explore whether you have evidence to embark upon registration or determine what gaps you might have to inform a development plan for the UKPHR portfolio route
- horizon scan, keep abreast of local and national politics, key legislation and policies. Be curious and aware of the current key drivers and the importance of embedding such legislation, and understand the value of benchmarking locally and nationally
- explore the evidence; subscribe to publications and evidence registries
- build your network of contacts and sources of information across the systems"

Jackie Irwin, registered principal public health practitioner
November 2021
Reproduced with permission

Health promotion practitioner registration

An alternate route is to register as a health promotion practitioner through the International Union for Health Promotion and Education (IUHPE) Accreditation System (Barry *et al.*, 2012). There are two pathways to becoming a registered health promotion practitioner in the UK:

- completion of an undergraduate or a post-graduate qualification which has been assessed against the *CompHP Competencies and Professional Standards* and accredited by IUHPE. The course will have a high health promotion content. Individuals submit evidence of successful completion of the qualification to the IUHPE to become registered

- completion through self-assessment is available to individuals who may have qualifications in health promotion but which are not IUHPE accredited, and they have significant health promotion work experience. Individuals submit a self-assessment of their practice, experiences and relevant training/education, mapped against the CompHP competencies and professional standards, along with references. The IUHPE decides whether the individual is eligible for registration

The UKPHR is the approved national accreditation organisation for the UK and for those in the UK wishing to register with IUHPE. Individuals, located elsewhere in Europe, wishing to be recognised for their health promotion practice need to apply directly to the IUPHE or through their own country's national accreditation organisation. A person may have dual registration with another profession.

Dual registration

A person, like the midwife who moved to a community development role discussed above, may choose to have dual registration. Dual registration is illustrated by the case study in Box 2.3. Note that 'chartered' means someone has attained a high degree of competence in a profession; it is different from registration.

Box 2.3 Registered psychologist and registered public health specialist

Tell us about your route into public health.

"After a completing a BSc Psychology and an MSc Health Psychology, I ended up using my qualifications to work in smoking cessation and sexual health promotion; it was here that I discovered public health. Alongside these roles, I completed the British Psychological Society's Stage 2 in Health Psychology to receive chartered status and I remain a registered psychologist with the Health Professionals Council.

"My next role, leading an NHS primary care trust's health inequalities programme, shaped my whole career. I realised that I wanted to use my skills in influencing systems to help the people who rarely have a voice. I had a wide portfolio which included ethnic minorities, new entrants to the UK, homelessness, domestic violence and those in touch with the criminal justice system. When primary care trusts were dissolved in 2013, I took up a regional role in Public Health England (PHE) focussed on health and justice. When I had worked in public health for about seven years, and gained a breadth of experience at senior level, I decided to complete my public health specialist registration with UKPHR through the portfolio route.

"During this time, I took up the role of leading Public Health England's (PHE) international health and justice programme. PHE was the only World Health Organization (WHO) Collaborating Centre for the Health in Prisons Programme at that time. In this role, I worked with international partners linked to the Worldwide Prison Health Research and Engagement Network to develop a minimum public health dataset on prison health, now held at the Global Health Observatory, and I contributed to several publications.

"My dual registration as a psychologist and a public health specialist has been a huge asset to my current role as a global public health consultant. Although I have often felt different to my traditionally trained public health colleagues, it is this difference which has enhanced my practice."

Please describe your current role.

"Today, I am a global public health consultant with the UK Health Security Agency (UKHSA), leading on public health programmes for the UK Overseas Territories, funded directly by the Foreign and Commonwealth Development Office. I am currently working on the health of people in contact with the justice system, which involves considering of all aspects of public health for people with some of the worst health outcomes. I also lead the co-ordination of UKHSA's input into managing chemicals and radiation hazards to ensure compliance with the International Health Regulations, and I am bringing my experience of working with local authorities to bear on a Joint Strategic Needs Assessment for St Helena, to understand the population's health needs and plan for future service provision.

"I work in a small team of people that spans both UKHSA and the Office for Health Improvement and Disparities in the UK's Department of Health and Social Care. We generally lead and deliver our own work programmes with some joint working, within an overall strategic approach. Having your own professional networks really helps with ensuring you are up to date with evidence-based practice and you can draw on other people's expertise – public health is definitely a collaborative discipline.

"I continue to provide support to the WHO and am looking to expand my role in mentoring with Health Education England. Public health skills are required across a broad range of settings and often public health consultants will work across different organisations and be contracted to advise on different projects. This allows me to develop a diversity of interests – work is certainly never boring!"

What advice would you give to someone who is thinking about a career in public health?

"Connecting your personal values to your career fuels a satisfying work life. My work with people in prison, who suffer some of the worse health inequalities, often as a result of the failings of the wider system, spoke directly to my need to address injustices in the world. This has helped to create a personal 'mission,' shaping my career and professional choices.

"Public health is all about the long game, both in terms of outcomes and developing the right skills and competencies to make a difference. It's a career, not a job, and you have to commit to continually learning and working with others. Once you realise that it's about the journey and the process, rather than the destination of becoming qualified or getting a consultant job, it becomes one of the most fulfilling life experiences."

Sunita Sturup-Toft
Global public health consultant, registered psychologist and registered public health specialist
November, 2021
Reproduced with permission

Individuals can work towards becoming a registered public health practitioner (UKPHR), a registered public health specialist (UKPHR, GMC or GDC) or a registered health promotion practitioner (IUHPE). The UKPHR and local public health teams can provide advice and support.

Continuing professional development, re-registration and revalidation

All professions are expected to engage in their own continuing professional development (CPD), which means participating in regular learning activities to enhance their competencies and ensure their practice remains up to date. Providing evidence of CPD is mandatory for all registered professionals who want to re-register, that is the application process to remain on their respective registers. Public health practitioners, registered with the UKPHR, need to re-register every five years. This includes providing evidence of recent CPD, appraisal and a personal development plan. Health promotion practitioners, registered with the IUHPE, need to re-register every three years.

Revalidation is a similar, but more formal process than re-registration. It provides stronger assurance to the public that professionals are safe, ethical and fit to practise. In addition to re-registration, public health specialists who are registered with the UKPHR must revalidate every five years. Those registered with the General Medical Council (GMC) are required by law to revalidate every five years. The UKPHR revalidation scheme requires evidence of professional appraisal, personal development planning, a declaration about the professional's health and conduct, professional indemnity insurance, mandatory CPD, evidence of quality improvement and a referee to confirm the presented evidence is true and accurate (UKPHR, 2022). UKPHR is planning to introduce a revalidation scheme for public health practitioners.

Registration, revalidation and continuing professional development help to assure the public that the public health workforce work to rigorous, safe and ethical standards.

Examples of career routes

Table 2.6 summarises the diverse entry and progression points in health promotion and public health careers, a field that is sometimes discovered or rediscovered mid-career.

Thinking point:

Consider the type of career and job roles that align with your values, skills and interests. Contact your local public health professionals, perhaps starting with the local public health team/department, to begin a discussion about your next career move.

Table 2.6 Examples of career routes

	BSc (Hons) Public health	Dip H.E. Sport and exercise management	Health promotion team administrator	BSc (Hons) Sustainable development	BSc (Hons) Nutrition	BA (Hons) Human geography	BSc (Hons) Public health practitioner degree apprenticeship (v)	BSc (Hons) Biomedical science	BSc (Hons) Nursing
Examples of starting points									
Examples of next steps	Community development worker (NHS Scotland) (i)	Health and fitness instructor (local business)	Black and ethnic minority (BME) substance misuse worker (local authority)	Research assistant (air quality) (university)	Public health nutritionist (NHS Trust)	MSc Transport	Health improvement practitioner (health inequalities) (civil service) MSc Public health and community wellbeing (p/t)	Research assistant (UK charity)	Staff nurse (NHS hospital)
	Senior community development specialist (NHS Scotland)	Assistant leisure centre manager (local business) BSc (Hons) (top-up) Health, wellbeing and exercise (p/t)	Adolescent health worker (charity)	Health intelligence analyst (Public Health Wales) (i)	MSc Health promotion and public health	Transport policy manager (local authority)	Health improvement principal (local authority)	Health protection practitioner (local authority) (iv)	PGDip Specialist community public health nursing (OH)
	Regional communities manager (NHS Scotland)	Health improvement practitioner (physical activity) (local authority)	Sexual health promotion specialist (local authority)	International research and development officer (international charity)	Health improvement practitioner (healthy eating) (local authority) (iv)	City transport planner (local authority)	Public health speciality training programme (vi)	Research fellow in epidemiology (university) MSc Public health (p/t)	Occupational health nurse (local business)
	Director of a charity to support the homeless	MSc Public health	Regional networks and learning manager (civil service) MSc Health promotion and public health (p/t) (iii)	Field epidemiology training programme	Senior health advisor (UK charity)	Assistant head of transport and environment (local authority) PGDip Public health (p/t) (iv)	Public health consultant (local authority)	Senior health protection officer (local authority)	Senior occupational health nurse (local business) MSc Public health (p/t)

(*Continued*)

Table 2.6 Examples of career routes (Continued)

Examples of starting points	BSc (Hons) Public health	Dip H.E. Sport and exercise management	Health promotion team administrator	BSc (Hons) Sustainable development	BSc (Hons) Nutrition	BA (Hons) Human geography	BSc (Hons) Public health practitioner degree apprenticeship (v)	BSc (Hons) Biomedical science	BSc (Hons) Nursing
		Lecturer/senior lecturer in public health (university) PhD (p/t) (iv)	Head of public health service (NHS Community Trust)	Senior epidemiology scientist (civil service)	Public health speciality training programme (vi)	Assistant director of transport (local authority)	Assistant director of public health (local authority)	Public health speciality training programme (vi)	Deputy health of occupational health and wellbeing (large business) (i)
		Principal lecturer and public health team leader (university)			Public health nutrition consultant (international organisation)		Director of public health (local authority)	Health protection consultant (Public Health Wales)	Head of occupational health and wellbeing (large business)

Notes: p/t = part-time.

(i) At this point, they might map their own competencies against the WHO-ASPHER Competency Framework and use this summary within their application for a more senior or international job.

(ii) At this point, they might map their own competencies against the UKPHR public health specialist standards as part of the evidence for their retrospective portfolio. If successful, they can add 'registered public health specialist' to their qualifications.

(iii) At this point, they might self-assess their own competencies against the CompHP competencies and professional standards and apply to the IUHPE. If successful, they can add 'registered health promotion practitioner' to their qualifications.

(iv) At this point, they might map their own competences against the UKPHR Practitioner Standards for Registration as part of the evidence for their retrospective portfolio. If successful, they can add 'registered public health practitioner' to their qualifications.

(v) On successful completion, they will have met the UKPHR Practitioner Standards for Registration and can add 'registered public health practitioner' to their qualifications.

(vi) On successful completion, they will have met the UKPHR public health specialist standards and can add 'registered public health specialist' to their qualifications.

Summary

This chapter has:

- described the structure of the UK public health workforce with examples of job roles
- outlined four competency frameworks that support the public health workforce and explained why and how they are used
- explained the process of professional registration for the public health workforce
- discussed the importance of re-registration, revalidation and continuing professional development
- provided several examples of career pathways into and within the public health workforce

Further reading

Sim, F. and Wright, J. (2015) *Working in public health. An introduction to careers in public health.* London: Routledge

Useful websites

Faculty of Public Health. Available at: www.fph.org.uk
International Union for Health Promotion and Education (IUHPE). Available at: www.iuhpe.org
Public health (careers). Available at: www.healthcareers.nhs.uk/explore-roles/public-health-careers
UK Public Health Register (UKPHR). Available at: https://ukphr.org

References

Barry, M. M., Battel-Kirk, B., Davison, H., Dempsey, C., Parish, R., Schipperen, M., Speller, V., van der Zanden, G., and Zilnyk, A. on behalf of the CompHP Partners (2012) *The CompHP project handbooks. International union for health promotion and education (IUHPE).* Available at: https://www.iuhpe.org/images/PROJECTS/ACCREDITATION/CompHP_Project_Handbooks.pdf. (Accessed 4th April 2022)

Centre for Workforce Intelligence (2015) *Understanding the wider public health workforce.* Available at: https://assets.publishing.service.gov.uk/government/uploads/system/uploads/attachment_data/file/507752/CfWI_Understanding_the_wider_public_health_workforce.pdf (Accessed 4th April 2022)

Department of Health (2012) *Healthy lives, healthy people: towards a workforce strategy for the public health system. Consultation document.* Available at: https://www.gov.uk/government/uploads/system/uploads/attachment_data/file/164228/consultation_doc.pdf (Accessed 4th April 2022)

Faculty of Public Health (2020) *Functions and standards of a public health system.* Available at: https://www.fph.org.uk/media/3031/fph_systems_and_function-final-v2.pdf (Accessed 4th April 2022)

Professional Standards Authority (2021) *UK public health register.* Available at: https://www.professionalstandards.org.uk/what-we-do/accredited-registers/find-a-register/detail/uk-public-health-register (Accessed 4th April 2022)

Public Health England (2019) *The wider public health workforce. A review.* Available at: https://assets.publishing.service.gov.uk/government/uploads/system/uploads/attachment_data/file/783867/The_wider_public_health_workforce.pdf (Accessed 4th April 2022)

Public Health England/Public Health Agency/Public Health Wales/NHS Scotland (2016) *Public health skills and knowledge framework 2016.* Available at: https://assets.publishing. service.gov.uk/government/uploads/system/uploads/attachment_data/file/584408/public_ health_skills_and_knowledge_framework.pdf (Accessed 4th April 2022)

Skills for Health (2004) *National occupational standards for the practice of public health guide.* Available at: http://www.wales.nhs.uk/sitesplus/documents/888/englishnos.pdf (Accessed 4th April 2022)

UK Public Health (2020) *People in UK public health.* Available at: https://ukphr.org/wp-content/uploads/2020/11/Report-PinUKPH-to-Select-Committees-Nov-2020.pdf (Accessed 4th April 2022)

UK Public Health Register (2014) *UKPHR code of conduct.* 2nd edn. Available at: https:// ukphr.org/registration/code-of-conduct (Accessed 4th April 2022)

UK Public Health Register (2020) *Public health practitioner standards for registration.* Available at: https://www.ukphr.org/wp-content/uploads/2014/08/UKPHR-Practitioner-Standards-14.pdf (Accessed 4th April 2022)

UK Public Health Register (2022) *Guidance. Revalidation of UKPHR's specialist registrants.* 4th edn. Available at: Revalidation-Guidance-Specialist-registrants-March-2022-edition-4.pdf (ukphr.org) (Accessed 4th April 2022)

WHO-ASPHER (2020) *WHO-ASPHER competency framework for the public health workforce in the European region.* Available at: https://www.euro.who.int/__data/assets/pdf_ file/0003/444576/WHO-ASPHER-Public-Health-Workforce-Europe-eng.pdf (Accessed 4th April 2022)

Yorkshire and Humber Public Health Network (2021) *Public health careers.* Available at: https://www.yhphnetwork.co.uk/links-and-resources/public-health-careers (Accessed 4th April 2022)

Part II
Disciplines and fields of study

3 Epidemiology

Rajeeb Kumar Sah and Gail Sheppard

Key points

- Introduction
- Defining epidemiology
- History of epidemiology
- Measures of disease frequency and deaths
- Cause and effect
- Epidemiological study designs
- Screening
- Summary

Introduction

The chapter will introduce the principles and practice of epidemiology. It begins by defining epidemiology, outlining the history of epidemiology and explaining some of the most common measures of disease and death such as mortality and morbidity rates. It discusses how epidemiologists try to find 'cause and effect', by identifying associations between health exposures and outcomes such as diseases. The chapter describes epidemiological research study designs, grouped as observational studies and experimental studies, with some of their strengths and limitations. Finally, the chapter discusses screening tests as one example of the many nuances that need to be considered when presenting epidemiological data.

Defining epidemiology

The word 'epidemiology' is constructed from three Greek words: 'epi', a prefix which means 'on, upon or befalls'; 'demos', a root or core word that means 'people'; and 'logos', a suffix which means 'the study of'. Medical terminology dictates that the suffix is read first, then the prefix and lastly the root. Taken literally, 'epidemiology' means the study of something that befalls the people. It is the study of the determinants and distribution of disease and death in human populations. *Demography* is the study of populations. A population may be defined as fixed when the membership is relatively permanent, such as when people share a common experience or an event such as surviving a disaster. Alternatively, a population may be dynamic, meaning the membership is transient. For example, people may move into a city and become city residents for a few years before moving away. Demographers are interested in the

DOI: 10.4324/9780367823696-5

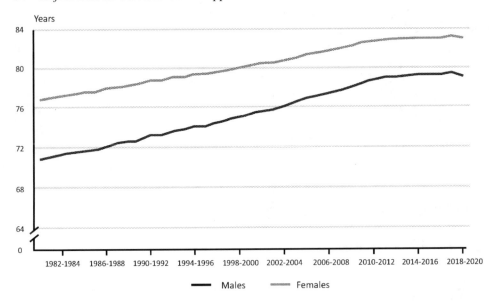

Figure 3.1 Life expectancy for males and females in the UK between 1980 to 1984 and 2018 to 2020

Source: ONS, 2021. Reproduced under the terms of the Open Government Licence v3.0

causes and consequences of changes in populations, so they collect population data such as age, sex, gender, ethnicity, income, fertility, length of life, migration figures and life expectancy (Figure 3.1). Life expectancy is a measure of the average number of years people are expected to live beyond their current age. Demographers also produce population pyramids to illustrate the structure of a population (Figure 3.2).

Demography underpins and interacts with epidemiology. *Epidemiology* is,

> "The study of the occurrence and distribution of health-related states or events in specified populations, including the study of the determinants influencing such states, and the application of this knowledge to control the health problem."
>
> (Porta, 2014, p. 95)

It is used to inform and develop public health policy and to guide which methods may be implemented to control a disease and/or maintain optimum levels of health in a population. An epidemiologist is,

> "A professional who to different degrees strives to study and control the factors that influence the occurrence and distribution of disease and other health-related conditions and processes in defined groups, populations and societies, has an expertise in population thinking and epidemiological methods, and is knowledgeable about public health and causal inference in health."
>
> (Porta, 2014, p. 95)

For example, epidemiologists examined the life expectancy data shown in Figure 3.1, noting life expectancy has been steadily rising for the last forty years. They noted that

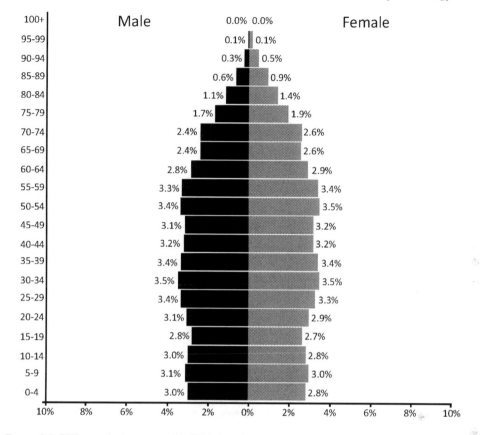

Figure 3.2 UK population pyramid, 2020 (*n* = 67,886,004)

Source: Populationpyramid.net, 2020. Reproduced under the terms of the Open Government Licence v3.0

the COVID-19 coronavirus pandemic in 2020 had caused a greater number of deaths than usual. This explains why life expectancy in females stalled and the life expectancy in males declined.

Epidemiology is situated within the positivist paradigm of research, which is explained in Chapter 4. It works with the medical model of health and illness and a negative definition of health, that is health being defined as an absence of disease (see Chapter 1). In the context of health promotion and contemporary public health, where we work with more holistic and positive understandings of health including the role of the social determinants of health, classical epidemiology remains valuable but also limited. This is one reason for the rise of *social epidemiology* over the last four decades, a branch of epidemiology that focuses on understanding how social factors influence a population's health. Professor Sir Michael Marmot is probably the most well known social epidemiologist who has argued that the structure of society, its policies for employment, income, housing, early childhood, climate change and so forth, significantly influences who suffers most disease and early death within a population (Marmot *et al.*, 2020). This chapter describes some core understandings that are relevant to all branches of epidemiology.

Disease outbreaks, epidemics and pandemics

The data collected by epidemiologists will identify whether cases of disease are described as an outbreak, endemic, an epidemic or pandemic. An *outbreak* of disease occurs suddenly within a confined geographical area; it is defined as,

> "An epidemic limited to localised increase in the incidence of a disease e.g. in a village, town or closed institution."
>
> (Porta, 2014, p. 206)

An *epidemic* is where the occurrence of cases of a disease are clearly above what would normally be expected within a defined population or within a geographical area over a given period. In contrast, an *endemic* is where a disease is regularly found among a particular population or within a specific geographical area. Although most epidemics capture the media and public attention, the significant burden of communicable diseases are endemic. In 2017, there were approximately 219 million cases of malaria across the world, and 200 million (92%) were in the African region of the World Health Organization (WHO, 2021). Malaria is endemic in the African region. A *pandemic* is when a disease crosses national boundaries and affects large numbers of people worldwide. The outbreak of COVID-19 coronavirus has been classified as a pandemic (Box 3.1).

Box 3.1 From outbreak to pandemic: COVID-19 coronavirus

The event

On December 31st 2019, the local health authority in Wuhan in China reported an outbreak of pneumonia with symptoms of fever, a dry cough, fatigue and occasional gastrointestinal symptoms. On January 30th 2020, the World Health Organization declared a public health emergency of international concern and later named the cause of the disease COVID-19, a type of coronavirus. The pathogen causing the outbreak was identified as a novel beta-coronavirus (2019-nCoV). The world remembered another beta-coronavirus which had caused Severe Acute Respiratory Syndrome in 2003, called SARS-2003. In 2012, Middle East Respiratory Syndrome (MERS) had also been caused by a novel coronavirus. The COVID-19 outbreak was significantly more worrying and severe than these.

Descriptive epidemiology

The initial COVID-19 outbreak affected 66% of the staff working at the Wuhan human seafood wholesale market. Soon the disease spread to many other provinces around China and by February 2020 it had reached 25 countries around the world including Japan, the Republic of Korea, Thailand, Germany and the United States of America. The World Health Organization declared the disease to be a pandemic on March 11th 2020. By March 31st 2022, 490 million cases and six million deaths had been reported across the world. In the UK, the first two cases were reported on January 29th 2020. By March 31st 2022, the UK reported 21 million cases and 165,000 deaths within 28 days of a positive test.

(Source: John Hopkins University, 2022; Shu *et al.*, 2021;
UKHSA, 2022; Wu *et al.*, 2020)

For an outbreak of disease to occur, it requires an agent, a host and an environment that is conducive to both (see Figure 10.1 p.250).

- An *agent* may be physical, chemical or biological. For example, allergens, drugs, poisons and nutrients are chemical agents; heat, light, noise and radiation are physical agents and bacteria, viruses, fungi and protozoa are examples of biological agents. In most natural habitats there are biological agents that are infectious to humans, and human behaviours often contribute to the spread of infectious diseases. A natural habitat of *infectious agents,* or *pathogens,* is called a *reservoir.* Infectious agents vary in their *infectivity,* meaning their ability to enter and multiply in the host and cause disease
- A *host* may be a human or another living animal including birds and arthropods. The host's reaction to an infection by an agent varies according to the dose of the agent as well as the host's personal characteristics such as their behaviours, immune status or genetic predisposition
- An *environment* will affect the existence and survival of a disease-causing agent. Environments can comprise physical, biological, social, economic and political elements. For example, malaria occurs in tropical and sub-tropical climates, influenza in the winter months of temperate climates; cholera thrives in dirty water and many diseases thrive in overcrowded, urban environments

The transmission of an infectious agent, or pathogen, occurs directly and indirectly. *Direct transmission* is transfer through close personal contact with another human or animal, such as touching, kissing, biting or through the direct projection of droplets released when coughing, speaking or sneezing. *Indirect transmission* suggests there is an intermediary mechanism. These may be

- *vehicle-borne*, meaning the pathogen is transmitted via a non-moving object such as water, food, soiled bedding, clothes or utensils
- *vector-borne*, meaning they are transmitted by animals including living insects such as the tick or mosquito which cause Lyme disease and malaria
- *airborne*, meaning the air carries small respiratory droplets released when sneezing, coughing or laughing such as tuberculosis or the COVID-19 coronavirus. The infectious agent remains in the air or holds onto surfaces for a long period of time. It can travel along the air currents across relatively long distances

Purpose of epidemiology

Epidemiology informs the practical steps which are taken to investigate an outbreak of a disease. These are discussed in Chapter 10. Epidemiologists provide the data that help to answer questions such as

- what are the health problems in this population?
- who suffers from this health problem?
- where do most cases of this disease occur?
- how many people have this condition?
- why do these health problems occur?
- when is the condition most common?

- what interventions have been tried, and what were the results?
- what trends in disease can be seen over time within a population?
- how does the health status of one population compare to another?
- what helps to prevent, manage or reduce this disease?

In turn, the answers to these questions can help to provide answers to an individual's questions, such as

- if I smoke, will I get cancer?
- how much physical activity must I do to keep healthy?
- how many units of alcohol are bad for my health?
- what might have caused my illness?

Jeremy Morris was a well-known Scottish epidemiologist. In the 1950s he suggested seven uses for epidemiology.

- Historical study – by understanding the rise and fall of diseases in a population over time, it may be possible to make future projections
- Community diagnosis – to diagnose the presence, nature and distribution of health and disease among a population, taking into account that society and health problems change
- Operational research – by researching a population's needs, the available resources and analysing local health services in action, epidemiologists build the evidence to recommend what they ought to do next
- Individual's chances – by understanding the common experience of a health problem in a population, it is possible to assess the risks for the average individual
- Completes the clinical picture – collected data from populations provide much broader information than hospital statistics alone can offer, e.g. information about the sex and age at which a disease is most likely to strike
- Identifies syndromes – by studying the patterns and causes of disease in populations, doctors learn more about their characteristics, such as the same disease being caused by different factors or showing previously unknown connections between factors
- Clues to causes – discovering groups in the population who have high or low rates of disease can illuminate the causes of disease and therefore directions for future prevention

(Morris, 1955)

Epidemiology is a population-based science which examines and reports the occurrence and distribution of deaths, diseases and health-related events.

History of epidemiology

The first epidemiologist might have been Hippocrates (460 BC–377 BC) who described disease as having natural origins, as opposed to supernatural ones, in his three books *Epidemic I, Epidemic III* and *On Airs, Waters and Places*. He noted the importance of the environment, diet and other behaviours as causes of disease; described cases of disease with their symptoms and causes; and noted the age, sex and location of the patient (Kayali, 2017). Ign An-Nafis, a medical and religious scholar in Egypt, wrote a *Commentary on Hippocrates* in 1215 and compared his study of cases of disease with those described by Hippocrates (Kayali, 2017).

John Graunt (1620–1674), a draper living in London in the 17th century, has been described as the founding father of both demography and epidemiology, replacing conjecture with evidence (Connor, 2022). In the mid-1600s, it was claimed several million people lived in London, yet Graunt was sceptical as he had noted a maximum of 15,000 burials each year. Assuming three out of every 11 households experienced a death each year, he estimated the total population of London would be about 381,338. He also used the number of baptisms each year to estimate the number of births. Women usually had a child every other year. From this, he calculated the number of women aged between 16 and 40 years old and then estimated there were 48,000 women of all ages in London. As the average household comprised eight people, there were about 384,000 people living in London. Clearly the population of London was between 381,000 and 384,000, not in the millions. He also calculated life expectancy and suggested that out of 100 babies born,

- 64 would be alive by the age of six
- 25 would be alive by the age of 26
- 10 would be alive by the age of 46
- three would be alive by the age of 60
- none would be alive after the age of 80

(O'Donnell, 1936)

Graunt used these demographic skills to understand more about the causes and patterns of disease and death. In the late 16th century, weekly bills of mortality were introduced to London (Figure 3.3). Boyce (2020) explains how the Worshipful Company of Parish Clerks would produce this single sheet of paper which listed the number of deaths and the causes of death for individuals living in each of the 130 parishes in London. These bills were an early warning system for infectious disease outbreaks and a source of revenue for the Worshipful Company. The process comprised

- collecting the data on the causes of death by searchers. These were often older women with local knowledge who were paid to find out what happened and report back to the local parish clerk
- collating the information
- printing the bills
- distributing the bills

The bills of mortality were seen as an essential warning of deadly infectious diseases such as plague. John Graunt analysed the bills produced between 1604 and 1660. An example is shown in Figure 3.4. He

- critiqued the accuracy and completeness of the data and identified sources of error
- presented, several large volumes of aggregated numbers in the form of tables. This is the first known record of health-related data being presented in this way
- interrogated the data using mathematical principles associated with double book-keeping

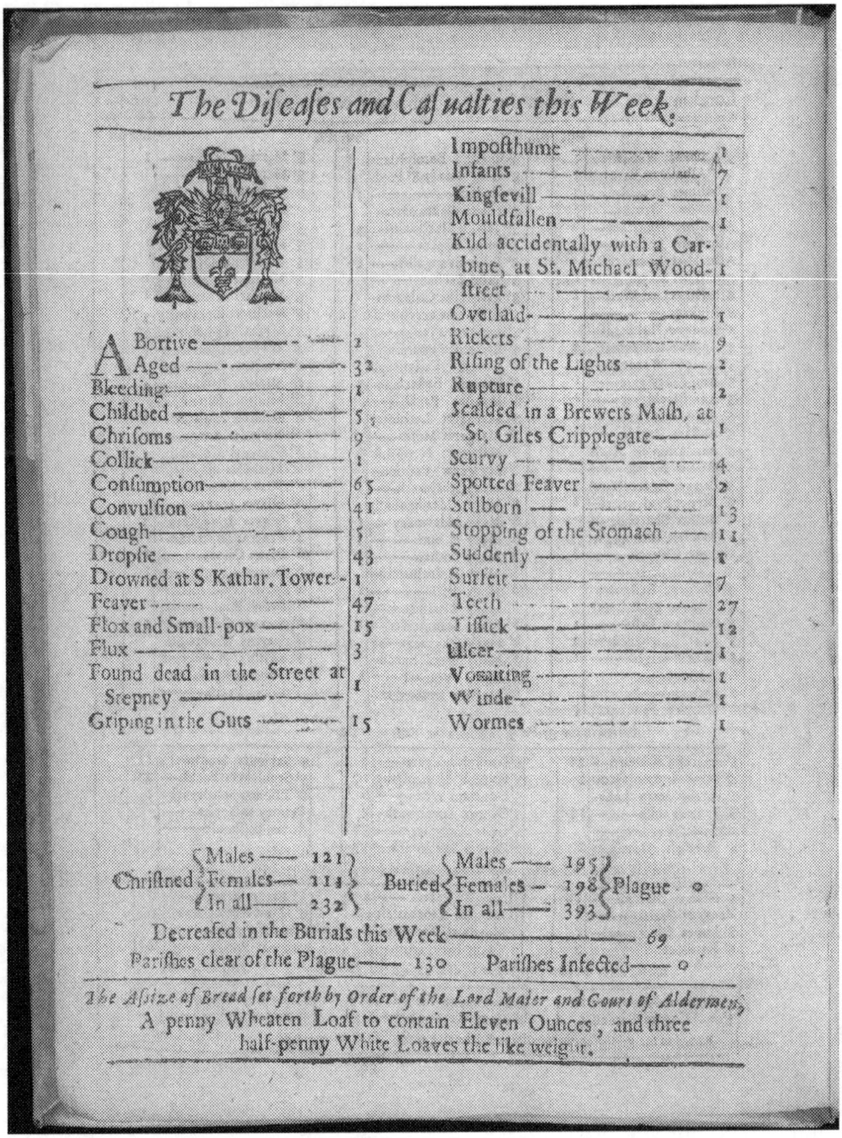

The Diseases and Casualties this Week.

Abortive	2	Imposthume	1
Aged	32	Infants	7
Bleeding	1	Kingsevill	1
Childbed	5	Mouldfallen	1
Chrisoms	9	Kild accidentally with a Carbine, at St. Michael Woodstreet	1
Collick	1	Overlaid	1
Consumption	65	Rickets	9
Convulsion	41	Rising of the Lights	2
Cough	5	Rupture	2
Dropsie	43	Scalded in a Brewers Mash, at St. Giles Cripplegate	1
Drowned at S Kathar. Tower	1	Scurvy	4
Feaver	47	Spotted Feaver	2
Flox and Small-pox	15	Stilborn	13
Flux	3	Stopping of the Stomach	11
Found dead in the Street at Stepney	1	Suddenly	1
Griping in the Guts	15	Surfeit	7
		Teeth	27
		Tissick	12
		Ulcer	1
		Vomiting	1
		Winde	1
		Wormes	1

Christned	Males	121	Buried	Males	195	Plague 0
	Females	111		Females	198	
	In all	232		In all	393	

Decreased in the Burials this Week — 69

Parishes clear of the Plague — 130 Parishes Infected — 0

The Assize of Bread set forth by Order of the Lord Maior and Court of Aldermen,
A penny Wheaten Loaf to contain Eleven Ounces, and three half-penny White Loaves the like weight.

Figure 3.3 A bill of mortality February 21st to 28th 1664

Source: Wellcome collection made available under a CC BY 4.0 licence

- grouped data according to age, sex, season, parish, year and so forth
- grouped data using the term 'acute' for disease that struck suddenly and 'chronic' for those that lasted a long time
- formulated hypotheses and then tested them
- searched for errors and inconsistencies in the data
- checked his conclusions by using different methods
- recorded his methods openly, inviting others to check his work

(Connor, 2022)

The Table of CASUALTIES.

The Years of our Lord	1647	1648	1649	1650	1651	1652	1653	1654	1655	1636	1635	1634	1633	1632	1631	1630	1629	1660	1659	1658	1657	1656	1651 1652 1653 1654	1655 1656 1657 1658	1647 1648 1649 1650	1629 1630 1631	1633 1634 1635	1636	1629 1649 1659	In 20 Years
Abortive and Still-born	335	329	327	351	389	381	384	433	483	573	597	475	500	445	410	439	499	544	421	467	463	419	1587	1832	1342	1793	2205	573	1247	8559
Aged	916	835	889	696	780	834	864	974	743	714	597	623	671	889	661	579	999	1095	909	800	869	892	3452	3680	3336	2473	2814	714	2377	15759
Ague and Fever	1260	884	751	970	1038	1212	282	1371	689	2360	1622	1279	953	1108	1115	1091	956	2148	2303	1800	999	875	4903	4393	3865	4418	6235	2360	4910	23784
Apoplex and Suddenly	68	74	64	74	106	111	118	86	92		26	35	17	17		36	22	67	91	138	113		421	445	286	85			177	1306
Bleach				3	1																	1							15
Blasted	4	5	2	2	7	6	3	2	4	4	6	3	6	5	10	2	13	8	6	5	4	1	9	14	12	54	14	4	16	99
Bleeding	4	5	5	2	3	3	3	5	7		2	4	6	7	10	8	13	2	12	13	11	2	12	19	11	16	7		17	65
Bloody Flux, Scouring and Flux	155	176	802	289	833	762	200	386	168	339	346	512	278	348	352	438	449	251	346	233	362	368	2181	1161	1422	1587	1466	339	1597	7818
Burnt and Scalded	3	6	10	5	11	8	5	1	5	3	12	3	1	5	7	10	3	6	6	4	7	5	31	26	24	25	19	3	19	125
Calenture	1			1			1																		2					13
Cancer, Gangrene and Fistula	26	29	31	19	31	53	36	37	73	30	24	30	27	28	23	14	52	52	63	35	24	31	157	150	105	85	112	30	114	609
Wolf																									8		8			13
Canker, Sore-mouth and Thrush	66	28	54	42	68	51	53	44	81	74	79	54	72	18	4	6	19	68	73	27	44	19	244	161	190	190	79	74	133	689
Child-bed	161	106	114	117	206	213	158	192	177	230	163	143	132	171	112	150	194	157	226	225	236	201	760	839	498	599	668	230	499	3364
Chrisoms and Infants	1359	1254	1065	990	1237	1280	1050	1343	1089	1895	2080	2315	2268	2035	1713	2378	2596	1123	858	1144	1162	1393	4910	4788	4578	9277	8453	1895	4519	32106
Colick and Wind	103	71	85	82	76	102	80	101	85	50	37	54	45	55	51	57	48	167	116	179	113	120	359	497	341	105	87	50	247	1380
Cold and Cough								36	21	57	00	54			1	58	10	24	31	58	30	58	77	140		174	207	57	43	598
Consumption and Cough	2423	2200	2388	1988	2350	2410	2286	2868	2606	2477	2080	1955	1754	1797	1713	1910	1827	3414	2982	3610	2757	3184	9914	12157	8999	5157	8266	2477	7197	44487
Convulsion	684	491	530	493	569	653	606	828	702	709	418	386	221	241	18	87	52	1031	742	841	807	1027	2656	3377	2198	498	1734	709	1324	9073
Cramp		1			1						2			5	1	4		4	6	4				13	01	01	00			38
Cut of the Stone			2				1	2	4	389								872	646	931	631	706	6	10	6	6	10		47	9623
Dropsie and Tympany	185	434	421	508	444	556	617	704	660	389	329	250	266	280	279	157	235	872	646	931	631	706	2321	2982	1538	1048	1734	389	1302	9623
Drowned	47	40	30	27	49	50	53	30	43	45	32	32	37	34	34	33	43	48	57	60	49	63	182	215	144	139	147	45	130	827
Excessive drinking					1																					2				2
Executed	8	17	29	43	24	12	19	21	19	13	13	13	13	18	12	13	19	18	7	18	20	22	76	79	97	62	52	13	55	384
Fainted in a Bath																														2
Falling-Sickness	1	2	2	183	1	4	4	2	4	6	6	5	7	7	58	10	3	5	6	7	10	7	8	13	10	27	21	6	47	74
Flox and small Pox	139	400	1190	139	525	1279	139	812	1294	127	293	1354	701	531	701	40	72	354	1523	499	835	823	2755	3361	1913	1048	1846	127	2785	10576
Found dead in the Streets	6	6	9	8	21	20	14	4	3	24	24	8	13	12	20	33	18	43	51	11	9	4	34	27	29	83	69	24	29	243
French-Pox	18	29	15	18	21	20	20	4	29	22	12	17	7	12	20	12	18	31	51	80	25	23	81	139	80	48	53	22	83	392
Frighted	4	4	4	1	1	2	2	1	1	3		1			3			2	3		1		5	7	3	3	3		3	22
Gout	4	5	12	7	7	7	11	6	8	20	7	17	14	4	4	20	14	9	14	13	10	7	36	28	28	14	24	20	28	134
Grief	12	13	16	14	17	14	11	17	10	7	58	11	7	7	11	5	2	2	13	13	10	7	59	45	55	71	56	7	47	279
Hanged, and made-away themselves	11	10	13	14	9	14	15	9	14	2	8	3			3	20	18	36	11	18	24	13	47	72	48	37	18	2	32	222
Head-Ach							1	6	6												4	4	4	14			6		46	51
Jaundice	57	35	35	49	41	43	57	71	61	63	54	45	35	43	35	59	47	43	35	77	46	41	212	225	180	184	197	63	188	998
Jaw-faln	1			1	3			6	2	11	4	10	50	88	73	16	10	21	9		3		14	14	6	47	35	11	10	95
Imposthume	75	61	65	59	80	105	79	90	92	130	73	62	10	74	73	76	58	96	105	134	80	122	35	428	260	282	315	130	228	1639
Itch																									01		10			11
Killed by several Accidents	27	57	39	94	47	45	57	58	52	60	51	41	49	46	47	55	54	47	55	47	52	43	207	194	217	202	201	60	148	1021
King's Evil	27	26	22	19	22	20	26	26	27	69	20	20	35	38	18	25	16	54	28	28	23	24	94	102	94	97	150	69	66	537
Lethargy	3	4			4	4	3	2	10				1					4	2	2	4	4	7	21	13	7			9	67
Leprosie		1		1	1	1	1											1			1	1	1		1					6
Liver-grown, Spleen and Rickets	53	46	56	59	65	72	67	65	50	99	98	77	82	87	96	12	94	15	55	51	38	50	269	191	213	392	356	99	158	1421
Lunatick	12	18	6	12	8	22	9	12	12	22	24	18	4	5	20	11	18	14	28	11	7	12	39	31	47	24	28	22	26	158
Meagrom	12	13	3	5	5			9	3	12		17	21	2	2	2		4	6	7	7		7	5	13	12	22	12	05	12
Measles	5	92	3	33	33	62	1	52	11	07	27	33	80	80	24	3	42	74	3	80	15	153	155	259	133	01	83	07	51	757
Mother	5	1	5	3	3	3	1	3	2	8	00	2	9	2	9	2	8	8	9	7	6	6	10	8	13	01	19	8	02	18
Murdered	3	2	4	4	4	3	30	3	58	14	5	6	8	7	10	10	4	43	46	7	5	6	123	215	17	34	46	14	77	86
Overlaid and Starved at Nurse	27	21	19	28	28	29	29	36	58	17	25	14	14	25	13	23	17	21	36	22	44	23	123	215	111	82	77	17	86	529
Palsie	25	21	67	15	23	16	6	16	9	82	10	21	8	7	13	10	4	14	36	14	17	23	61	87	53	34	77	82	53	423
Plague	3597	611	67	19	23	6	30	16	87	10400	17	21	14	25	274	23	17	402	253	14	4	315	142	844	4290	1599	10401	10400	253	16384
Plague in the Guts	30	26	13	7	23	19	32	23	10	24	45	21	21	36	26	24	26	14	12	87	17	9	72	33	89	112	90	24	51	415
Pleurisie		3	3				17																							415
Poisoned		1		1	1	1		3	1	1	1	1							1						1	1				14
Purples and Spotted Fever	145	47	43	65	54	69	75	89	56	397	245	125	24	38	58	58	32	146	368	126	56	290	278	290	300	186	791	397	243	1845

Figure 3.4 John Graunt's data based on the bills of mortality 1647 to 1659

Source: Graunt, 1676, cited in Petty, 1899, pp. 406, 407. Made available under a CC0 1.0 licence

James Lind (1716–1794), a Scottish surgeon, was concerned about scurvy among Royal Navy sailors. Scurvy caused ulcers, blackened gums, fatigue and sometimes death. In 1747, after eight weeks at sea, there were between 30 and 40 sailors with scurvy on HMS Salisbury. Sutton (2003) describes how Lind chose 12 sailors who had similar symptoms of putrid gums and weakness. He put them into six pairs and each pair was given: cider, elixir of vitriol (diluted sulphuric acid), vinegar, sea water, two oranges and lemons or a purgative (laxative) mixture. About a week later, the two sailors given the citrus fruit had almost recovered. This experimental study was followed by further research where Lind asked classic epidemiological questions about the causes of scurvy as well as when and where it occurred. His work confirmed that eating citrus fruit could prevent and cure scurvy.

The term 'epidemiology' began to be used in the 19th century. Dr John Snow (1813–1858), an anaesthetist, was interested in the cause and spread of cholera in London. He conducted many years of ground-breaking work to test his hypothesis that cholera was a waterborne, not an airborne, disease. In 1854, he drew a street map, marking the houses where cases of cholera had been identified. In the centre was the Broad Street water pump. On having the pump handle removed so it could not be used, the cases of cholera reduced, thus demonstrating the contaminated water was the cause of the cholera (Snow, 1855). Snow's work demonstrated 'cause and effect' and he, also, is often credited as being one of the first and most well-known epidemiologists.

We often think of Dr John Snow as the first epidemiologist, but some of the core concepts of epidemiology can be traced back to Hippocrates.

Measures of disease frequency and deaths

Epidemiologists use specific terminology to describe and present the amount of disease or death in a population. *Mortality* means death and *morbidity* means disease or illness. The Office for National Statistics is a reliable source of UK mortality and morbidity data. For example, between 2001 and 2018, most females in the UK died from dementia and Alzheimer's disease, and most males died from ischaemic heart disease (Figure 3.5) (ONS, 2020). A *rate* means the frequency that an event occurs. It is often expressed as a proportion of the population, for example 'per 1,000' of the population or 'per 100,000' of the population. Rates may be

- *crude rates*, which relate to the whole population. For example, a crude mortality rate means the number of people who died per 1,000 of the population
- *specific rates*, for example those relating to a specific age group or sex. For example, age-specific mortality rate means the number of people, per 1,000 of the population, who died within a specific age group. Cause-specific mortality rates mean the number of people, per 1,000 of the population, who died from a specific cause, such as dementia
- *infant mortality rates*, which record the number of deaths under one year per 1,000 live births. Infant mortality rates are an important indicator of a whole population's health
- *standardised rates*, where an epidemiologist wants to compare two or more populations and they 'remove' certain variables so that they are comparing like with like. For example, they may wish to compare men with prostate cancer in

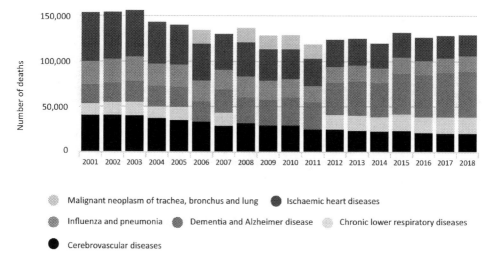

Malignant neoplasm of trachea, bronchus and lung ● Ischaemic heart diseases

Influenza and pneumonia ● Dementia and Alzheimer disease ● Chronic lower respiratory diseases

● Cerebrovascular diseases

Figure 3.5 Number of male deaths in the UK by the leading causes, 2001 to 2018

Source: ONS, 2020. Reproduced under the terms of the Open Government Licence v3.0

Box 3.2 Some epidemiological calculations

$$\text{Crude mortality rate} = \frac{\text{number of deaths during the year} \times 1000}{\text{total population mid} - \text{year}}$$

$$\text{Age-specific mortality rate} = \frac{\text{number of deaths aged e.g. 60 to 70 years}}{\text{total mid-year population aged e.g. 60 to 70 years}}$$

$$\text{Infant mortality rate} = \frac{\text{number of deaths in the first year of life} \times 1000}{\text{number of live births in the population}}$$

$$\text{SMR} = \frac{\text{observed number of deaths} \times 100}{\text{expected number of deaths in the population}}$$

$$\text{Incidence rate per 1000} = \frac{\text{number of new cases of a disease} \times 1000}{\text{number of people at risk of developing the disease}}$$

$$\text{Prevalence rate per 1000} = \frac{\text{total number of cases of a disease} \times 1000}{\text{number of people at risk of developing the disease}}$$

Wales with those in England, but England has a greater number of men at an older age and so the epidemiologist will 'standardise' the data, they remove the difference that age may make before comparing both nations

- Sometimes epidemiologists calculate a *standardised mortality ratio* (SMR) when comparing different populations. They divide the observed number of deaths by the expected number of deaths in each population. If the SMR is greater than 100, it means the mortality in the population is higher than expected; if it is lower than 100, the mortality in a population is lower/better than expected

Thinking point:

> Consider why infant mortality rate is an indicator of the health of a whole population.

Incidence means the number of new cases of disease or death, per 1,000 of the population during a specific period of time. *Prevalence* means the number of people, per 1,000 of the population, with a disease over an interval of time. This is the number of new and existing cases, meaning the total number of people living with a disease. It will depend on the incidence of the disease and its duration from onset to recovery or death. Prevalence is useful for assessing the health status of a population and for planning healthcare services. It is less useful for identifying risk factors for diseases or diseases of short duration such as diarrhoea.

Demographers have used population pyramids to demonstrate *demographic transitions*, that is how the structure of populations change over time. For example, the UK's population has moved from being a country with a high birth rate and high (early) death rate to one with a very low birth rate and a low death rate over a period of 350 years. It has a much larger older population than in the past. This is attributed to changes in society, industrialisation and technological advances including improvements in public health. Epidemiologists study the changing patterns of populations over time alongside the rates and causes of mortality. Omran (1971) described the *epidemiological transition*. In essence, it states that as a country transitions from being a developing nation to a developed one, death rates from communicable/infectious diseases such as tuberculosis fall and death rates from non-communicable diseases/chronic diseases such as cardiovascular disease and cancer rise (Table 3.1). The concept of the epidemiological transition is being challenged by the discovery that some non-communicable diseases can be caused by infections and criticisms that the model was originally based on only four countries (Ciccacci *et al.*, 2020; Mercer, 2018).

Table 3.1 Most common causes of female deaths in the UK, 1915 to 1975

Age (years)	1915	1935	1955	1975
20–24	Pulmonary tuberculosis	Pulmonary tuberculosis	Pulmonary tuberculosis	Motor accidents
30–34	Pulmonary tuberculosis	Pulmonary tuberculosis	Pulmonary tuberculosis	Breast cancer
40–44	Pulmonary tuberculosis	Pulmonary tuberculosis	Breast cancer	Breast cancer
50–54	Heart valve disease	Gastrointestinal cancer	Breast cancer	Breast cancer
60–64	Bronchitis	Gastrointestinal cancer	Coronary heart disease	Heart attack
70–74	Bronchitis	Heart failure	Coronary heart disease	Heart attack

Source: ONS, 2017.

Cause and effect

Epidemiology is based on two fundamental assumptions

- human disease and its absence are not distributed randomly. Some people are healthier not by chance, but by factors that can be measured and potentially controlled
- the factors which cause or prevent a health problem can be identified by systematically investigating the population

A core task of epidemiology is to be able to prove, reliably, that a factor causes an outcome. A *cause* is,

> "... an event, condition or characteristic (or a combination of these factors) that plays an essential role in producing an occurrence of the disease."
>
> (Rothman, 1976, p. 588)

and,

> "... something that makes a difference in the outcome (or the probability of the outcome) when it is present compared with when it is absent, while all else is held constant."
>
> (Parascandola and Weed, 2001, p. 906)

An *outcome* is a health problem such as physical or mental disease, an injury or death. There are three types of causes:

- a *sufficient cause* is a factor, or more usually a combination of several factors, that will inevitably produce disease
- a *component cause* is a factor that contributes towards the cause of disease, but it is not sufficient to cause disease on its own
- a *necessary cause* is any agent, or component cause, that is required for the development of a given disease e.g. the specific infectious agent/pathogen

(Merrill, 2017)

Causation is a term used when we know that a certain event will always cause another event, for example universal laws of nature. It is not always possible to measure everything in the real world, much less carry out perfect scientific experiments, so epidemiologists often measure associations. An *association* means there is a link between a health exposure and an outcome. A *health exposure* means an individual is exposed to a physical, chemical or biological agent. For example, we may observe an association between a type of air pollution and a respiratory disease. This is not implying that one causes the other. More research is needed to make this claim. Epidemiologists also use the term *risk factors*. A risk factor is a characteristic that is associated with an increased probability of an outcome. Risk factors include inherited genes, contact with an agent/health exposure and health-related behaviours. For example, a person with the risk factor of having a high percentage of body fat has an increased risk of developing type 2 diabetes. Typically, one risk factor is not sufficient to cause a health problem; people usually become ill due to a combination of risk factors. There are two types of causal association:

- *direct causal association* means there is a direct line from exposure to outcome. For example, trauma to the skin results in a bruise
- *indirect causal association* means the line is indirect because there are other intermediate factors in play. For example, poor diet and stress together may lead to high blood pressure which leads to cardiovascular disease

Aside from something like a major disaster or a nuclear explosion, it is difficult to identify a single factor that is the cause of a disease. The example of tobacco smoking illustrates these points. It is well established that smoking is a risk factor for developing lung cancer (Doll and Hill, 1950;1954). This does not mean that every person who smokes will always develop lung cancer; neither does it mean that people who develop lung cancer are always smokers. It means that a smoker has a higher risk/probability of developing lung cancer compared to non-smokers.

In 1882, John Stuart Mill introduced three methods of thinking when considering cause and effect. These can be a useful starting point when considering associations and planning what research might be fruitful.

- *Method of difference.* The rate of disease varies in different situations. If a risk factor can be identified in one situation but not in another situation, it may be that this risk factor is the cause of the disease. Alternatively it may be the absence of the exposure that causes the disease. For example, we may identify rates of sunburn as lower in Edinburgh than Margate. We note one difference is the greater sunshine in Margate
- *Method of agreement.* If there are high rates of a disease in many different situations and all these situations have something in common, perhaps high rates of physical inactivity, this suggests physical inactivity may be the cause of the disease
- *Method of concomitant variation.* When the frequency or strength of an effect, such as increased rates of food poisoning, varies with the frequency of an exposure, such as increased consumption of a type of meat, this may suggest that the meat is causing the food poisoning

Sir Austin Bradford Hill presented a paper to the Royal Society of Medicine in 1965. He explained when we consider an association between two variables, such as a potential health exposure and an outcome, we should focus on nine features:

- strength of the association, e.g. in Hill's research, death rates from lung cancer in cigarette smokers were nine to ten times that of non-smokers
- consistency of the association means whether the association is seen in different places, times and situations
- specificity, e.g. consider whether the association is only seen in a specific group of workers or widespread across the population
- temporality, e.g. does the diet lead to the disease or does the disease change the diet?

- biological gradient means if a factor is associated with a disease, we would expect to see higher rates of disease when exposure to the factor is increased
- plausibility means if the association is supported by current biological knowledge, it makes the idea of causation more plausible
- coherence means that cause and effect is less plausible if it contradicts current knowledge
- experiment, e.g. if we think the dust in a workplace is associated with a disease, the disease should reduce if we remove the dust
- analogy means examining similar evidence relating to similar variables

(Hill, 1965)

If an epidemiologist thinks there might be a strong association between a health exposure and an outcome, the next step is to conduct research to test the hypothesis.

Epidemiologists present data about mortality and morbidity and then analyse it to show potential associations between a health exposure and its consequences.

Epidemiological study designs

Epidemiologists carry out research to measure the occurrence of outcomes such as deaths, diseases and injuries or to establish if there is an association between a health exposure and an outcome (Munnangi and Boktor, 2021). They mostly use quantitative methodology and questionnaires, but also use qualitative interviews and case studies, and occasionally clinical tests. These are discussed in Chapter 4. The design of epidemiological studies falls into two categories, observational studies and experimental studies.

Observational studies

Observational studies take place in the natural environment (Figure 3.6). An investigator observes health exposures, such as those in nature or people's behaviours, and outcomes. They may observe *prospectively*, observing outcomes in real time for as long as the study is active, or *retrospectively*, meaning they examine information about the past. Observational studies can be *individual-based*, meaning the study is trying to explain variations between individuals within the same population, or *population-based*, meaning they are not; they are trying to explain what is happening to the population as a whole. Observational studies are either descriptive or analytical.

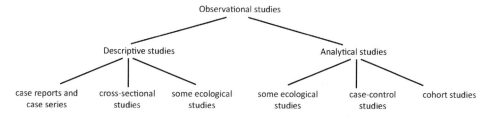

Figure 3.6 Observational studies

Descriptive studies

Descriptive studies aim to measure the frequency of outcomes in a population. Sources of descriptive data include the Census and other routinely collected data such as birth and death registers, disease registers and hospital records. From these, an investigator may propose an idea or a hypothesis about what exposures may be associated with the outcomes. These findings will inform strategies, such as public health interventions, to prevent or manage a health problem. This type of study can also be used to evaluate the effectiveness of a strategy. Descriptive data will only provide information about the frequency and distribution of a health exposure or an outcome; it cannot make comparisons or find associations. Descriptive studies will collect data on the variables of person, place and time, that is 'who, where and when'.

- *Person variables* include the attributes of age, sex, genetic predispositions, race, ethnicity, culture, religion, marital status, level of education, occupation, socio-economic status, etc. They also include health-related behaviour such as smoking, alcohol consumption, dietary practices and physical activity. Age and sex are probably the most important personal characteristics associated with variations in disease outcomes. Figure 3.7 shows the age-specific incidence rates, that is the age at which new cases are diagnosed, for all forms of cancer for males and females (Cancer Research UK, 2021). Descriptive studies have shown that the occurrence of most diseases increases with age, and some are more common among males and others among females
- *Place variables* are the characteristics of the environment in which people live, work and stay. These include geographical places such as a street, town, city, county or country; physical environments such as air, water, soil or climate; and

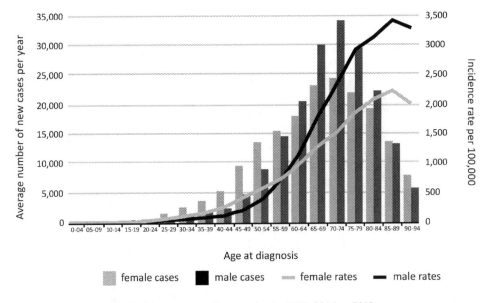

Figure 3.7 Age-specific incidence rates of cancer in the UK, 2016 to 2018

Source: Cancer Research UK, 2021. Reproduced with permission from Cancer Research UK

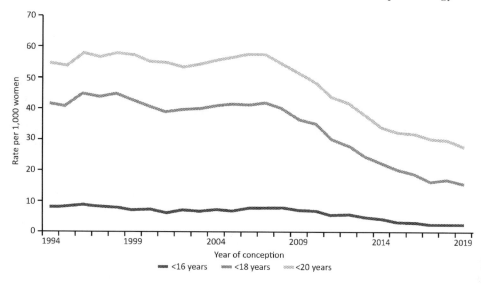

Figure 3.8 Teenage pregnancies in Scotland by age at conception, 1994 to 2019

Source: Public Health Scotland, 2021. Reproduced under the terms of the Open Government Licence v3.0

environmental factors such as rural or urban settings, economic development and social disruptions. A place can influence the prevalence of a health exposure and how susceptible the local people are to it

- *Time variables* include the seasons, month, day, time and duration of exposure and time of diagnosis. It can be measured as days, weeks, months, years or decades. For example, Figure 3.8 presents data from 1994 to 2019 to show the falling trends in pregnancies among those under 20 years old in Scotland

There are three types of descriptive studies: case reports and case series, cross-sectional studies and ecological (descriptive) studies.

CASE REPORTS AND CASE SERIES

A case report describes a case, where a *case* is a single occurrence of a noteworthy outcome, perhaps an unusual disease, or a health-related event. Once the facts have been researched, they are presented in chronological order. A case series is a collection of cases, perhaps a small group of people with a similar diagnosis. Case reports and case series may indicate the emergence of a new disease or an epidemic.

CROSS-SECTIONAL STUDIES

Cross-sectional studies, also known as prevalence surveys, take place with a sample of individuals from the population of interest at one point in time, measuring *point prevalence*, or over a period of time, measuring *period prevalence*. There is no follow-up period. The investigator collects data to measure the prevalence of an outcome and the prevalence of an exposure simultaneously. Therefore it is difficult to infer that a certain outcome was caused by a certain exposure. However, cross-sectional surveys can reveal associations between health exposures and population characteristics such as age, gender, marital status, ethnicity, education and occupation, and thus reveal possible health risks to specific populations.

The advantages of cross-sectional studies include they can be used to study several associations at once, they can be conducted over a short period of time, they are relatively inexpensive, they can be used to develop a hypothesis and they can provide evidence to demonstrate a need for an analytic study to test a hypothesis. Cross-sectional studies are best used for measuring the prevalence of chronic outcomes, for example the prevalence of long-term pain or sedentary behaviour. Although it can be relatively easy to conduct a cross-sectional study with a large random sample of individuals who are representative of a population, it is not possible to establish whether an exposure preceded or followed a health outcome, for example whether the population's diet caused the weight loss and fatigue, or whether the weight loss and fatigue changed what people ate. Cross-sectional studies are also prone to recall or response bias; for example individuals who are answering a questionnaire may not remember accurately or they bring their own biases into their answers. Also, cross-sectional studies are not suitable for studying rare diseases.

ECOLOGICAL STUDIES

An ecological study compares the frequency, meaning the incidence or prevalence, of an outcome and an exposure at a population level, where the population represents a group of individuals with a shared characteristic such as ethnicity, socioeconomic status, employment or gender. Data on outcome and exposure may be collected at an individual level and then aggregated at a population level; for example the Census collects data from individuals, and then collates it together. However, we cannot say that an exposure will cause a disease in one person, because the data from an individual is not the same as the data from a population. Drawing conclusions about individual-level associations from a population-level study is known as an *ecological fallacy*. The ecological fallacy, a type of confounding that is specific to ecological studies, assumes that an association seen in the aggregate (the population) is true for individuals, which is a false assumption. For example, the data may suggest an association between unemployed people in one town and a higher-than-average incidence of depression, but we cannot suggest there is an association between an individual who is unemployed and an increased likelihood of being diagnosed with depression. One of the main reasons for conducting an ecological study is when individual-level data is not readily available but population-level data is, or when an exposure can only be measured at the population level. Ecological studies are inexpensive and comparatively easy to carry out using routinely collected data, but they are prone to bias and confounding. An ecological study can be used to analyse time trends or make large-scale comparisons such as comparing countries or regions. In such circumstances, it would normally be described as an 'analytic' (not descriptive) ecological study.

Analytical studies

Analytical studies aim to measure the association between a health exposure and an outcome, such as a disease. Most studies begin with one or more hypotheses about what might be causing what outcome. To test a hypothesis, the investigator sets up an analytical study. There are two types of commonly used analytical studies: case-control studies and cohort studies.

COHORT STUDIES

Cohort studies, also called incidence studies, begin with a cohort of interest (Figure 3.9). A cohort refers to a group of people with shared characteristics such as being born at the same time, students who graduate in a particular year, factory workers or people who have a common health-related behaviour. Investigators begin by identifying a cohort, the defined population who are free from the outcome; for example they do not have the disease of interest. The study follows the experiences of all the individuals in the cohort over a period of time. The investigators note whether anyone coming into contact with an exposure of interest develops the disease. This allows the investigators to observe the natural progression of the disease in real time from the point of exposure. Normally, a cohort study often involves comparing the group of individuals from a cohort that are 'exposed' to a group that has not been exposed. An investigator follows both groups for a period of time and collects data on the health outcomes of individuals within those groups. The like-to-like comparisons are a core feature of cohort studies; without them, the incidence of the outcomes could be due to factors other than the exposure. These 'other factors' are called *confounders*, and this phenomenon is known as confounding.

In a *prospective cohort study*, events are yet to occur. The investigators follow up the cohort to measure the incidence of the disease among the exposed and unexposed groups. Selecting a cohort carefully is key to the success of a prospective cohort study because withdrawals and non-responses will increase the potential for 'selection bias'. In a *retrospective cohort study*, the investigators observe events from the past. Retrospective data can be obtained from a variety of sources such as anonymised medical records; vital records systems, which include records of life events such as births and marriages; or a surveillance system, meaning ongoing systems for collecting health or disease-related data in the population. As these studies use existing records, they can be completed relatively rapidly and economically. *Retrospective cohort studies* start by selecting a cohort, following the recorded data for the cohort for a period of time, and then comparing the incidence rates (the incidence proportion of the disease) among the exposed and unexposed groups.

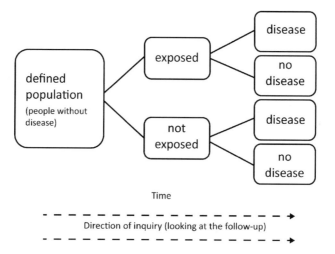

Figure 3.9 Cohort study design

In cohort studies, the *relative risk* (RR), also known as the *risk ratio*, is used to measure the association between the frequency of exposure and the frequency of outcome. Relative risk is the ratio of the incidence of a disease in an exposed group to the incidence of the disease in a non-exposed group. It can also be understood as the ratio of the risk of finding the outcome among people who are in contact with the health exposure compared to those who are not. An RR value of

- one (1) indicates the risk of the disease among the exposed is not different from the risk of disease among the non-exposed
- more than one (>1) indicates the risk of the disease among the exposed is higher than the risk of disease among the non-exposed
- less than one (<1) indicates the risk of the disease among the exposed is lower than the risk of disease among the non-exposed

The advantages of cohort studies lie in their ability to study the natural history of an outcome and to establish the time sequence of events. Although the study is not focused on a specific health exposure, it will reveal the incidence of several outcomes, perhaps several diseases, at the same time. The disadvantages of cohort studies include being complicated, expensive, time consuming and the problem that cohort participants might leave mid-way through the study. There are sometimes problems with investigator bias when selecting cases, and of misclassifying who is to be, or was, in contact with the health exposure.

CASE-CONTROL STUDIES

Case-control studies start by identifying *cases* (Figure 3.10). Cases are individuals from a defined population who have already experienced an outcome of interest, such as a disease. These cases should be representative of the population and are often identified from sources such as anonymised hospital records, health clinics or

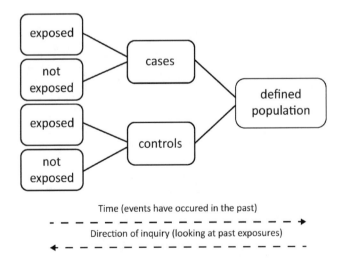

Figure 3.10 Case-control study design

government sources. Next, the investigator selects a *control group*, that is a group of individuals from the same population, with similar characteristics, who have not had the disease. Investigators use a *retrospective* approach, meaning they ask people to recall the past or examine available records. Information on people's exposure should be collected in the same way; for example investigators may use questionnaires, interviews or medical records for both the cases and the control group to avoid bias. The investigators might obtain information from employers, spouses or siblings as part of their research. The odds of exposure to the cases are compared to the odds of exposure to the controls.

In case-control studies, the *odds ratio* (OR) is used to measure the strength of the association between the frequency of exposure and the frequency of outcomes. Odds ratio is the ratio of the odds of the exposure among the cases to the odds of the exposure among the controls. An OR of

- one (1) indicates there is no association between the health exposure and the outcome
- less than one (<1) indicates a decreased risk that the health exposure is associated with the outcome
- more than one (>1) indicates an increased risk that the health exposure is associated with the outcome

The advantages of case-control studies include they are effective for studying rare outcomes and they require less time and money than a cohort study. It is possible that a case-control study could simultaneously identify an association between multiple exposures and a single outcome. As a case-control study does not measure the frequency of an outcome, such as the incidence of a disease, and it does not examine the natural history of an outcome in real time, it is less effective than a cohort study at establishing timelines and the sequence of events. Case-control studies can also be prone to bias in terms of the selection of cases and their reliance on people's memories (recall bias), as well as potential investigator bias.

Experimental studies

Experimental studies are also called intervention studies. They have similarities with classic scientific experiments carried out in laboratories but are modified because we are dealing with people. Here, an investigator plays an active role in allocating some people to the health exposure and watching what happens. Experimental studies include clinical trials and community trials (Figure 3.11).

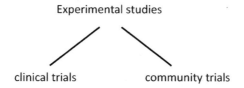

Figure 3.11 Experimental studies

Clinical trials and community trials

CLINICAL TRIALS

Clinical trials are used to evaluate the efficacy and safety of a new drug, diagnostic procedure or screening test. In a clinical trial, an investigator takes a group of individuals who have some key characteristics in common, perhaps of similar age and health status. The investigator randomly divides the group into two groups: an intervention and a control group. The intervention group receives the new treatment or new procedure, while the control group receives an existing one or a placebo. The results from both groups are compared to find out which group has the better outcome. *Randomisation* is the process where everyone has an equal chance of being allocated to the intervention group or the control group. Randomisation and 'blinding' play a crucial role in minimising bias and confounding. A *single blind trial* means the participants do not know which group they are in. A *double blind trial* means neither the participants nor the investigators know who is in the intervention group or the control group. Clinical trials are extremely expensive, time consuming and complex to conduct, but the rigour of the procedures produces evidence that is considered of such high quality that it is often called 'the gold standard'.

COMMUNITY TRIAL

A community trial investigates the effect of exposing a community or group to a health exposure, perhaps in a workplace or a village. A community trial is often used to test the impact of introducing an educational or social intervention. It may investigate changes in knowledge or behaviour by, for example, a 'nudge' (see Chapters 5 and 6) and seek to understand the costs and benefits of the intervention. The investigator does not randomly assign individuals from the same community to a control group and an intervention group, as in a classic experimental design, for practical, political and ethical reasons. Investigators adopt quasi-experimental designs such as selecting several communities which have similar features in terms of size, population characteristics and level of urbanisation. Part of the community becomes the intervention group, such as being exposed to a campaign, and the remainder is seen as the control group. The intervention is evaluated over a period of time, and then investigators compare the results to find out which group has the better outcome.

Thinking point:

> Consider the ways in which epidemiological study designs could be prone to different forms of bias.
>
> *Epidemiologists carry out observational and experimental research studies to measure the occurrence of an outcome and/or to establish an association between a health exposure and an outcome.*

Screening

Epidemiologists not only report data, but they must understand and explain some of the nuances that lie behind data. One example is the reporting of population-based screening test results. Screening is the process of identifying healthy people who have a higher risk of having a particular condition or health problem so they can be offered information to help them make informed decisions about potential treatment (NHS, 2021). Screening is an example of secondary disease prevention. Screening test results are collated by epidemiologists and the data provides evidence which helps to inform public health policy and practice related to controlling major chronic diseases such as cancer and the safeguarding of mothers and babies during pregnancy and after birth. The UK screening programmes are regulated by the independent UK National Screening Committee (UKNSC) which advises the National Health Service and government ministers. It is internationally respected as providing a model of best practice for national, population-based screening programmes (Seedat *et al.*, 2014). Types of screening and examples of screening programmes in the UK are discussed in Chapter 10.

If a screening programme is to be useful, the screening test needs to be accurate, meaning it corresponds to the true state of the disease being measured. Tests are never completely accurate in the real world, and accuracy varies across different diseases in different situations. We measure accuracy by considering the test's reliability and validity (Friis, 2018).

- *Reliability* means the test will give a consistent measure each time it is used; it is a precise test
- *Validity* means the measure will be accurate, it is true and it will distinguish accurately between people who have the disease and those who do not

Reliability and validity are interrelated terms; it is possible for a measure to be reliable, consistent, but be untrue, invalid. It is not possible for a test that produces unreliable, inconsistent measures to be valid, true. Therefore validity is important, and we measure it by examining a test's sensitivity, specificity, positive predicted value and negative predicted value, as shown in Table 3.2.

- *Sensitivity* is the ability of a screening test to identify true positives, where the test correctly identifies all individuals who 'actually' have the disease. Having 100% sensitivity means all the people who receive a positive test result have the disease
- *Specificity* is the ability of a screening test to identify true negatives, where the test correctly identifies all individuals who 'actually' do not have the disease. Having 100% specificity means all people who receive a negative test result do not have the disease

Table 3.2 Validity of a screening test

	Disease is present	*Disease is absent*
Total number of positive screening tests = a+b	Number of true positives (a)	Number of false positives (b)
Total number of negative screening tests = c+d	Number of false negatives (c)	Number of true negatives (d)
Total number of screening tests = a+b+c+d	Sensitivity (a measure of those who have the disease) = a/(a+c)	Specificity (a measure of those who do not have the disease) = d/(b+d)
Positive predictive value = a/(a+b)		
Negative predictive value = d/(c+d)		

Source: Adapted from Bonita *et al.*, 2006, p. 112.

- *Positive predictive value* is the proportion of people who are known to have the disease who receive a positive test result. It is the ratio of people diagnosed with the disease, true positives, to all those who received a positive test, which will include some people without the disease. It is a measure of the number of people correctly identified as having the disease
- *Negative predictive value* is the proportion of people who are known to have the disease who receive a negative test result. It is the ratio of people who do not have the disease, true negatives, to all those who received a negative test, which will include some people who were incorrectly identified as having the disease. It is a measure of the number of people correctly identified as not having the disease

There is a balance between sensitivity and specificity. Increased sensitivity often comes at the expense of reduced specificity; it is likely to produce more false positives leading to potential worry and unnecessary treatment. Increased specificity often means reduced sensitivity; it is likely to produce more false negatives which may delay diagnosis and treatment. Epidemiologists are aware of the accuracy of screening tests, and the margins of error, and need to make these clear in their reporting of data which is used to inform public health strategies.

Epidemiologists need to understand the nuances that lie behind data, such as margins of error.

Summary

This chapter has

- defined epidemiology and outlined its history
- described common measures of mortality and morbidity used in epidemiology
- explained how epidemiologists seek to find causal associations between health exposures and outcomes
- discussed various epidemiological study designs with their advantages and disadvantages
- used the example of screening tests to illustrate some of the nuances that epidemiologists need to consider when reporting data

Further reading

Bhopal, R.S. (2016) *Concepts of epidemiology: integrating the ideas, theories, principles, and methods of epidemiology.* 3rd edn. Oxford: Oxford University
Carneiro, I. (2017) *Introduction to epidemiology.* 3rd edn. Maidenhead: Open University Press
Celentano, D.D. and Szklo, M. (2019) *Gordis epidemiology.* 6th edn. London: Elsevier
Webb, P., Bain, C., and Page, A. (2020) *Essential epidemiology: an introduction for students and health professionals.* 4th edn. Cambridge: Cambridge University Press

Useful websites

Gapminder. Available at: https://www.gapminder.org
Office for National Statistics. Available at: https://www.ons.gov.uk
United Kingdom Health Security Agency. Available at: https://www.gov.uk/government/organisations/uk-health-security-agency

References

Bonita, R., Beaglehole, R. and Kjellström, R. (2006) *Basic epidemiology*. 2nd edn. Geneva: World Health Organization

Boyce, N. (2020) 'Bills of mortality: tracking disease in early modern London', *The Lancet*, 395(10231), pp. 1186–1187

Cancer Research UK (2021) *Cancer incidence by age*. Available at: https://www.cancerresearchuk.org/health-professional/cancer-statistics/incidence/age#heading-Zero (Accessed 14th April 2022)

Ciccacci, F., Orlando, S., Majid, N. and Marazzi, C. (2020) 'Epidemiological transition and double burden of diseases in low-income countries: the case of Mozambique', *The Pan African Medical Journal*, 37(49) doi:10.11604/pamj.2020.37.49.23310

Connor, H. (2022) 'John Graunt F.R.S. (1620–74): the founding father of human demography, epidemiology and vital statistics', *Journal of Medical Biography*, 30 doi:10.1177/09677720221079826

Doll, R. and Hill, A. (1950) 'Smoking and carcinoma of the lung in physicians', *British Medical Journal*, 2(4682), pp. 739–748

Doll, R. and Hill, A. (1954) 'The mortality of doctors in relation to their smoking habits', *British Medical Journal*, 1(4877), pp. 1451–1455

Friis, R.H. (2018) *Epidemiology 101*. Burlington: Jones and Bartlett

Graunt, J. (1676) *Natural and political observations made upon the bills of mortality*. 5th edn. London: Royal Society

Hill, A. (1965) 'The environment and disease: association or causation?', *Proceedings of the Royal Society of Medicine*, 58(5), pp. 295–300

John Hopkins University (2022) *COVID-19 Dashboard*. Available at: https://coronavirus.jhu.edu/map.html (Accessed 31st March 2022)

Kayali, G. (2017) 'The forgotten history of pre-modern epidemiology: contribution of Ibn An-Nafis in the Islamic golden era', *Eastern Mediterranean Health Journal*, 23(12), pp. 854–857.

Marmot, M., Allen, J., Boyce, T., Goldblatt, P. and Morrison, J. (2020) *Health equity in England: the Marmot review 10 years on*. London: Institute of Health Equity

Mercer, A.J. (2018) 'Updating the epidemiological transition model', *Epidemiology and Infection*, 146(6), pp. 680–687

Merrill, R.M. (2017) *Introduction to epidemiology*. 7th edn. Burlington: Jones and Bartlett

Morris, J.N. (1955) 'Uses of epidemiology', *British Medical Journal*, 2(4936), pp. 395–401

Munnangi, S. and Boktor, S.W. (2021) *Epidemiology of study design*. StatPearls publishing. Available at: https://pubmed.ncbi.nlm.nih.gov/29262004 (Accessed 14th April 2022)

National Health Service (2021) *NHS Screening*. Available at: https://www.nhs.uk/conditions/nhs-screening (Accessed 14th April 2022)

O'Donnell, T. (1936) 'History of life insurance in its formative years. By Terence O'Donnell (pp.844 American conservation company, Chicago. 1936)', *Journal of the Staple Inn Actuarial Society*, 7(3), pp. 182–184

Office for National Statistics (2017) *Causes of death over 100 years*. Available at: https://www.ons.gov.uk/peoplepopulationandcommunity/birthsdeathsandmarriages/deaths/articles/causesofdeathover100years/2017-09-18 (Accessed 10th April 2022)

Office for National Statistics (2020) *Leading causes of death, UK: 2011 to 2018*. Available at: https://www.ons.gov.uk/peoplepopulationandcommunity/healthandsocialcare/causesofdeath/articles/leadingcausesofdeathuk/2001to2018 (Accessed 10th April 2022)

Office for National Statistics (2021) *National life tables – life expectancy in the UK: 2018 to 2020*. Available at: https://www.ons.gov.uk/peoplepopulationandcommunity/birthsdeathsandmarriages/lifeexpectancies/bulletins/nationallifetablesunitedkingdom/2018to2020 (Accessed 14th April 2022)

Omran, A.R. (1971) 'The epidemiologic transition. A theory of the epidemiology of population change', *The Milbank Memorial Fund Quarterly*, 49(4), pp. 509–538

Parascandola, M. and Weed, D. (2001) 'Causation in epidemiology', *Journal of Epidemiology and Community Health*, 55(12), pp. 905–912

Petty, W. (1899) *The economic writings of Sir William Petty (volume 2). Edited by Hull C.H.* Cambridge University Press. Available at: https://oll.libertyfund.org/title/hull-the-economic-writings-of-sir-william-petty-vol-2 (Accessed April 10th 2022)

Populationpyramid.net (2020) *Population pyramids of the world from 1950 to 2100.* Available at: www.populationpyramid.net/united-kingdom/2020 (Accessed 10th April 2022)

Porta, M. (ed.) (2014) *A dictionary of epidemiology.* Oxford: Oxford University Press

Public Health Scotland (2021) *Teenage pregnancies. Year of conception, ending 31 December 2019.* Available at: https://publichealthscotland.scot/publications/teenage-pregnancies/teenage-pregnancies-year-of-conception-ending-31-december-2019/#:~:text=The%20teenage%20pregnancy%20rate%20in,28%20per%201%2C000%20in%202019 (Accessed 14th April 2022)

Rothman, K.J. (1976) 'Causes', *American Journal of Epidemiology*, 104(6), pp. 587–592

Seedat, F., Cooper, J., Cameron, L., Stranges, S., Kandala, N., Burton, H. and Taylor-Phillips, S. (2014) *International comparisons of screening policy-making: a systematic review.* Available at: https://assets.publishing.service.gov.uk/government/uploads/system/uploads/attachment_data/file/444227/FINAL_REPORT_International_Screening.pdf (Accessed 14th April 2022)

Shu, Y., He, H., Shi, X., Lei, Y. and Li, J. (2021) 'Coronavirus disease-2019 (review)', *World Academy of Sciences Journal*, 3(2) doi:10.3892/wasj.2021.83

Snow, J. (1855) *On the mode of communication of cholera.* London: John Churchill

Sutton, G. (2003) 'Putrid gums and "dead men's cloaths": James Lind aboard the Salisbury', *Journal of the Royal Society of Medicine*, 96(12), pp. 605–608

United Kingdom Health Security Agency (2022) *Coronavirus (COVID-19) in the UK.* Available at: https://coronavirus.data.gov.uk (Accessed March 31st 2022).

World Health Organization (2021) *Malaria.* Available at: https://www.afro.who.int/health-topics/malaria#:~:text=Most%20were%20in%20the%20WHO,%2C%20and%20Uganda%20(4%25) (Accessed 14th April 2022)

Wu, Y., Chen, C. and Chan, Y. (2020) 'The outbreak of COVID-19: an overview', *Journal of the Chinese Medical Association*, *83*(3), pp. 217–220

4 Research methods and evidence-based practice

Elisabetta Corvo, Joanne Cairns and Sally Robinson

Key points

- Introduction
- Research and evidence-based practice
- Searching and reviewing literature
- Research philosophies
- Methodology and methods
- Validity and reliability
- Sampling
- Research ethics
- Summary

Introduction

This chapter explains some of the important factors to consider when planning to undertake research which can support evidence-based health promotion and public health practice. It begins by defining research and evidence-based practice before describing how to search and review literature in preparation for a research study. It distinguishes between quantitative, qualitative and mixed method research, and examines common research methods such as questionnaires, interviews and focus groups with their advantages and disadvantages. The chapter discusses validity and reliability, sampling and research ethics.

Research and evidence-based practice

Every day someone conducts research to better understand the world. They are trying to understand 'reality'; what, how and why things exist or existed. All research starts from observation and wondering why things work in a certain way. We are driven by a curiosity to find answers; to understand a situation, an aspect of something or a mechanism; or to learn about the connections between events. In 1543, Copernicus demonstrated that the earth revolves around the sun and published the work in *De Revolutionibus Orbium Coelestium*. It marked the moment that science moved from merely observing reality and theorising the past, to carrying out experiments to try to understand the past. Philosophers of science such as Descartes, Bacon and Hobbes

DOI: 10.4324/9780367823696-6

crystallised the procedures which became known as the scientific method, a formal way of gathering data to try to answer a question about reality.

- 'Question' means the research question we want to investigate
- 'Formal' means using a scientific, rigorous and logical investigative process
- 'Data' refers to all those elements that are collected during an investigation

Research may be primary, secondary, empirical or theoretical.

- Primary research is carried out by observing and collecting data, such as an experiment, a survey or an interview
- Secondary research uses a pre-existing body of knowledge such as documents and published research papers
- Empirical research means the research is concerned with that which can be observed or experienced, e.g. observing a crowd, interviewing a group or conducting an experiment
- Theoretical research is that carried out by thinking; there are no practical procedures

Primary research begins with an observation; for example we note that students are eating more chocotreats than last year. Some research is framed by a simple aim and objectives, for example

> Aim: To understand the rise in consumption of chocotreats among students over the last year
>
> Objectives:
>   i   to describe what students know about chocotreats today compared to one year ago
>   ii to explore students' attitudes towards chocotreats today compared to one year ago

Research, at its most rigorous, begins with a hypothesis; for example students eat chocotreats because they think they contain vitamins.

- A hypothesis generates a prediction that is capable of being tested, e.g. if we provide information to students about the nutritional content of chocotreats, which do not contain vitamins, they will eat less
- Research is designed in a way that will test whether the hypothesis has a foundation/is real/is true, e.g. we will give one group of students information about the nutritional content of chocotreats and one group will receive no information. We will measure how many bags of chocotreats each group eats over a month
- If the group with the nutritional information eats fewer chocotreats, we say the research confirms the hypothesis and the research has generated a theory. A theory tries to explain why something happens, e.g. we have a research-based (evidence-based) theory that if students are given information about the nutritional content of chocotreats they will eat fewer than students who are not given this information
- Many research studies, testing the same hypothesis but using different research designs, can help to confirm the theory as real/true/valid. Alternatively, if they obtain different results, they will challenge the theory and/or point to a new theory

Table 4.1 Glossary of research terms

Research term	Definition
Critical appraisal	Assessing the trustworthiness and quality of research in a systematic way
Data analysis	Inspecting research data in a systematic/rigorous way to describe, summarise and illustrate what has been found
Deductive	Developing a hypothesis based on existing theory, testing a theory or a preconception
Empirical	Concerned with what can be observed or experienced; not theoretical
Evaluation	Research which aims to judge or describe something such as the effectiveness of a project to improve health. It may be ongoing or carried out at the end
Generalisability	The extent to which research findings can be applied to other settings
Inductive	Generating new theory which emerges from data; there is no preconception of what will emerge
Interpretivism	Philosophical approach which sees reality as complex and multi-variate
Narrative literature review	An overview or summary in the form of a logical story or persuasive argument based on reading and analysing existing literature. Narrative reviews are published in academic and professional journals and books. They also preface research studies, providing a summary of what is known and not known and presenting the argument for what is to be researched
Objectivity	Being impartial in research; neutrality; focussed on external perspectives
Pilot study	A small, preliminary trial of the research carried out before the main study to check the research will be feasible, practical, acceptable and whether anything needs to be modified before the main study begins
Positionality	How the researcher and researched are positioned in terms of the social, historical or political context of the research; this includes real and perceived power differences between the researcher and their respondents
Positivism	Philosophical approach based on the idea that only one reality exists, and it can be observed and understood through measurement
Qualitative research	A research methodology or approach that seeks to understand something by analysing people's words and images, their subjective views and experiences. Uses methods such as interviews and focus groups
Quantitative research	A research methodology or approach that seeks to understand something by measuring/counting data; looks for 'cause and effect'; objective. Uses methods such as questionnaires (polls and surveys) and scientific experiments
Reflexivity	The researcher being self-aware and recognising how their own beliefs, appearance and role will affect the research process and outcomes
Reliability	The extent to which the same research design and methods produces the same results; consistency
Replicate	To be able to reproduce research because the processes are clearly explained/transparent
Research	Using procedures, based on the scientific method, to find out about and understand reality/realities
Research article/ paper	An original piece of research that is usually published in a peer-reviewed academic or professional journal. It often includes headings such as literature review or introduction, methods, results or findings, discussion and references
Research design	A succinct, overall plan of the whole research study which may comprise multiple strands, methods and analysis
Subjectivity	Focussed on internal perspectives; recognising and valuing individuals' values, feelings, opinions and experiences; recognising research is influenced by the internal perspectives of the researcher as well as the researched

(Continued)

Table 4.1 Glossary of research terms *(Continued)*

Research term	Definition
Systematic review	A research methodology that aims to answer a specific research question by examining all/most research studies that have addressed this question. The research methods include selecting and reviewing relevant research studies; using and then reporting the logical/systematic and explicit process that is used to critically review each one; and finally drawing conclusions that take into account the rigour of the studies
Theoretical	Based on ideas, thoughts, arguments and concepts; not empirical
Validity	True, accurate and meaningful
Variable	The person, place, object or phenomenon in which the researcher is interested. The independent variable is the factor which does not change, like a control group, and the dependent variable is the factor which changes

Evidence-based practice

Research produces evidence. Evidence refers to the knowledge that emerges from rigorous research. Using current evidence about what improves and damages people's health is central to health promotion and public health practice. We use evidence to inform every communication or social intervention designed to improve people's health. Then we evaluate the impact of the intervention, what change it made, by doing research again. We collect and analyse evidence to find out how successful the intervention was. This evidence will inform the next intervention. Evidence-based practice is the process that supports practitioners when making decisions, and it is the way in which we demonstrate that practice is effective, safe and cost-effective (Dileo and Bradt, 2009). Rychetnik and colleagues (2004) define evidence-based public health as,

> "… a public health endeavour in which there is an informed, explicit, and judicious use of evidence that has been derived from any of a variety of science and social science research and evaluation methods."
>
> (p. 538)

Rigorous research, using the scientific method, provides the evidence that informs health promotion and public health practice.

Searching and reviewing literature

Research often starts by searching for what has already been written about a topic, the current evidence. Reviewing the literature means finding, reading and analysing it. We apply the evidence to practice and/or use it to write a literature review. We will outline where to search for literature, how to search in a logical way, how to assess the quality of the literature and how to approach writing the review.

Where to search for literature

There are numerous online databases which contain literature relevant to health promotion and public health. Some are listed in Table 4.2. Many are purchased by university libraries. When searching for evidence-based studies, which include published

Table 4.2 Useful databases for searching for health promotion and public health evidence

Database	Description
ASSIA	Social science including social services, psychology, sociology, economics, politics and education literature
CENTRAL	A register of Cochrane biomedical clinical trials
CINAHL	Nursing and allied health-related literature
Cochrane Library	Systematic reviews of health-related interventions
Embase	Biomedical literature including European and Asian journals
ERIC	Education literature
PubMed	Biomedical and public health literature
PsycINFO	Psychology and psychiatry literature
ScienceDirect	Scientific, medical and health literature
Sociological Abstracts	Sociological literature
Web of Science	Science, social science, arts and humanities literature

research articles and literature reviews, it is important that peer-reviewed sources are consulted where possible. Peer review means the article is read critically and approved by academic and/or professional peers before it can be published (Box 4.1). Most academic and some professional journals include a system of peer review, but not all. It is stated in the description of the journal and it is a mark of quality. Some databases may include 'grey literature,' meaning literature that has not been published through formal channels. Grey literature includes unpublished conference abstracts, reports, theses, policy documents, working papers and media. These are not normally peer reviewed but may be useful. For example, we may need to understand the political or social context of a topic. Avoid using generic search engines, such as Google, as

---

Box 4.1 From researcher to student

- Indira carries out her research, analyses her results and draws conclusions
- Indira sends her research article to the journal Health Promotion International
- The editor asks two academics to review and comment on Indira's article
- The two academics report the research is robust, the article is well written and they recommend it should be published
- Indira's article is published in Health Promotion International
- The databases Web of Science, PubMed and ScienceDirect always include articles published in Health Promotion International, so they add the current edition to their databases which includes Indira's article
- Max is a student using the university's library resources. He enters his key search terms into the PubMed database. The title of Indira's article appears
- He clicks on 'download pdf' or 'full text' and can read the whole article
- He thinks Indira's research is good quality and he notes it was peer reviewed
- He cites Indira's results in the short narrative literature review which will preface, and provide a rationale for, his own research
- Max carries out his own research and writes up his dissertation
- Later, he writes a research article based on his dissertation
- Max sends his research article to a journal to be peer reviewed and hopes it will be accepted for publication

this will generate a lot of irrelevant content that has not been peer reviewed, and the credibility of the work is unknown. However, Google Scholar can be useful if it is not possible to access recommended databases. Searching multiple databases will ensure a comprehensive search has been undertaken.

How to search for relevant literature

Searching for literature in the databases begins by identifying key search terms, the words or phrases that are most central to the research question and are likely to appear in relevant published titles or abstracts. For example, using the advanced search function in Google Scholar we searched for published articles about smoking and deprivation. It is helpful to think about synonyms for the search terms such as smoking, tobacco or cigarette, and then use the AND/OR Boolean operators. An asterisk (*) can be used as a wild card to find words that start with the same letters but have different endings, such as deprivation or deprived. We asked the database to

find articles
with *all* of the words smoking OR tobacco OR cigarette
with the *exact phrase* depriv* OR disadvantage

The database produced a list of titles, authors and a very short extract of text. For example,

[PDF] Socioeconomic status and **smoking**: a review

R Hiscock, L Bauld, A Amos, JA Fidler ... Annals of the New York ..., 2012 researchgate.net ... primary metabolite of nicotine, are strongly associated with a genetic risk factor for heavy **smoking** than self-reported daily **cigarette** consumption (Munsafo ... Objective measures of tobacco use, such as co-tinine concentrations, may give us greater insight into the social ...

There were 2,220 results, too many to search through manually, so the next step is to filter the results. It can be helpful to clarify what is to be *included* in a search, and what is to be *excluded*. This idea is borrowed from the research methodology called a systematic review. These are called inclusion and exclusion criteria. For example, if we are searching for published articles about smoking and deprivation, we may clarify that we will be including

- studies carried out inside the UK
- between 2011 and 2023
- written in English

and excluding

- studies carried out outside of the UK
- before 2011 or after 2023
- those not written in English

Databases often have a separate advanced function which enables the researcher to filter the results by year or language. This will reduce the results to a more manageable number. Keeping a record of search terms and the inclusion and exclusion criteria, and including these when writing up the research, helps the work to be transparent and replicable.

How to assess the quality of literature

We can consider the quality of literature, and therefore the quality of the evidence it reports, by noting

- the expertise/job role of author(s)
- whether the work was peer reviewed
- any links to an organisation, for example if a research study received funding from a source that might suggest a potential lack of neutrality
- whether it is primary or secondary literature. Primary sources are those that report individual pieces of original work, such as empirical research studies that used interviews or questionnaires. A secondary source is one where a person has read a number of research studies and interprets, analyses, summarises or comments on what they have read (Houser, 2016), such as a narrative literature review. Primary sources are better because we are reading the words of the original author(s), whereas secondary sources may distort or only partially report the original content and we are less certain of its accuracy
- whether research studies received ethical approval before the research commenced

When assessing the quality of a research study, it may be helpful to use a critical appraisal tool such as the one shown in Table 4.3. This is also a useful checklist for researchers when writing up their own research.

Table 4.3 A critical appraisal tool

Topic	Question	Yes/No
1 Purpose	a Is the knowledge sought readily available? b Is there an important reason for the research to be undertaken? c Are the potential outcomes of the study realistic? d Is the researcher(s) appropriately qualified/ supported to undertake the research? e Are there any concerns about the funders of the research in relation to the process of research described?	
2 Research question(s)	a Is the problem significant and researchable and have all the potential ways of solving the problem been considered? b Are all the research questions and hypotheses developed directly from the problem?	
3 Literature search	a Was there a search of a good range of literature using named databases and key search terms? b Was the review balanced and not biased? c Was the literature critically appraised? d Was any conflicting evidence clearly presented? e Did the literature review provide a rationale and direction for the research? f Were any limitations of the literature identified?	

(Continued)

Table 4.3 A critical appraisal tool *(Continued)*

Topic	Question	Yes/No
4 Sample selection	a Was an appropriate sampling strategy used? (e.g. random sampling) b Were any biases in the sample group identified? c Was the target population identified in a quantitative study? d Was there a clear account of how participants were recruited and selected to take part in the study? e Was there any coercion in recruiting participants? f Was there clear evidence that participants gave informed consent? g Were all the participants accounted for throughout the study, i.e. did the numbers add up?	
5 Research design and data collection	a Was the design of the study appropriate to the research questions? b Was an appropriate method of data collection used? c Were the data gathered by appropriate people? d Was the researcher's role and relationship with the participants fully considered? e Were the data authenticated in qualitative studies?	
6 Results and analysis of findings	a Were the results and analysis linked back to the original research questions? b Were the results and analysis manipulated in order to favour particular findings? c Was there any evidence of lost data? d Was there evidence of a statistician's input into complex quantitative analysis?	
7 Conclusions, recommendations and limitations	a Were the conclusions and recommendations based on the results of the study? b Was it clear that there was no intention to mislead or give false conclusions? c Was the sample selected considered in relation to the recommendations? d Did the research acknowledge any limitations? e Were limitations of the findings of the study identified, as well as limitations of the study design and techniques?	
8 Ethical issues	a Was the research reviewed by a Research Ethics Committee? b Were the participants protected from physical and psychological harm? c Did the research place unethical or unrealistic demands on participants? d If the participants were vulnerable, has this been clearly considered in the study?	

Source: Adapted from Hek and Moule, 2006, pp. 160–161.

Literature review

The two main types of literature reviews are narrative and systematic. Both can

- be stand-alone summaries of the current evidence, including current understandings, about a topic
- be used to preface a research study, where their purpose is to present the context and rationale for the research
- help the researcher to clarify their research question, the aim of the research
- help to identify gaps in knowledge and/or identify which research methods have previously been used to investigate similar topics, and which have not

Reviews that preface a research study are usually narrative reviews. These are evidence-based arguments which take the reader through the context of the topic, what is currently known about this topic, what has been researched and what has not. It is a well-referenced rationale for this research study. It justifies the study's aim, or research question, and objectives. The reader should be persuaded that this research study is important and will add something new to current knowledge. A systematic review is quite different and beyond the scope of this chapter.

> *The rationale for the research study, and the research question, is summarised and justified in a literature review.*

Research philosophies

The main philosophical approaches to scientific, including social scientific, research are positivism and interpretivism. A researcher uses these philosophies to guide which research methodologies and methods they are going to use.

Positivism

Positivism holds that there is only one truth, one reality. This reality can be measured. The researcher uses research methods that are standardised, objective and neutral so as not to influence the observed reality in any way. A positivist approach dominated research during the 19th century and the first half of the 20th, a time when research was mostly focussed on natural science. Positivism,

> "… assumes that phenomena are measurable using the deductive principles of the scientific method."

> (Bowling, 2014, p. 132)

A positivist researcher answers questions such as, "What?", "How much?" and "What is the relationship between this aspect of reality and another?" The main criticism of positivism is that reality cannot be simplified to laws, numbers, axioms (statements which are accepted as the established truth) or postulates (assumptions that something is established as fact), but it is much richer and more complex.

Interpretivism

Interpretivism claims there is not one objective reality; there are many subjective realities. Each person creates their reality based on their individual thoughts and experiences.

The different realities must be understood, analysed and compared. The interpretivist researcher answers questions such as, "Why?" According to Gray (2013),

> "Interpretivism asserts that natural reality (and the law of science) and social reality are different and therefore require different kinds of [research] method."

(p. 23)

Methodology and methods

Philosophy informs which methodology will be used for the research.

Quantitative and qualitative methodology

The methodology is the broad approach we take to selecting research methods. The two main methodologies are quantitative, derived from positivism, and qualitative, derived from interpretivism.

- Quantitative methodology involves the collection of quantities, that is measurable data. A typical quantitative question may be, "How frequently do people play tennis each week?"
- Qualitative methodology collects descriptive data in words or images. A typical qualitative question may be, "Why do some people never play tennis?"
- Mixed methods research means researchers combine quantitative and qualitative methods

Research may incorporate creative activities to elicit information such as taking photographs, drawing, sculpting clay or movement. A researcher chooses the methodology and then the best methods that will answer their research question, keeping in mind the types of data that will emerge and how these will need to be analysed and presented (Table 4.4). For example, data may include numbers, statistics, quotes, visual images and/or lengthy passages of writing.

Table 4.4 Philosophy, methodology, methods and question types

Philosophy	Methodology	Common methods	Types of questions
Positivism	Quantitative	Experimental research Questionnaires	Mostly structured/closed or semi-structured questions

Interpretivism	Qualitative
	  e.g. Ethnography
	  Narrative research
	  Phenomenology
	  Grounded theory
		Interviews
		Focus groups
		Observation
		Case study
		Documentary analysis
			Mostly unstructured/open or semi-structured questions

Pragmatism	Mixed methods	Combinations of both
		  quantitative and
		  qualitative methods
			Combinations of types of questions

Table 4.5 Types of questions

Structured/closed questions	Semi-structured questions	Unstructured/open questions
Can only choose from a very restricted number of options. A dichotomous question allows for two e.g. yes or no/ agree or disagree	Multiple choice Ranking e.g. from 1 to 5 Rating scale e.g. strongly agree to strongly disagree	Questions begin with What, Where, Why, When, Who or How. There are no restrictions on the answer. Sometimes used to illicit further clarification about a preceding structured/ semi-structured question

Quantitative methods

We can collect data by carrying out experimental research, typically in a laboratory, using a controlled experiment and an intervention, and measuring the difference. In health promotion and public health, we are normally working with people, and the most common type of quantitative research is carried out using a questionnaire. A questionnaire comprising only one or two questions is a poll; a questionnaire administered to many is a survey. Chapter 3 discusses how we use different types of study designs to collect epidemiological data from populations. A questionnaire may be administered face-to-face, online or by post. A questionnaire seeks to answer the research question through a series of questions. The questionnaire may be described as structured or semi-structured according to the types of questions included (Table 4.5). The main advantage of this type of questionnaire is that a large amount of data can be collected from a sample of people in a relatively short time and once the data has been analysed, it may be possible to generalise the results to a larger population. The main disadvantages are that the answers to the questions may be superficial as they will not illuminate or explain an answer and, like all research methods, participants may not answer questions honestly.

Developing and analysing a structured or semi-structured questionnaire

When developing a questionnaire, it is important to focus on answering the research question and to think carefully about the sequence of questions; they should be logical and may be divided into sections. Often, questionnaires will start or end with demographic data, that is information about the person's characteristics. Some tips for planning a questionnaire for quantitative research include

- set out the research question/aim e.g. to find out what university students know about the impact of smoking on health
- set out objectives. These are specific and collectively address the aim of the research, e.g. to find out what students know about
  - smoking and respiratory disease
  - smoking and cancer
  - smoking and pregnancy
  - smoking and bones
  - second-hand/passive smoking

- the objectives will guide the content of the questions. The questions will seek to elicit answers that will answer the objectives
- questions need to be specific, simple, short and focussed
- questions should not lead, that is assume an answer or viewpoint; they need to be neutral
- consider the types of questions, structured or semi-structured, with a rationale for the choice
- consider asking the same thing in different ways, perhaps reversing the sense of the question (see Box 4.2 Question 3h and 7). This will enhance the internal validity of the questionnaire
- carry out a pilot study to test how well the questions are understood, how long it takes to complete the questionnaire – very long questionnaires can be off-putting, work through how the data is to be collated, analysed and presented

---

Box 4.2 Example of a questionnaire

University students' knowledge about smoking and health

1 Does smoking increase a person's risk of developing cancer?

Yes   No

2 Does smoking increase a person's risk of developing cancer?

Yes   No

3 Which of these health conditions are more likely to develop among regular smokers compared to non-smokers? (circle as many as you wish)

   a Heart disease
   b Cancer
   c Influenza
   d Stroke
   e Impotence
   f Chronic obstructive pulmonary disease
   g Tuberculosis
   h Bone fractures
   i Common cold

4 Rank the following diseases according to how strongly they are associated with smoking. Score 1 for the most strongly associated with smoking and score 6 for the least associated with smoking.

Oral cancer _____
Bowel cancer _____
Skin cancer _____
Lung cancer _____
Prostate cancer _____
Stomach cancer _____

5 To what extent do you agree or disagree with the statement 'Smoking in pregnancy harms the foetus'?

Strongly agree   Agree   Neutral   Disagree   Strongly disagree

6 Which of the following may be encouraged by smoking during pregnancy? (circle as many as you wish)

   a Miscarriage
   b Premature birth
   c Kidney problems in the mother
   d Weight gain in the mother
   e Low birth weight baby
   f Sudden infant death syndrome (SIDS)

7 Smoking can damage the health of bones.
True   False

8 To what extent do you agree or disagree with the statement 'Passive smoking, that is inhaling second-hand smoke, is as dangerous as active smoking'.

Strongly agree   Agree   Neutral   Disagree   Strongly disagree

A quantitative questionnaire, comprising mostly structured or semi-structured questions, will produce data that can be quantified. The data may be analysed manually, or with the help of a simple Excel spreadsheet or software package such as Statistical Package for the Social Sciences (SPSS). The data may be presented as descriptive statistics such as simple percentages, for example '60% strongly agreed that smoking in pregnancy harms the foetus'. Statistical tests may be applied to provide more insight into what the data shows.

Qualitative methodology

Five qualitative methodologies, or approaches, include ethnography, narrative research, phenomenology, grounded theory and case study. Over time, each of these has evolved giving rise to variations.

Ethnography

The word ethnography is derived from the Greek ἔθνος (people) and γράφω (writing), meaning 'the writing of a given population'. Ethnography means the researcher closely studies the behaviour of a population, usually by living among them. They often focus on a particular sample of people, geographical area or theme. This 'participant observation' allows the researcher to describe both the people, the actors and their actions. In addition, researchers often carry out interviews. Ethnography is a method that generates questions. The questions propel further observation and interviews, as the researcher's knowledge, understanding and curiosity increase. Recently, due to the rise of online research, a variation of ethnography called 'netnography' has emerged to describe what happens in virtual environments and to understand online social experiences (Kozinets, 2015).

Narrative research

There is no agreed definition of narrative research, but it aims to capture individuals' stories, in words or images, to illuminate their understandings of their reality. Research methods may include asking individuals to complete diaries, studying documents, interviews and/or observing the individuals' environments, such as a workplace. The findings are inductively analysed to allow the stories and their meanings to emerge. What the researcher captures is accepted without judgement, and we often see a plethora of different understandings of reality, a range of realities.

Phenomenology

Phenomenology is concerned with describing the phenomena, the actions and experiences, of people's everyday lives (Grønmo, 2020). It seeks to find out, "What is this experience like?" and uses methods such as in-depth interviews, focus groups and asking people to keep diaries or write essays.

Grounded theory

Grounded theory is based on the principle that the observation of a phenomenon, and the development of the theory that underlies/explains this phenomenon, develop at the same time. Researchers repeatedly interact with participants, collecting and analysing data over time, using a range of methods. There are variations of grounded theory, but constant elements include

- simultaneously collecting and analysing data, e.g. from interviews, observations or documents
- data analysis is called 'coding'. It involves sorting and labelling the data, such as words or phrases, as codes (themes)
- comparative method, meaning making constant comparisons between data and codes, e.g. comparing new interview transcripts with the themes that have already been identified, to reveal differences and similarities
- writing memos, meaning making short notes which capture relationships between codes. In this way, a picture of what the coding shows in terms of concepts, key issues or the researcher's own assumptions, can emerge
- continual checking and reviewing to ensure the emerging theory is supported by the evidence

(Silverman, 2011)

Case study

A case study is a flexible way to explore a phenomenon. A case refers to a person, place, group, event, problem, process or activity which has some interesting, perhaps unique, characteristics. The case is studied *per se* using a range of methods; it is not a sample of a larger population. A case study can be used as a first step to generate a tentative theory which is subsequently tested by further research studies (DePoy and Gitlin, 2020).

Qualitative methods

Commonly used qualitative research methods include interviews, focus groups, observation and documentary analysis. Qualitative research can be very time consuming, and therefore potentially costly, to carry out and to analyse. Questionnaires can be qualitative if they comprise mostly open questions, but this necessitates a lot of writing for the respondent. Qualitative researchers prefer to use the term 'findings' for their results, rather than 'data'. Unlike quantitative research, with its emphasis on aiming for objectivity and detachment, qualitative research is inherently subjective. The person conducting the research cannot be completely invisible; they influence the research. Researchers need to be aware of their own biases. Some biases are unconscious, which is why qualitative researchers learn about positionality and reflexivity and bring awareness of these into their research process. Positionality refers to a person's position in society, their social status, age, gender, ethnicity, culture and so forth. Gregory and colleagues (2009) explain how a researcher's position affects,

"... the questions they ask; how they frame them ... their relations with those they research ... in the field or through interviews; interpretations they place on empirical evidence; access to data, institutions and outlets for research dissemination; and the likelihood that they will be listened to and heard."

(p. 556)

Mann (2016) defines reflexivity in terms of self-awareness and examining one's assumptions, beliefs and 'conceptual baggage'. Being a reflexive researcher supports good quality research. In practice, this includes keeping field notes, or a diary, during the research process as these can help a researcher to recognise their own assumptions and how these may influence the research and/or their interpretation of the findings. The COVID-19 coronavirus pandemic, which started in late 2019, led to more qualitative research, normally carried out face to face, being carried out online. Several advantages and disadvantages emerged (Table 4.6).

Table 4.6 Advantages and disadvantages of online qualitative research

Advantages	Disadvantages
Can reduce research costs and time e.g. travelling to sites to conduct an interview	May exclude those who do not have access to technology or who are not digitally literate
Greater reach to more people and areas	
Some online platforms, such as Zoom and Microsoft Teams, have built-in transcription	May be hard to establish a relationship, especially when researcher and participant meet for the first time
Convenient for the research participants who can fit their participation around other commitments e.g. childcare	Harder to have eye contact and to see body language
Participants may feel more comfortable as they can be in their own homes	Poor internet connection
	Data security may be compromised unless settings are applied correctly

Interviews

Interviews are useful for gathering an in-depth understanding of human behaviour, experiences and viewpoints. Interviews can be carried out with individuals or a group face to face, online or by telephone. Building rapport and establishing trust with participants is a key ingredient to the success of the interview (Denzin and Lincoln, 2005). Interviews usually comprise unstructured/open and/or semi-structured questions depending on how much breadth and depth the researcher wants. An interview guide, which is a type of questionnaire, may comprise a simple list of the themes the interviewer wants to ask about, or it may comprise questions like the example shown in Box 4.3.

Box 4.3 Example of an interview guide

Mental health among university students

Opening

Welcome participant, introduce yourself, outline the aims of the research and how long the interview will roughly take. Provide any other information such as a participant information sheet detailing ethical approval, anonymity, no right or wrong answers, and then gain their consent to take part.

Demographic questions

 1 How old are you?
 2 How would you describe your ethnicity?
 3 How would you describe your gender?
 4 What course are you studying at university?
 5 Which year are you in?

Topic specific questions

 6 How would you describe your mental health?
 7 Has your mental health changed since starting university?

If so, how has it changed? Why do you think this is? If not, go to Q8

 8 How comfortable do you feel/would you feel about talking to others about your mental health concerns?
 9 What sources of support for students with a mental health problem are available in the university? Name as many as you can think of.
10 If you have received mental health support during your time at university, could you describe the type of support you received and how you felt about it? (If participant has not received support, go to Q11)
11 What other types of support would you like to see offered by the university? Why?

Closing

Do they have any questions? Have information about mental health services to hand in case the participant needs follow-up support. Be prepared to sit with participant for a while post-interview.

Questions need to be simple and specific, and leading questions should be avoided. Sometimes a question may have follow-on questions, depending on the answer. Interviews might invite a participant to create their answer as a visual image which may, or may not, be a starting point for a verbal interview.

Thinking point:

> Consider the interview in Box 4.3. In what ways might your own position and assumptions influence this research?

Interviews may be recorded and transcribed, or the researcher may make field notes during or after the interview. Thematic analysis means researchers read the data several times and highlight the key words or phrases that appear often. They look for patterns and themes out of the complexity of the participants' accounts (Green and Thorogood, 2018). This is an inductive approach. Deductive would mean the researcher was looking for certain themes. Software such as NVivo can be used to aid this process.

Interviews have many advantages. They enable researchers to find out information that cannot be accessed using other methods such as questionnaires or observations (Blaxter *et al.*, 2006). This might include highly sensitive research topics such as personal sexual behaviour. Interviews can provide in-depth, rich information and the researcher can check they have clearly heard and understood what the participant(s) is saying alongside seeing non-verbal communication. However, interviews can be time-consuming and the quality of the interview is dependent upon a good rapport between the interviewer and participant.

Focus groups

While a group interview is characterised by the interviewer asking a group of people to answer a question, in turn, a focus group is where the interviewer introduces and encourages a dynamic discussion among the group. Participants may be homogenous, sharing similar characteristics such as gender, or heterogeneous, meaning they are chosen because they are dissimilar, perhaps people of different ethnicities. Focus groups may be set up online, such as a Facebook group or a forum made up of people with a common interest. The main advantage of focus groups is that group conversations enable rich information, insights, feelings and emotions to emerge, from which researchers can gain a deeper understanding compared to other research methods (Kitzinger, 1995). The disadvantages are, due to the nature of group dynamics, some voices may be silenced by the more dominant participants in the room. When discussing sensitive issues, some individuals may be less inclined to contribute in a group setting. Those with more shy or timid personalities might feel less inclined to be honest and resort to more socially desirable answers. The researcher needs to be skilled and able to give space to all participants. Focus groups are time consuming, though less so than a series of interviews with individuals. The focus group findings are usually analysed in the same way as interviews.

Observation

According to Bowling (2014) observation is,

> "… a research method in which the investigator systematically watches, listens to and records the phenomenon of interest."
>
> (p. 453)

Observation is more than merely looking at the world/phenomenon; it is a critical appraisal of what the phenomenon reveals to the researcher. There are two types of observation:

- participant observation, where the researcher situates themselves within the phenomenon such as becoming an active member of the group being studied
- structured observation, where the researcher looks for certain features, perhaps behaviours

The observation of reality is 'translated' via/through the researcher, who keeps research notes or journals/diaries from which rich findings can emerge. Or, if the researcher decides to focus on specific aspects of interest, they may develop an instrument, such as a check list. The latter is more deductive and may be designed to collect descriptive or quantifiable data.

Researchers may observe a phenomenon, such as how a group of people interact online. Some online forums are completely open, so the researcher can enter and observe what happens without asking for any formal permission and without revealing who they are. This is known as covert observation. Covert observation is both interesting and ethically highly controversial. The researcher should seek permission to access such forums and to observe what happens. However, once the participants know they are being observed, they may modify their attitudes and behaviours.

The advantages of observation are that data is collected directly when and where the event happens; it is incisive. The method does not rely on participants' willingness to adhere to a certain situation, nor are they asked to remember situations or emotions. The researcher can choose what they observe and how to record. The researcher, through observation, sees the world as it is and draws their own conclusions. However, observation can be quite a restrictive research tool in that the quality of the research is dependent on the way an individual carries out the research and records the findings. Avoiding personal bias and the influence of the observer on the phenomenon are two of the main dangers. Observation is time-consuming and therefore costly, and the method may not reveal why participants behave in a certain way.

Documentary analysis

Documents are socially produced materials that include written records such as diaries, letters or formal records and statements; photographs, audio or video recordings; and online blogs and other social media. Documentary analysis can be a quantitative or qualitative research method depending on whether the researcher is looking for entries to be counted or for illumination and insight (Moule and Goodman, 2009).

Mixed methods

Mixed methods research means blending qualitative and quantitative research methods. In philosophical terms, this is often referred to as pragmatism. For example, a researcher may carry out a large survey to understand the quantity of a phenomenon, such as how many over 60s use cannabis, and then conduct 20 interviews with older cannabis users to find out why, when and how they use it. Together we gain a fuller picture of cannabis use.

Researchers decide whether they wish to find out measurable/quantitative data, descriptive/qualitative views, experiences and insights or both. They choose the methods and questions that will answer their research objectives.

Validity and reliability

Both quantitative and qualitative research needs to be carried out robustly and have a high degree of validity and reliability if we are to confidently draw conclusions from the research findings and use the evidence to make recommendations.

- Validity means the research results are accurate, meaningful and true. Internal validity refers to how well the study is conducted, whether it is carried out correctly and properly without bias, and how well it addresses the research objectives. External validity is the degree to which the results are applicable to the real world/are true and includes whether they can be generalised to wider populations or to other situations
- Reliability refers to the consistency of results, e.g. in quantitative research, this is whether we would get the same results if we repeated the research

There are many ways to increase the validity and reliability of research such as minimising bias, keeping objective, keeping participants anonymous to encourage truthfulness, and having a second researcher check the data analysis and the conclusions drawn. Triangulation is where a researcher uses more than one method to answer the same research question, for example asking the same question but in different ways. This allows the responses to be compared, and if they match the response is reliable (consistent). Researchers often report the steps they took to enhance the validity and reliability of their research when writing up their work.

Sampling

Sampling refers to how the researcher selects a sample of the population that interests them. The population, and therefore the sample, may comprise people with certain characteristics, cases – such as cases of disease, objects, interventions or events. Quantitative researchers often work with larger samples because they want to be able to report results that can be extended, or generalised, to the population. Qualitative researchers select smaller samples, focussing on the quality not the quantity of the sample, and may keep adding to their sample until they reach 'saturation', that is when no new themes are emerging from their findings. Sampling strategies include convenience, probability or random, strategic and snowballing.

Convenience sample

Convenience sampling is one where a relatively small number of participants/cases are chosen because they are convenient to access. A convenience sample is often used for small-scale student research projects, qualitative studies and for pilot studies. A convenience sample will not allow the researcher to generalise the conclusions to a population.

Probability or random sample

Probability, or random, sampling is mainly used in quantitative research where the researcher wants to generalise the results to the population. The sample needs to represent the population from which it is drawn, and each person/case has an equal chance of being selected. For example, if we want to investigate the wearing of glasses among older people living in the UK, we may choose every tenth person on an alphabetical list of older people who wear glasses for the sample. A statistical test can confirm whether the sample will be large enough to allow the researcher to generalise the results to the population. Sometimes we want to ensure that the sample will include certain characteristics. For example, we may want to ensure that we collect some data from older people within ethnic minorities. A stratified random sample means we would divide the population into strata, such as White British/Irish, Black/African/Caribbean/Black British, Asian/Asian British, Mixed Ethnic Heritage and Other Ethnic Group. Then we choose the tenth person from each list.

Strategic sample

Strategic samples are used mainly for qualitative studies which aim to develop a theory or hypothesis, or an understanding of a specific community. Grønmo (2020) defines this as sampling,

> "… based on strategic and systematic assessment of which units [of the population] are most relevant and most interesting from a theoretical perspective."
>
> (p. 158)

For example, a researcher may choose older people with diabetes who wear reading glasses.

Snowball sampling

A snowballing technique, also called chain sampling, is a way of recruiting particularly marginalised members of the population, for example gypsy/travellers or illegal migrants. The researcher starts with a few key contacts who can recommend others who might participate in the research. In turn participants recommend others, and the sample grows. This type of sample is unlikely to be representative of the population.

Recruitment

Recruiting a research sample of people can present challenges.

- For a large, representative sample, it may be possible to work with a market research company that has access to a wide range of people with a variety of social and demographic characteristics
- To engage with 'seldom heard'/marginalised/vulnerable people, it is worth considering contacting stakeholders, meaning those who have a particular interest in the research, and/or gatekeepers, those who can gain access to these people e.g. a charity or a profession
- Attending existing community groups, to build relationships and rapport, may facilitate access to potential research participants e.g. the researcher joining a local sports team or Women's Institute

Public involvement (PI) means conducting research 'with' the public, or research that is conducted 'by' members of the public, as opposed to conducting research 'for' them. It is an international initiative adopted within UK healthcare, public health and social care research led by the National Institute for Health Research (NIHR) Centre for Engagement and Dissemination. It makes recommendations about how to make research relevant, acceptable and impactful, along with ideas about how to recruit participants from marginalised groups.

Research ethics

When carrying out research, researchers must

- consider the costs and benefits. Research should be worthwhile, robust, provide value and be beneficial (beneficence)
- avoid causing harm and respect people's privacy (non-maleficence)
- respect the right of individuals to make their own decisions (autonomy)
- treat individuals equally, fairly and respectfully (justice)

(Beauchamp and Childress, 2019; BPS, 2021)

For these reasons, researchers are strongly advised, and often required, to submit their research proposal, their plans, to an ethics committee to review and approve before starting the work. Universities and workplaces with appropriate expertise offer this service. Gaining ethical approval for a well-written research proposal is often straightforward unless the focus of the research is highly sensitive in nature, as many health topics are, and/or involves researching people who may be vulnerable such as children, sick people, people with disabilities, pregnant women or patients/ service users. Guardians, parents or others might need to provide support during the research. Researchers who hope to conduct research in a UK healthcare setting will need ethical approval from the Health Research Authority.

Informed consent

Giving informed consent means the participant(s) is fully informed about the research, understands what taking part will involve and then agrees to participate. Informed consent should always be obtained unless the research is being conducted covertly, and this ethical dilemma would be discussed as part of the ethical approval process. To be fully informed, an individual needs to be given

- 'a participant information sheet' which outlines the study and its procedures. It may include the research question, what the participant is being asked to do, e.g. complete a questionnaire, how long the task is expected to take and how the participant's data will be used and stored. All participants should be made aware of their right to withdraw from the study at any point without having to give a reason
- 'a consent form' to be signed by the participant (or the guardian/parent if agreed as part of the ethical approval). The form would include consent to the researcher taking photographs or make recordings if these are part of the research. Sometimes researchers seek consent to use data, anonymously, in future research publications

General Data Protection Regulation (GDPR)

The UK General Data Protection Regulation (UK-GDPR) took effect from January 2020. The law aims to protect the privacy of every citizen, so they have certainty that their data is protected and treated transparently. Everyone who is responsible for using personal data must follow the data protection principles. They must make sure the information is

- used fairly, lawfully and transparently
- used for specified, explicit purposes
- used in a way that is adequate, relevant and limited to only what is necessary
- accurate and, where necessary, kept up to date
- kept for no longer than is necessary
- handled in a way that ensures appropriate security, including protection against unlawful or unauthorised processing, access, loss, destruction or damage

(Gov.UK, 2021)

Some personal characteristics have stronger legal protection such as an identified person's race, ethnic background, political opinions, religious beliefs, trade union membership, genetics, biometrics (where used for identification), health, sex life and sexual orientation. In summary, the data obtained for a research project must be requested for a specific reason, be treated with respect, must not be kept for longer than necessary and be processed knowing these are private data and must not be disclosed at any stage of the research.

Researchers consider how to increase the reliability and validity of their research, the type of sample that will enable them to answer their research question and work within ethical guidelines.

Summary

This chapter has

- explained how rigorous research produces evidence that supports practice
- detailed how to search for evidence to support the rationale for a research study

- outlined different research philosophies and methodologies
- discussed a selection of commonly used research methods
- identified a range of research terms including validity and reliability
- explained different sampling strategies
- highlighted important features of ethical research practice

Further reading

Bowling, A. (2014) *Research methods in health: investigating health and health services.* 4th edn. Maidenhead: Open University Press
Greetham, B. (2019) *How to write your undergraduate dissertation.* Basingstoke: Macmillan
Thomas, G. (2017) *How to do your research project: a guide for students.* London: Sage

Useful websites

Centre for Health Promotion Research (CHPR). Leeds Beckett University. Available at: www.leedsbeckett.ac.uk/research/centre-for-health-promotion
National Institute for Health Research. Available at: www.nihr.ac.uk

References

Beauchamp, T.L. and Childress, J.E. (2019) *Principles of biomedical ethics.* 8th edn. Oxford: Oxford University Press
Blaxter, L., Hughes, C. and Tight, M. (2006) *How to research.* 3rd edn. New York: McGraw-Hill Education
Bowling, A. (2014) *Research methods in health: investigating health and health services.* Maidenhead: Open University Press
British Psychological Society. (2021) *BPS code of human research ethics.* Available at: https://www.bps.org.uk/sites/www.bps.org.uk/files/Policy/Policy%20-%20Files/BPS%20Code%20of%20Human%20Research%20Ethics.pdf (Accessed 26th April 2022)
Denzin, N.K. and Lincoln, Y.S. (2005) *The sage handbook of qualitative research.* 3rd edn. London: Sage
DePoy, E. and Gitlin, L.N. (2020) *Introduction to research. Understanding and applying multiple strategies.* 6th edn. London: Elsevier Mosby
Dileo, C. and Bradt, J. (2009) 'On creating the discipline, profession and evidence in the field of arts and healthcare', *Arts and Health*, 1(2), pp. 168–182
Gov.UK. (2021) *Data protection.* Available at: www.gov.uk/data-protection (Accessed 26th April 2022)
Gray, D.E. (2013) *Doing research in the real world.* London: Sage
Green, J. and Thorogood, N. (2018) *Qualitative methods for health research.* 4th edn. London: Sage
Gregory, D., Johnston, R., Pratt, G., Watts, M. and Whatmore, S. (2009) *The dictionary of human geography.* 5th edn. Chichester: Wiley-Blackwell
Grønmo, S. (2020) *Social research methods: qualitative, quantitative and mixed methods approaches.* London: Sage
Hek, G. and Moule, P. (2006) *Making sense of research. An introduction for health and social care practitioners.* London: Sage
Houser, J. (2016) *Nursing research: reading, using and creating evidence.* 4th edn. Burlington: Jones and Bartlett Learning
Kitzinger, J. (1995) 'Qualitative research: introducing focus groups', *BMJ*, 311(7000), pp. 299–302

Kozinets, R.V. (2015) 'Netnography: understanding networked communication society', in Quan-Haase, A. and Sloan, L. (eds) *The sage handbook of social media research methods*. Available at: www.researchgate.net/publication/319613944_Netnography (Accessed 26th April 2022)

Mann, S. (2016) *The research interview: reflective practice and reflexivity in research processes*. London: Palgrave Macmillan

Moule, P. and Goodman, M. (2009) *Nursing research. An introduction*. London: Sage

Rychetnik, L., Hawe, P., Waters, E., Barratt, A. and Frommer, M. (2004) 'A glossary for evidence-based public health', *Journal of Epidemiology and Community Health*, 58(7), pp. 538–545

Silverman, D. (ed.) (2011) *Qualitative research*. London: Sage

5   Health psychology

Murray Allen

Key points

- Introduction
- What is psychology?
- Health psychology
- Theories and models of behaviour change
- Summary

Introduction

Understanding the factors that influence people's health-related behaviours is important for those working in health promotion and public health because behaviours shape the population's health. This chapter will provide an overview of the key areas of psychology before focussing on health psychology. It will describe, apply and critique six theories and models of health psychology, demonstrating their relevance to primary and secondary disease prevention and health promotion. These include the health belief model, the theory of reasoned action, the theory of planned behaviour, the transtheoretical model, the common-sense model and nudge theory.

What is psychology?

The word 'psychology' derives from the Greek words 'psyche' referring to the spirit or soul and 'logia' meaning to study. The American Psychological Association defines psychology as the study of mind and behaviour (APA, 2022), while the British Psychological Society defines it as,

> "The scientific study of the mind and how it dictates and influences our behaviour from communication and memory to thought and emotion."
>
> (BPS, 2022a)

Despite psychology being a relatively new science, with most advances occurring in the twentieth century, ancient civilisations engaged in philosophical discussions about the mind. For example, Greeks such as Socrates, Plato and Aristotle studied subjects which are now established within the field of psychology (Shields, 2020). During the 19th century, there were two main perspectives on how the brain worked; a structuralist approach and a functionalist approach (McLeod, 2019). Structuralism was pioneered by Wilhelm Wundht (1832–1920), and it focused on how mental processes could be

DOI: 10.4324/9780367823696-7

broken down into their basic components. The mind could be analysed in an objective and measurable manner. This structuralist approach began to separate psychology from philosophy. William James (1842–1910) disagreed and developed functionalism. He argued that conscious experience is not structured because it is constantly changing. He focussed on the function and purpose of the brain. These early perspectives developed into many different approaches to psychology including Sigmund Freud's (1856–1939) theory of psychoanalysis, which became the dominant theory of the early twentieth century. As the century progressed, other perspectives emerged including behavioural, humanistic, developmental and social psychology.

The British Psychological Society was formed in 1901. It continues to set professional standards and promotes public understanding of the field of psychology (Jackson, 2019). This broad and rapidly changing field is reflected in the varied roles that psychologists perform and the numerous protected professional job titles that are endorsed by the Health and Care Professions Council. These include clinical psychologist, occupational psychologist, sport and exercise psychologist, forensic psychologist, counselling psychologist, practitioner psychologist, educational psychologist, registered psychologist as well as health psychologist (HCPC, 2022). The British Psychological Society website provides information for both the public and professionals about their work and the varied career pathways available within the field of psychology (BPS, 2022b). These include:

- forensic psychology
- health psychology
- clinical psychology
- educational psychology
- sport and exercise psychology
- neuropsychology
- occupational psychology
- counselling
- academia, research and teaching

Health psychology

The medical model was the predominant model of health and illness for much of the 20th century until it was challenged by, among others, Engel who noted that the medical model, with its emphasis on biology, did not account for the psychological or social dimensions of illness. He proposed his biopsychosocial model in 1977 (see Chapter 1). The second half of the twentieth century saw a shift from most ill-health being caused by communicable diseases to non-communicable diseases. The biopsychosocial model was used to try to better understand health and illness including their psychosocial dimensions and related behaviours. This, in turn, led to the increased role of psychology in the field of health, the development of the discipline of health psychology and in 1986 the British Psychological Society created its Division of Health Psychology (BPS, 2022c). Today, the American Psychological Association claims psychology is important for promoting people's health through its role in disease prevention and addressing health inequalities. The British Psychological Society describes the health psychologist as an expert in the application of evidence and psychological theory to promoting changes in people's health-related behaviour.

Data from the Global Burden of Disease Study (Murray *et al.*, 2020) showed that 13.5% of female deaths were attributed to poor diet and 20.3% to high blood pressure. In males, 21.4% of deaths were attributed to using tobacco and 18.2% were linked to high blood pressure. In developed countries, smoking, poor diet and physical inactivity alone are thought to cause one-third of preventable deaths (Hardman and Stensel, 2009). In England, 40% of deaths are thought to be attributable to poor diet and tobacco smoking (PHE, 2017). Consequently, the maintenance of positive health-related behaviours and tackling negative health-related behaviours is a central theme in many UK reports and policies as part of the wider aim to reduce health inequalities and to ensure the National Health Service can cope with the challenges of funding, staffing and an ageing population (HM Government, 2010; DHSC, 2018; The King's Fund, 2018; Marmot *et al.*, 2020). This is a vital element in the primary prevention of disease with healthy populations as well as secondary and tertiary disease prevention, where changing behaviour can help to reduce symptoms and the deterioration of health (NHS, 2019). Health psychology contributes to public health because it can identify, target and change people's health-related behaviours by using behaviour change techniques (PHE, 2018).

Thinking point:

List the factors that you would consider when deciding whether to

- have a new vaccine
- stop a behaviour which you know is health-damaging, e.g. smoking or chewing tobacco
- adopt a new healthy behaviour, e.g. a type of physical activity

Psychology comprises multiple specialities including health psychology. Health psychology concerns understanding and changing people's health-related behaviours.

Theories and models of behaviour change

This section provides a brief overview of six of the most widely used theories and models used in health psychology with examples of their application to practice. Theories and models seek to explain and predict health-related behaviour and can therefore inform and shape interventions designed to change behaviour. They tend to be based at the individual rather than the societal level. There is often disagreement about the exact date when a certain theory or model came into use because they have often been developed over a period of time. We will describe the health belief model, the theory of reasoned action, the theory of planned behaviour, the transtheoretical model, the common-sense model and nudge theory.

The health belief model

The origins of the health belief model (HBM) go back to the 1950s. The model tried to explain why people did not take action to prevent disease, for example attending screening tests for conditions such as tuberculosis (Rosenstock, 1974). The model was developed by social psychologists, including Irwin Rosenstock, at the American Public Health Service. Rosenstock's seminal paper 'Why people use health services', published in 1966, outlined the development of the model and how it could be used to predict health-related decision making (Rosenstock, 1966). Rosenstock updated the work, alongside Becker in 1974, and the model was used to explain and predict preventative health-related behaviours across a wide range of conditions (Janz and Becker, 1984).

In essence, the HBM suggests that an individual weighs up how susceptible they are to a disease or other negative health event and how severe it may be against the benefits they may gain from making the change in behaviour and the barriers, or costs, of making the change. Turning the decision into action is often due to a 'cue to action' which may be an event, a conversation or an experience. For example, here is the model with its five dimensions applied to an individual who is considering stopping smoking.

> Perceived susceptibility – the individual's own assessment of their risk of disease e.g. their chances of getting lung cancer through smoking

> Perceived severity – how serious the individual considers the condition to be e.g. how badly might lung cancer affect them

> Perceived benefits – what might an individual gain by changing behaviour e.g. by giving up smoking would they save money or feel better?

> Perceived barriers – what might get in the way or discourage an individual from changing behaviour e.g. anticipating they would feel irritable without smoking or no longer feel a member of a group of friends who smoke

> Cue to action – an internal or external cue that prompts the decision to be turned into action e.g. developing a smoker's cough or advice from a doctor or a health promotion campaign

A critical review of research studies from 1974 to 1984 concluded the HBM could explain and predict preventative health-related behaviours in individuals (Janz and Becker, 1984). An individual's perceived barriers and their perceived susceptibility were identified as the strongest predictors of behaviour. The model was further amended in 1988 to reflect the evidence that self-efficacy, an individual's belief that they have the capacity to carry out a behaviour successfully, was an important dimension of health-related behaviour. It also included modifying variables which were thought to influence perceptions about susceptibility, seriousness, benefits and barriers. These include the individual's demographic characteristics such as their age, sex and ethnicity; their psychosocial characteristics such as personality and social class; and structural characteristics such as general knowledge about the health issue (Figure 5.1) (Rosenstock *et al.*, 1988).

Application of the model to the prevention and early detection of breast cancer

One example of the HBM being used successfully has been in the prevention and early detection of breast cancer. Damghanian and colleagues (2020) conducted a clinical trial with 80 Iranian women who had a family history of breast cancer. All the participants completed a questionnaire before and after four educational sessions based on the HBM, but only half received the education. The questionnaire asked about risk

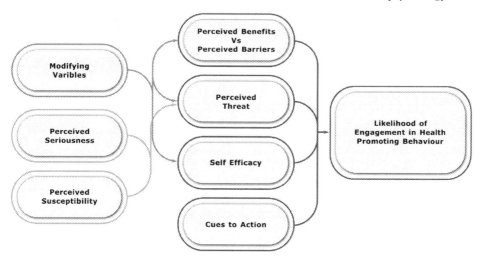

Figure 5.1 The health belief model

Source: Graphic Grid/Shutterstock.com

factors for breast cancer; perceived sensitivity, perceived severity; perceived benefits of screening behaviours; perceived barriers; self-efficacy and questions about personal health-related behaviours which included the individual's physical activity and diet (as weight is a risk factor) and alcohol consumption. The four sessions included the participants' familiarity with breast cancer; its symptoms and complications; risk factors; breast screening (mammography and breast self-examination); health-related behaviours; effective behaviours in confronting breast cancer; and finally a discussion about barriers to health-related behaviours. The researchers found significant improvements in the knowledge, beliefs and health-related behaviours related to the prevention and early diagnosis of breast cancer among the women who had received the education. Also in Iran, Ghaffari and colleagues (2019) found similar results when they provided education about breast screening behaviours, attending for mammograms and breast self-examination, to 240 healthy female volunteers. Compared to their control group of 240 women who did not receive the education, those who had received the education significantly improved their knowledge about their perceived susceptibility, severity, benefits and barriers, as well as their self-efficacy and behavioural intention related to attending for mammography and breast self-examination. This difference persisted two months later.

In the United States of America, Guilford and colleagues (2017) gave a questionnaire to college women which asked about their breast cancer knowledge, health motivation, perceived susceptibility to breast cancer, perceived severity of breast cancer, perceived benefits and barriers towards screening activities, self-efficacy and their breast self-examination behaviour. The researchers found the women had low levels of believing themselves to be susceptible to breast cancer and low levels of breast self-examination, despite breast cancer being the second leading cause of death in American women. They found having greater knowledge, lower perceived barriers and stronger self-efficacy were associated with more self-examination. They recommend breast health education may be more effective at promoting healthy behaviours if it focuses on increasing women's knowledge about their susceptibility to breast cancer; enhances their self-efficacy, that is their belief that they can successfully carry out breast cancer screening activities; and reduces their perceived barriers.

Limitations of the model

Research has suggested there are limitations to the HBM. For example, Carpenter (2010) analysed 18 studies looking at the ability of the dimensions to accurately predict positive changes in behaviour. He found their predictive power was weakened over time, and so he recommended using the HBM for this direct purpose should be discontinued. Jones and colleagues (2014) reviewed 18 research studies where the HBM was used in the design of interventions to improve health-related behaviours. They concluded that success was unrelated to the model, and so the model should not be used for this purpose. Recently, Tong and colleagues (2020) tested whether the HBM could predict whether people would adopt precautionary measures such as wearing face masks, proper hand washing and social distancing shortly after the outbreak of the COVID-19 coronavirus pandemic in Macau, China. This was before measures were enforced by law. The authors found a correlation between the health-related behaviours and all the dimensions of the HBM except for perceived susceptibility. However, they also acknowledged that the dimension of social norms is not included in the HBM and they had observed those people with a mistrust of authority, 'social cynicism', was associated with less hand washing and face mask wearing. It appears the HBM has its uses in explaining and predicting health-related behaviour, but it also has its limitations. Perhaps it still receives attention due to its longevity and the sheer volume of studies conducted over the last half century.

The theory of reasoned action and the theory of planned behaviour

The theory of reasoned action (TRA) was introduced by Fishbein and Ajzen in 1975. The theory was widely used to predict behaviour and to inform strategies for changing behaviours (Madden *et al.*, 1992). The TRA suggests an individual's intention to carry out a behaviour will predict whether they will carry it out. An individual's intentions are influenced by their attitude towards the behaviour and their subjective beliefs about 'norms' in their social world (Figure 5.2). The theory assumes that the individual's behaviour is under their voluntary control and there is a strong relationship between attitude and behaviour (Madden *et al.*, 1992; Ajzen and Fishbein, 1977).

Later, Ajzen (1991) recognised that the TRA was limited because not all behaviours are under voluntary control. If intention cannot always predict action, the TRA has limited application (La Barbera and Ajzen, 2020). The theory of planned behaviour (TPB) was developed by Ajzen in 1985, as an extension of the earlier TRA. Ajzen (1991)

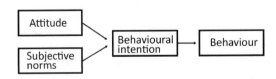

Figure 5.2 The theory of reasoned action

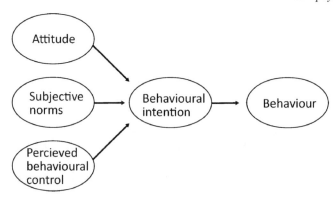

Figure 5.3 The theory of planned behaviour

noted that the more strongly an individual perceived they had the ability to perform a behaviour, the more likely they would carry it out. An individual's level of perceived behavioural control can be influenced by factors such as their time and financial resources, their motivation, the support they have from others and their skills. The TPB states an individual's intentions are influenced by their attitude towards the behaviour, their subjective beliefs about 'norms' in their social world and their perceived behavioural control (Figure 5.3).

Comparing the TPB to the TRA, Madden and colleagues (1992) concluded that by assessing an individual's perceived behavioural control over a behaviour, in addition to their attitude and subjective norms, we could more accurately predict their behaviour. This means that strategies designed to change behaviour can be enhanced by including an individual's perception of behavioural control. This explains why the TPB is described as,

> "… the dominant theoretical approach to guide research in health-related behaviour over the last three decades."
>
> (Sniehotta *et al.*, 2014, p. 1)

Application of the theory to colorectal cancer screening

An example of the TPB being used in practice is provided by Huang and colleagues (2020) who wanted to know whether the TPB could predict whether a large sample of 61 to 70 year olds in Hong Kong would take up invitations for colorectal cancer screening. They carried out a telephone survey using a questionnaire based upon the five variables.

- Behaviour – attending for screening
- Behavioural intention – how likely it was that the individual would attend for screening
- Attitude – the individual's overall evaluation of the screening programme, e.g. its accuracy and effectiveness at testing for cancer as well as the individual's feelings about the screening

- Subjective norms – the individual's perceptions of whether other people close to them would like them to join the screening programme, e.g. would they go for screening if a relative or friend suggested it, and would they go for screening if a relative or friend went for screening
- Perceived behavioural control – to what extent the individual feels able to go for screening, e.g. would it be easy and is it something they can decide for themselves

The authors concluded that the five variables were pertinent to whether individuals attended for screening. A positive attitude and a high level of perceived behavioural control were strongly associated with the intention to be screened and then the uptake of screening. The subjective norms variable did not play an important role. They recommend those who work in health promotion and public health could increase the uptake of colorectal screening by tailoring information about screening in a way that will encourage a positive attitude towards screening and increase perceptions of behavioural control.

Limitations of the model

The TPB continues to be reviewed by Ajzen and other researchers. Some have found, like the study in Hong Kong, that the variable of subjective norms seems to have only a weak influence on predicted behaviour, especially where an individual has high perceived behavioural control (Armitage and Connor, 2001; La Barbera and Ajzen, 2020). Others are interested in reverse causal relationships, that is whether a behavioural intention influences attitude, subjective norms and perceived behavioural control (Sussman and Gifford, 2019). Sniehotta and colleagues (2014) have suggested that making further amendments to the TPB is not helpful and propose the model is retired in favour of discovering better ways of explaining human behaviour.

The transtheoretical model

The transtheoretical model, also known as the stages of change model, was developed by Prochaska and Di Clemente (1982; 1983) who analysed the processes that smokers went through when stopping smoking, with or without various types of therapeutic support. They identified ten processes of change: consciousness raising, self-liberation, social liberation, self-re-evaluation, environmental re-evaluation, counterconditioning, stimulus control, reinforcement management, dramatic relief and helping relationships. These were grouped into five distinct stages of smoking behaviour: immotives, contemplators, recent quitters, long-term quitters and relapsers. As the model was subsequently applied to other concerning health-related behaviours, it was modified to the five stages that are commonly used today.

- Pre-contemplation – not considering making a change
- Contemplation – considering making a change
- Preparation – planning to take action or making small changes
- Action – actively engaging in the new behaviour
- Maintenance – continuation of the new behaviour

Beyond these five stages, an individual may reach *stable behaviour* whereby they are no longer tempted to engage with the unhealthy behaviour. Alternatively, an individual

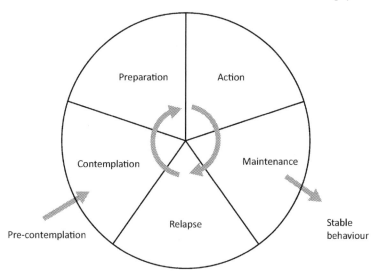

Figure 5.4 The transtheoretical model

may *relapse* and revert to their previous behaviour. Prochaska and Di Clemente (1982) acknowledged that individuals may stall at any stage, and the problems with maintaining smoking cessation varied considerably between recent and long-term smoking quitters before they experienced no difficulties at all with being a non-smoker. Like many of the other models discussed in this chapter, the transtheoretical model has evolved over time as it has been used in multiple fields. This has led to differing interpretations and representations of the stages. The model can be expressed as a spiral, ladder or a cycle (Figure 5.4) (Cahill *et al.*, 2010). Some versions incorporate time frames, for example

- pre-contemplation – has no intention of changing behaviour in the next six months
- contemplation – is considering making a change during the next one to six months
- preparation – is planning to take action in the next month
- action – has actively engaged in the new behaviour for up to six months
- maintenance – has continued the new behaviour for more than six months

Application of the model to helping rough sleepers trying to overcome alcohol and drug dependency

Weal (2020) explains how the transtheoretical model is often used in the UK as the basis for a person-centred approach to helping people who are sleeping rough and have alcohol and/or drug dependencies. He describes the *pre-contemplative* stage as when people do not view their alcohol or drug use as being harmful. Research carried out by St Mungo's charity to support the homeless, based in London and the south of England, shows how rough sleepers have often suffered multiple disadvantages including childhood and adult trauma (St Mungo's, 2016), and they are often unable or unwilling to engage with services such as mental health services, drug and alcohol services or housing support. To begin to engage rough sleepers in the *pre-contemplation* stage, St Mungo's outreach workers try to build trusting, supportive relationships with rough sleepers and then, together, they work out what the individual needs and begin to work towards solutions. As the rough sleepers' lives can be very chaotic, each encounter may only present a ten-minute window in which to try to work together. One rough sleeper said,

> "… [outreach] is probably the best service I've ever encountered. They come to you on the street, they find you."
>
> (Greg quoted in Weal, 2020, p. 39)

Once the outreach worker feels they have built a trusting relationship, they aim to encourage the individual to reach the stage of *contemplation*, that is, to consider harm reduction or harm minimisation (see Chapter 12). This is the next step because rough sleepers who are dependent on alcohol and/or drugs are at high risk of death (NRS, 2021). Rough sleepers with heroin dependency who have reached the stage of *contemplation* may prepare to accept a 'script', a prescription, for methadone as a safer substitute for heroin. This can help to stabilise their lives and simultaneously begin to bring them into contact with health and other services. It is vital that scripts are available in a timely manner for those who have reached *preparation* and are now ready to take *action*. If the scripts are delayed, the opportunity may be lost. St Mungo's survey, undertaken in 2019, showed three-quarters of rough sleepers had to wait more than three days, and some waited more than three weeks (Weal, 2020). *Maintenance*, that is regularly taking the methadone, often requires attending for set appointments which is a significant challenge in the context of very limited services for individuals who often don't have an alarm clock, diary or phone. It is not surprising that many *relapse* and the charity is fighting for improved services. One individual said,

> "I must have gone to maybe 20-25 appointments in the last two months, and I've only achieved script and support once … I've got nothing to show for any of it …"
>
> (Greg quoted in Weal, 2020, p. 41)

Limitations of the model

In 2005, criticisms of the transtheoretical model were raised. West (2005) stated that the definitions of stages were 'arbitrary lines in the sand' and it was erroneous to assume that an individual's plans to change behaviour were always stable and coherent. Although it appealed to practitioners, West recommended the model should be discarded. He was formulating his own alternative model at the time. Adams and White (2005) argued that using the stages as the basis for designing interventions, in the context of physical activity, was not effective. They cited the complexity of physical activity as a behaviour; the problems with stages being identified purely on subjective, non-measurable self-assessment; the limitations of a model which focuses on decision-making and self-efficacy whilst not including wider factors that can influence how someone approaches changing their behaviour; the lack of evidence that using an individualised staged approach is any better than not using one; the lack of evidence that changes in behaviour are long lasting and concerns that focusing on progressing through stages does not necessarily lead to a change in behaviour. Brug and colleagues (2005) critiqued these arguments and concluded that using the model to promote physical activity was very challenging, but some stage-based interventions had shown promising results and therefore further research was warranted.

A year later, Prochaska (2006) defended the model by explaining it does not assume that decision-making is a rational and conscious process. There was a lack of research in this field before the model was published as well as little support for individuals with multiple problems who lacked the motivation to change their health-related behaviour. He argued that the model had helped to progress this field of study and it had allowed a more inclusive approach to the practice of supporting people who needed to change their health-related behaviour. Later, he emphasised the importance of assessing the individual's stage of change and then tailoring interventions accordingly (Prochaska *et al.*, 2013).

Today, the transtheoretical model is widely used in the field of changing health-related behaviour such as increasing physical activity and fruit and vegetable consumption, weight management and smoking cessation. For example, it was successfully used to understand and then advance vaping cessation programmes among American college students (Martinasek *et al.*, 2021). It has also been incorporated into some clinical guidelines (Cahill *et al.*, 2010). The National Institute for Health and Care Excellence has raised concerns that that the model has been incorporated into UK health professional training programmes as a basis for behaviour change interventions despite it not being able to predict and explain behaviour change with sufficient accuracy (NICE, 2014). The enduring appeal of the model seems to be partly because its critics have not yet improved upon it.

The common-sense model

The common-sense model is also known as the self-regulatory model or Leventhal's model, after its developer Howard Leventhal (Figure 5.5). The model was not developed at a single moment, rather it evolved during the late 1970s and early 1980s. Leventhal wrote his seminal publication 'The common-sense representation of illness danger' in 1980. This model provides a framework for examining the processes through which an individual becomes aware of a health threat and formulates a plan to manage their response (Leventhal *et al.*, 2016). It can be described as a model of the processes which underlie common-sense managements of everyday threats to health (Leventhal *et al.*, 2011). There are three stages of self-regulation:

- stage one: interpretation of the threat, e.g. perception of symptoms and social messages
- stage two: formulation of a coping strategy, e.g. to avoid or to approach coping
- stage three: appraisal of the consequences of the strategy, e.g. whether it was effective

In stage one, Leventhal and colleagues (2016) suggest that changes to the individual's normal functioning, discussing their illness with others, past experiences and treatments will generate mental representations of, or beliefs about, the threats to their health in five cognitive (thinking) dimensions. These are:

- identity – the label or name given to the illness
- perceived cause of illness, e.g. poor health-related behaviour or infection
- timeline – how long the illness is expected to last
- consequences – the impact of the illness on the individual's life
- cure and/or control – whether the illness can be cured or managed

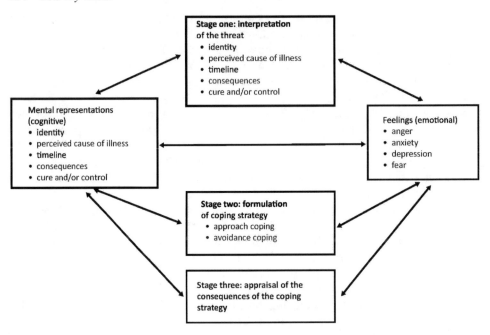

Figure 5.5 The common-sense model

Source: Adapted from McGuire and Walsh, 2006, p.3

These mental representations affect, and are affected by, the individual's feelings about the illness. Feelings may include

- anger
- anxiety
- depression
- fear

In stage two, the individual adopts a coping response based on their beliefs and feelings. Coping may be

- approach coping, meaning they actively start to cope
- avoidance coping, meaning they are passive with a sense of helplessness

In stage three, the individual evaluates their coping response, such as whether it is helping them. This evaluation encourages them to consider their perception about the illness again. The process starts again.

The common-sense model is important within health promotion and public health because the rise of non-communicable and chronic diseases, such as cardiovascular disease, means there is a need to encourage people towards greater self-management of illness and away from overstretched healthcare systems (Hagger and Orbell, 2021). For example, 4.2 million people have diagnosed type 2 diabetes in the UK, and an estimated 13 million have undiagnosed diabetes or are at risk of developing it (Whicher *et al.*, 2020). Self-management means the regulation of blood glucose. In diabetes, the blood glucose levels are too high because the glucose cannot enter the cells of the body. This may be because the body does not produce enough insulin or because it cannot use the insulin that the body does produce. The excess glucose in the blood can cause a range of serious health problems including high blood pressure, blindness, gangrene and kidney failure (Robinson, 2021). The National Institute for Health and Care Excellence (2015) advises individuals to gain control over their blood glucose levels by adhering to advice about a good diet, physical activity and medication, and by self-monitoring their blood glucose levels. Self-monitoring of blood glucose is usually carried out by testing a finger-prick of blood. Continuous glucose-monitoring systems, based on the long-term insertion of a sensor into the body, provide a reading on a small monitor. Also, less precisely, urine tests can show high glucose levels in the body. Self-monitoring of blood glucose has no purpose if individuals do not make the appropriate behaviour changes in response to their readings (Breland *et al.*, 2013). People with diabetes, especially in the early phases, often display no symptoms and people rarely adopt new positive health-related behaviours when they experience no symptoms (Tanenbaum *et al.*, 2015).

Application of the model to type 2 diabetes

Fall and colleagues (2021) tested the common-sense model with a sample of 253 patients with type 2 diabetes in France. They completed questionnaires about their beliefs about diabetes, beliefs about medicines, their coping strategies, their current adherence to treatment, their general quality of life and their quality of life in relation to diabetes. Their blood glucose measurements were recorded. The researchers analysed all the direct and indirect pathways between the patients' cognitive and emotional perceptions of diabetes and its treatment; their coping strategies, including adherence or avoidance of the diabetes regime; and outcomes measured as achievement of blood glucose control and quality of life. They found that the patients' perceptions about diabetes and their coping strategies were significantly related to their adherence to their diabetes regime, that is the control of their blood glucose and their quality of life. This suggests if we address an individual's perceptions about type 2 diabetes and its potential to be controlled, or even go into remission, we can narrow the gap between a self-monitored blood glucose reading and the likelihood an individual will respond with the appropriate health-related behaviour. Therefore the authors endorse the common-sense model as a potentially useful framework when designing an intervention to change health-related behaviour, where the individual needs to be an 'active agent' in their own health.

Limitations of the model

Like other models, the common-sense model is used widely, but it has its critics. For example, Brandes and Mullan (2014) carried out a review of 30 research studies and found that the relationship between cognitive mental representations and adherence to a health-related behaviour in the context of chronic illness, was weak. Yet, when Leventhal and colleagues (2016) presented a review of their model's contribution to the self-management of illness for over 50 years, they appeared to ignore studies that found any negative findings (Doyle and Mullan, 2017). Hagger and Orbell (2021) proposed extending the model to include additional constructs which would explain the relationship between the cognitive mental representations, coping responses and outcomes more fully. Such suggestions illustrate how models of health-related behaviour are constantly being refined to try to achieve the 'perfect' model.

Nudge theory

Nudge theory was coined by Thaler and Sunstein in 2008. It concerns influencing people's decisions by designing their available choices in ways that acknowledge we often make decisions instinctively and irrationally, not always logically and rationally. It is often used in social marketing, as discussed in Chapter 6. Nudging is,

> "Any aspect of the choice architecture that alters people's behaviour in a predictable way, without forbidding any options or significantly changing their economic incentives."
>
> (Thaler and Sunstein, 2008, p. 6)

For those wishing to promote people's health, negative nudging is where supermarkets position unhealthy snacks such as crisps, chocolate or sugary drinks at or near to the checkout. All customers need to go to the checkout and may spend a long time in the queue where they can be influenced to make an impulse purchase of these products. Ejlerskov and colleagues (2018) conducted an experiment with the help of six supermarkets who agreed to move the display of 'unhealthy' items away from the checkout area to somewhere else in the stores. They noted a 17.3% reduction in the purchases of these items immediately, a finding that was maintained 12 months later. Customers could still purchase the items, they were not being denied a choice, but there was a reduction in their impulse buying.

Application of the theory to hospital food

Hospitals often sell unhealthy snacks despite their remit to promote health through healthcare, because the profits from cafeterias and vending machines are important to their business. In Australia, the Alfred Hospital in Victoria agreed to participate in research trials to nudge patients, visitors and staff towards healthier choices in their cafeteria. Halpern (2016) describes a trial where sugary drinks were moved to a less prominent position. Despite concerns from the cafeteria manager that revenue might fall, the 12% reduction in sales of high-sugar drinks was offset by sales in low and moderate sugar drinks, and so total revenue was not affected. In a second trial, from 2015 to 2016, the prices of high-sugar drinks sold in half the hospital's vending machines were increased by 20%. The prices of high-sugar drinks in the remaining machines were kept the same. Five percent fewer high-sugar drinks were sold from the machines with higher prices compared to those machines with standard pricing. However, there was no decrease in overall revenue as, again, the sales of low and moderate-sugar drinks compensated. Both trials showed it was possible to decrease the consumption of sugar without negatively impacting revenue through nudging.

This research influenced the Victoria State Government to modify their policies to encourage healthy eating in hospitals. The policies actively nudge staff, visitors and volunteers towards healthier food and drink choices by increasing their availability and promotion whilst also reducing unhealthy choices.

Thorndikeand colleagues (2012) report how the 'choice architecture' of the cafeteria in Massachusetts General Hospital, Boston, was modified. The refrigerators were re-arranged so that the healthier drinks were at eye level and the less healthy drinks were out of people's direct eye-line. Bottled water was also added at various points near to food stations throughout the cafeteria. The researchers reported an 11.4% decrease in unhealthy drinks sales and a 25.8% increase in bottled water sales due to this nudging intervention.

The Behavioural Insights Team, also known as The Nudge Unit, was formed by the UK Government in 2010 following the publication of Thaler and Sunstein's (2008) book. It became a UK independent company in 2014 and today it has offices around the world. It utilises international expertise to apply behavioural science across a wide range of fields including health and wellbeing. The Behavioural Insights Team have recently worked with the UK Local Government Association to reduce sugar consumption, especially from high-sugar drinks. In two Liverpool hospitals, 'stop' signs were placed near to high-sugar drinks on refrigerator shelves. There was a 7.3% reduction in the sales of high-sugar drinks with no overall change in revenue suggesting lower sugar drinks were purchased instead (LGA and BIT, 2019).

Halpern (2016) suggests that adding tax to an unhealthy product can act as a 'triple nudge'. The initial price rise nudges some customers to switch to a healthier food or drink; retailers are nudged to provide more healthy products and then manufacturers develop healthier alternatives, such as lower-sugar items. Changes in consumption and supply patterns further nudge other customers to buy more healthy products.

Limitations of the theory

Nudge theory is based on behavioural economics and psychology with little attention to how social interactions and the social context, such as culture, also influence behaviour. Ewert (2020) argues it is important to recognise that behavioural interventions have limitations because they do not help with tackling the underlying causes of the health problem. For example, the underlying causes of obesity include the factors which shape the obesogenic environment. These include the powerful food industry, poverty and deprivation as cheap, high calorie food is widely accessible. Nudges are 'top down' in keeping with the 'top down' social change model of health promotion discussed in Chapter 8. Nudges are usually designed by policymakers, the 'architects of the choices', with no reference to individuals' lay knowledge, their personal interests and priorities, or their empowerment. The covert nature of the nudge presents ethical concerns about openness and transparency; it is an easier form of regulation compared to the more costly, more comprehensive and holistic alternatives for dealing with the underlying structural causes behind negative health-related behaviours. Ewert suggests nudging may be part of the solution, but it needs to be used alongside other ways to promote health. Schmidt and Engelen (2019) agree but go further by rejecting nudging on the grounds of it being unethical. They discuss the role of digital nudging where companies collect data to shape behaviour, and smartphone apps and social media can prey on people's weaknesses for instant rewards, discouraging wider, more fulfilling choices. For the authors, nudging is manipulative, paternalistic, reduces people's freedom of choice and autonomy, it violates human dignity and it focuses on individuals rather than structural reform.

In response to criticisms, de Quintana Medina (2021) argues that there is a difference between what people want and what is right for them. For example, the UK Government introduced legislation for the wearing of seatbelts in cars and helmets when riding motorbikes with significant health benefits. Nudging may be paternalistic, but it may also be legitimate if it improves health, social welfare and reduces health inequalities. Nudges can be a tool to help with changing people's behaviour where traditional approaches have been unsuccessful; it can complement other tools. Critics suggest nudging exploits people's irrational choices, not their rational ones. Yet, even when people are making free autonomous choices, these are not always rational and conscious. Behaviour is not based only on rational choices. Getting people to agree to a nudge may be more ethical, but it is likely to undermine and restrict its implementation. In response to concerns that nudging is not transparent, de Quintana Medina argues nudges are designed in different ways. Some are designed to be noticed by individuals who then reflect on the choice they are being given; some are not. Although an individual may be unaware of how they are being nudged, they will be aware of their resulting behaviour. Individuals are being nudged all the time by policy-makers, businesses and so forth. The context of their choices is very influential, whether the choice is conscious, unconscious, intentional or not. She concludes that nudges are not intrinsically problematic, but we need to be clear about the rationale behind them and reflect carefully upon the ethics of each intervention.

Theories and models of behaviour change have evolved to explain and predict health-related behaviour. Each has its strengths and limitations.

Summary

This chapter has

- outlined the development of psychology and health psychology
- described key behaviour change models and theories
- provided examples of how these models and theories have been applied to the primary and secondary prevention of ill-health
- discussed some of the limitations of these models and theories

Further reading

Anisman, H. (2021) *Health psychology: a biopsychosocial approach*. 2nd edn. London: Sage
Ogden, J. (2019) *Health psychology*. 6th edn. London: McGraw-Hill Education

Useful websites

American Psychological Association. Available at: www.apa.org
British Psychological Society. Available at: www.bps.org.uk
The Behavioural Insights Team. Available at: www.bi.team

References

Adams, J. and White, M. (2005) 'Why don't stage-based activity promotion interventions work?', *Health Education Research*, 20(2), pp. 237–243

Ajzen, I. (1991) 'The theory of planned behaviour', *Organisational Behaviour and Human Decision Processes*, 50(2), pp. 179–211

Ajzen, I. and Fishbein, M. (1977) 'Attitude-behaviour relations: a theoretical analysis and review of empirical research', *Psychological Bulletin*, 84(5), pp. 888–918

American Psychological Association (2022) *APA dictionary of psychology*. Available at: https://dictionary.apa.org/psychology (Accessed 23rd February 2022).

Armitage, C.J. and Connor, M. (2001) 'Efficacy of the theory of planned behaviour: a meta-analytic review', *British Journal of Social Psychology*, 40(4), pp. 471–499

Brandes, K. and Mullan, B. (2014) 'Can the common-sense model predict adherence in chronically ill patients? A meta-analysis', *Health Psychology Review*, 8(2), pp. 129–153

Breland, J.Y., McAndrew, L.M., Burns, E., Leventhal, E.A. and Leventhal, H. (2013) 'Using the common sense model of self-regulation to review the effects of self-monitoring of blood glucose on glycaemic control for non-insulin treated adults with type 2 diabetes', *The Diabetes Educator*, 39(4), pp. 541–559

British Psychological Society (2022a) *What is psychology?* Available at: https://www.bps.org.uk/public/what-is-psychology (Accessed 23rd February 2022)

British Psychological Society (2022b) *Your journey into psychology*. Available at: https://careers.bps.org.uk (Accessed 23rd February 2022)

British Psychological Society (2022c) *Division of health psychology*. Available at: https://www.bps.org.uk/member-microsites/division-health-psychology (Accessed 23rd February 2022)

Brug, J., Conner, M., Harre, N., Kremers, S., McKellar, S. and Whitelaw, S. (2005) 'The transtheoretical model and stages of change: a critique', *Health Education Research*, 20(2), pp. 244–258

Cahill, K., Lancaster, T. and Green, N. (2010) 'Stage-based interventions for smoking cessation', *Cochrane Database of Systematic Reviews*, 11 doi:10.1002/14651858.CD004492.pub4

Carpenter, C.J. (2010) 'A meta-analysis of the effectiveness of health belief model variables in predicting behaviour', *Health Communication*, 25(8), pp. 661–669

Damghanian, M., Mahmoodzadeh, H., Khakbazan, Z., Khorsand, B. and Motaharinexhad, M. (2020) 'Self-care behaviours in high-risk women for breast cancer: a randomized clinical trial using health belief model education', *Journal of Education and Health Promotion*, 9(265) doi:10.4103/jehp.jehp_76_20

de Quintana Medina, J. (2021) 'What is wrong with nudges? Addressing normative objections to the aims and means of nudges', *Gestión y Análisis de Políticas Públicas*, 25, pp. 23–37

Department of Health and Social Care (2018) *Prevention is better than cure. Our vision to help you live well for longer*. Available at: https://assets.publishing.service.gov.uk/government/uploads/system/uploads/attachment_data/file/753688/Prevention_is_better_than_cure_5-11.pdf (Accessed 23rd February 2022)

Doyle, F. and Mullan, B. (2017) 'Does the CSM really provide a consistent framework for understanding self-management?', *Journal of Behavioural Medicine*, 40(2) doi:10.1007/s10865-016-9806-y

Ejlerskov, K.T., Harp, S.J., Stead, M., Adamson, A.J., White, M. and Adams, J. (2018) 'Supermarket policies on less-healthy food at checkouts: natural experimental evaluation using interrupted time series analyses of purchases', *PLoS Medicine*, 15(12) doi:10.1371/journal.pmed.1002712

Engel, G.L. (1977) 'The need for a new medical model: a challenge for biomedicine', *Science*, 196(4286), pp. 129–136

Ewert, B. (2020) 'Moving beyond the obsession with nudging individual behaviour: towards a broader understanding of behavioural public policy', *Public Policy Administration*, 35(3), pp. 337–360

Fall, E., Chakroun-Baggioni, N., Bohme, P., Maqdasy, S., Izaute, M. and Tauveron, I. (2021) 'Common sense model of self-regulation for understanding adherence and quality of life in type 2 diabetes with structural equation modelling', *Patient Education and Counselling*, 104(1), pp. 171–178

Ghaffari, M., Esfahani, S.N., Rakhshanderou, S. and Koukamari, P.H. (2019) 'Evaluation of health belief model-based intervention on breast cancer screening behaviours among health volunteers', *Journal of Cancer Education*, 34(5), pp. 904–912

Guilford, K., McKinley, E. and Turner, L. (2017) 'Breast cancer knowledge, beliefs, and screening behaviours of college women: application of the health belief model', *American Journal of Health Education*, 48(4), pp. 256–263

Hagger, M.S. and Orbell, S. (2021) 'The common sense model of illness self-regulation: a conceptual review and proposed extended model', *Health Psychology Review*, 1 doi:10.1080/17437199.2021.1878050

Halpern, D. (2016) *Behavioural insights and healthier lives. VicHealth's inaugural leading thinkers residency. A report by David Halpern.* Melbourne: Victorian Health Promotion Foundation. Available at: https://www.bi.team/wp-content/uploads/2016/04/2016-Behavioural-Insights-and-Healthier-Lives.pdf (Accessed 20th February 2022)

Hardman, A.E. and Stensel, D.J. (2009) *Physical activity and health: the evidence explained.* London: Routledge

Health and Care Professions Council (2022) *Professions and protected titles.* Available at: https://www.hcpc-uk.org/about-us/who-we-regulate/the-professions/ (Accessed 23rd February 2022)

HM Government (2010) *Healthy lives, healthy people. Our strategy for public health in England.* London: The Stationery Office

Huang, J., Wang, J., Pang, T., Chan, M., Leung, S., Chen, X., Leung, C., Zhang, Z.-J. and Wong, M. (2020) 'Does the theory of planned behaviour play a role in predicting uptake of colorectal cancer screening? A cross-sectional study in Hong Kong', *BMJ Open*, 10(8) doi:10.1136/bmjopen-2020-037619

Jackson, C. (2019) *A history of psychology in the United Kingdom. Meeting of minds – the road to professional practice.* The British Psychological Society. Available at: https://www.bps.org.uk/sites/www.bps.org.uk/files/History%20of%20Psychology/A%20History%20of%20Psychology%20in%20the%20United%20Kingdom%20-%20Claire%20Jackson.pdf (Accessed 6th April 2022)

Janz, N.K. and Becker, M.H. (1984) 'The health belief model: a decade later', *Health Education Quarterly*, 11(1), pp. 1–47

Jones, C.J., Smith, H. and Llewellyn, C. (2014) 'Evaluating the effectiveness of health belief model interventions in improving adherence: a systematic review', *Health Psychology Review*, 8(3), pp. 253–269

La Barbera, F. and Ajzen, I. (2020) 'Control interactions in the theory of planned behaviour: rethinking the role of subjective norm', *Europe's Journal of Psychology*, 16(3), pp. 401–417

Leventhal, H., Leventhal, E.A. and Breland, J.Y. (2011) 'Cognitive science speaks to the "common-sense" of chronic illness management', *Annals of Behavioural Medicine*, 41(2), pp. 152–163

Leventhal, H., Meyer, D. and Nerenz, D. (1980) 'The common-sense representation of illness danger', *Contributions to Medical Psychology*, 2, pp. 17–30

Leventhal, H., Phillips, A. and Burns, E. (2016) 'The common-sense model of self-regulation (CSM): a dynamic framework for understanding illness self-management', *Journal of Behavioural Medicine*, 39(6), pp. 935–946

Local Government Association and The Behavioural Insights Team (2019) *Using behavioural insights to reduce sugar consumption in Liverpool.* Available at: https://www.local.gov.uk/sites/default/files/documents/Liverpool%20City%20Council_BI_executive%20summary.pdf (Accessed 20th February 2022)

Madden, T., Ellen, P.S. and Ajzen, I. (1992) 'A comparison of the theory of planned behaviour and the theory of reasoned action', *Personality and Social Psychology Bulletin*, 18(1), pp. 3–9

Marmot, M., Allen, J., Boyce, T., Goldblatt, P. and Morrison, J. (2020) *Health equity in England: the Marmot review 10 years on*. Available at: http://www.instituteofhealthequity.org/resources-reports/marmot-review-10-years-on/the-marmot-review-10-years-on-executive-summary.pdf (Accessed 21st February 2022)

Martinasek, M., Tamulevicius, N., Gibson-Young, L., McDaniel, J., Moss, S.J., Pfeffer, I. and Lipski, B. (2021) 'Predictors of vaping behaviour change in young adults using the transtheoretical model: a multi-country study', *Tobacco Use Insights*, 14 doi:10.1177/1179173X20988672

McGuire, B. and Walsh, J.C. (2006) 'Diabetes self–management: facilitating behaviour change', *Diabeteswise*, 3(1), pp. 2–6

McLeod, S. (2019) *What is psychology?* Available at: https://www.simplypsychology.org/whatispsychology.html (Accessed 6th April 2022)

Murray, C.J., Aravkin, A.Y., Zheng, P., et al. (2020) 'Global burden of 87 risk factors in 204 countries and territories, 1990-2019: a systematic analysis for the global burden of disease study 2019', *The Lancet*, 396(10258), pp. 1223–1249

National Health Service (2019) *The NHS long term plan*. Available at: https://www.longtermplan.nhs.uk/publication/nhs-long-term-plan (Accessed 21st February 2022)

National Institute for Health and Care Excellence (2014) *Behaviour change: individual approaches*. Available at: https://www.nice.org.uk/guidance/ph49 (Accessed 25th April 2022)

National Institute for Health and Care Excellence (2015) *Type 2 diabetes in adults: management*. Available at: https://www.nice.org.uk/guidance/ng28 (Accessed 20th February 2022)

National Records of Scotland (2021) *Homeless deaths 2020*. Available at: https://www.nrscotland.gov.uk/files//statistics/homeless-deaths/20/homeless-deaths-20-report.pdf (Accessed 28th March 2022)

Prochaska, J.O. (2006) 'Moving beyond the transtheoretical model. Further commentaries on West (2005)', *Addiction*, 101(6), pp. 768–778

Prochaska, J.O. and Di Clemente, C.C. (1982) 'Transtheoretical therapy: toward a more integrative model of change', *Psychotherapy Theory, Research and Practice*, 19(3), pp. 276–288

Prochaska, J.O. and Di Clemente, C.C. (1983) 'Stages and processes of self-change of smoking – toward an integrative model of change', *Journal of Consulting and Clinical Psychology*, 51(3), pp. 390–395

Prochaska, J.O., Norcross, J.C. and Di Clemente, C.C. (2013) 'Applying the stages of change', *Psychotherapy in Australia*, 19(2), pp. 10–15

Public Health England (2017) *Health profile for England: 2017. Chapter 2: major causes of death and how they have changed*. Available at: https://www.gov.uk/government/publications/health-profile-for-england/chapter-2-major-causes-of-death-and-how-they-have-changed (Accessed 22nd February 2022)

Public Health England (2018) *Improving people's health: applying behavioural and social sciences to improve population health and wellbeing in England*. Available at: https://assets.publishing.service.gov.uk/government/uploads/system/uploads/attachment_data/file/744672/Improving_Peoples_Health_Behavioural_Strategy.pdf (Accessed 23rd February 2022)

Robinson, S. (2021) 'Diabetes', in Robinson, S. (ed) *Priorities for health promotion and public health*. London: Routledge, pp. 432–466

Rosenstock, I.M. (1966) 'Why people use health services', *Milbank Memorial Fund Quarterly*, 44(3), pp. 94–124

Rosenstock, I.M. (1974) 'Historical origins of the health belief model', *Health Education Monographs*, 2(4), pp. 328–335

Rosenstock, I.M., Strecher, V.J. and Becker, M.N. (1988) 'Social learning theory and the health belief model', *Health Education Quarterly*, 15(2), pp. 175–183

Schmidt, A.T. and Engelen, B. (2019) 'The ethics of nudging: an overview', *Philosophy Compass*, 15 doi:10.1111/phc3.12658

Shields, C. (2020) 'Aristotle's psychology', in Zalta, E.N. (ed) *Stanford encyclopaedia of philosophy*. Available at: https://plato.stanford.edu/entries/aristotle-psychology/ (Accessed 23rd February 2022)

Sniehotta, F.F., Presseau, J. and Araujo-Soares, V. (2014) 'Time to retire the theory of planned behaviour', *Health Psychology Review*, 8(1) doi:10.1080/17437199.2013.869710

St Mungo's (2016) *Stop the scandal: an investigation into mental health and rough sleeping*. Available at: www.mungos.org/publication/stop-scandal-investigation-mental-health-rough-sleeping (Accessed 28th March 2022)

Sussman, R. and Gifford, R. (2019) 'Causality in the theory of planned behaviour', *Personality and Social Psychology Bulletin*, 45(6), pp. 920–933

Tanenbaum, M.L., Leventhal, H., Breland, J.Y., Yu, J., Walker, E.A. and Gonzalez, J.S. (2015) 'Successful self-management among non-insulin treated adults with type 2 diabetes: a self-regulation perspective', *Diabetic Medicine*, 32(11), pp. 1504–1512

Thaler, R. and Sunstein, C. (2008) *Nudge: improving decisions about health, wealth, and happiness*. Connecticut: Yale University Press

Thorndike, A.N., Sonnenberg, L., Rills, J., Barraclough, S. and Levy, D. (2012) 'A 2-phase labelling and choice architecture intervention to improve healthy food and beverage choices', *American Journal of Public Health*, 102(3), pp. 527–533

The King's Fund (2018) *A vision for population health. Towards a healthier future*. Available at: https://www.kingsfund.org.uk/publications/vision-population-health (Accessed 23rd February 2022)

Tong, K.K., Chen, J.H., Yu, E.W. and Wu, A.M.S. (2020) 'Adherence to COVID-19 precautionary measures: applying the health belief model and generalised social beliefs to a probability community sample', *Applied Psychology: Health and Well-Being*, 12(4), pp. 1205–1223

Weal, R. (lead author) (2020) *Knocked back: failing to support people sleeping rough with drug and alcohol problems is costing lives*. London: St. Mungo's Broadway. Available at: www.mungos.org/app/uploads/2020/01/StM_Knocked_Back_DA_Research_Report_Final_2901.pdf (Accessed 28th March 2022)

West, R. (2005) 'Putting the transtheoretical (stages of change) model to rest', *Addiction*, 100(8), pp. 1036–1039

Whicher, C.A., O'Neill, S. and Holt, R.I.G. (2020) 'Diabetes UK position statements. Diabetes in the UK: 2019', *Diabetic Medicine*, 37(2), pp. 242–247

6 Communicating health

Sally Robinson

Key points

- Introduction
- Health communication
- World Health Organization's Strategic Communications Framework
- Health communication theories
- Health literacy
- Summary

Introduction

This chapter will define health communication, its scope, purpose and characteristics. It will explore different types of communication including intrapersonal, interpersonal and mass communication. It will explain how the process of health communication affects the outcomes one can expect and includes evidence-based guidelines for best practice when communicating to promote health. This includes the approach used by the World Health Organization for its own health-related communications. The chapter includes some brief examples of theories and models which can inform health communication and ends with a discussion about the importance of health literacy to understanding, as well as creating, health communications.

Health communication

Communication helps all species to survive, to reproduce and to feel they belong. It is easy to see why communication is vital to people's health. Communication is cognitive, thinking; affective, feeling; and behavioural. Communication always takes place within a context of culture, history, time and other constraints and it is often a medium through which personal and social power is expressed. Health communication comprises,

> "... interpersonal or mass communication activities focused on improving the health of individuals and populations."
>
> (Ishikawa and Kiuchi, 2010, p. 1)

DOI: 10.4324/9780367823696-8

Health communication includes

- communication between health practitioners and individuals, groups or populations
- individuals searching for and using health or illness-related information
- dissemination of information about health risks and how to prevent them, e.g. campaigns
- influencing attitudes and behaviours towards a health issue
- demonstrating a health-related skill
- correcting misunderstandings or misleading information about a health issue
- cultural images of health or illness, e.g. in the media
- information about how to access private and public health services
- the process of expressing health-related experiences

When communicating to promote the health of others, we consider

- the communication process – how clearly and effectively health-related messages are transferred to, between and from individuals, groups, organisations or populations
- how well the individual, group, organisation or population can understand and can act upon the communication

The purpose of health communication

The aims of health communication are usually educational; to achieve some health-related learning which can include

- cognitive, e.g. to raise awareness, to gain knowledge or to clarify understanding
- affective, e.g. to raise self-awareness, self-esteem or confidence
- conative, e.g. to clarify motivations, encourage self-direction or make a decision
- psychomotor, e.g. to learn a skill, change behaviour or to maintain a behaviour

and it can have the goal to bring about personal, social or environmental change. This is discussed further in Chapters 7 and 8.

Clear content

Once we have decided what we are trying to achieve, we need to clarify the message. This will be informed by a good understanding of the audience's needs and their assets, discussed in Chapter 8. It is important to 'start from where they are'. The message may be,

- "I'm here to support you"
- "We are going to work together to achieve your/our goal"
- to impart information that needs to be clear, unambiguous, contain no contradictions and, where possible, be tested to gain feedback, e.g. "Am I making this clear? Would you like me to go over anything again?" "What do you think is the key message in this leaflet?" or "Who do you think is the audience for this type of website?"

Box 6.1 Assessing readability

Writing that is to be read by others needs to be readable. There are many tests that can objectively calculate how readable a text is. Many can be accessed online along with calculators. Here are two.

The Simple Measure of Gobbledygook (SMOG) Index

The SMOG index was developed in 1969 by the psychologist G. Harry McLaughlin.

- Take a piece of writing that is 30 sentences or longer
- Highlight 10sentences near the beginning, 10 in the middle and 10 towards the end of the text
- Within these 30 sentences, count every word which has three or more syllables
- Square root the number of these long words, and round it to the nearest 10
- Add three to this figure

The higher the score, the more difficult the piece of writing is to read.

The Flesch Reading Ease Score

Rudolf Flesch initially developed his readability formula to support newspapers, and it was later used in marketing and policy reports.

- Count 100 words of the text
- Count the number of sentences in the 100 words
- Divide the total number of words (100) by the number of sentences
- Multiply the answer by 1.015 (this is A)
- Count the number of syllables in the 100 words
- Divide the total number of syllables by the total number of words (100)
- Multiply the answer by 84.6 (this is B)
- Subtract A from 206.835 to give C

  $$206.835 - A = C$$

- Subtract B from C

  $$C - B = \text{the Flesch score}$$

A Flesch score between 60 and 70 should be reasonably easy for an average adult to read. Higher scores suggest it is very easy to read; lower scores suggest the text is difficult to read.

(Source: Readable, 2022)

Communication process

We need to take time to understand the audience and how the communication is best delivered. Barriers to a good communication process include the following.

The communication may fail to take account of

- cultural or religious barriers, e.g. different attitudes to contraception, different family values or different understandings about health and illness
- environmental barriers, e.g. cold, noise or discomfort

- power imbalances between the communicator and their audience
- needs associated with a disability or impairment, emotional distress, poor memory or lack of self-worth
- language barriers including the use of jargon
- previous negative experiences which may induce fear; a lack of trust in the communicator or the message; or avoidance because it is too painful to re-visit and/or beliefs that there is nothing new to learn

and the communicator may

- have poor communication skills due to a lack of confidence or training, e.g. being vague or a poor listener
- deliberately withhold communication as an act of paternalism or a reluctance to demystify their professional knowledge
- make assumptions that they have pitched their communication appropriately and are being understood, without checking
- fail to illicit trust due to their appearance or manner
- feel it is not a priority, or work in a culture that does not consider communication to be a priority when time is short

One-way or two-way communication

Thinking about the direction of communication, one-way or two-way, is vital because it reflects the practitioner's

- understandings of what health means and who defines it
- views about the purpose of health education, health promotion and public health

One-way means the communication flows in one direction. There is no opportunity to respond or clarify understanding, and it cannot be accurately tailored to individuals' needs. One-way communication includes a talk, a poster or a website that provides information. Scriven (2017) suggests one-way communication may suggest a practitioner

- is not interested in, or does not value, individuals' knowledge or experience
- does not feel they have anything to learn from their audience
- wants to discourage questions or being challenged
- does not want individuals to learn from each other

Two-way communication suggests

- a partnership where a practitioner and individuals are working together
- an interest in individuals' views and opinions about health
- both are learning from each other
- an intention to try to understand and 'start from where the individuals are'

One-way communication is associated with the preventive, medical/behaviour change, model of health promotion and the social change model of health promotion.

Two-way communication is associated with the educational and empowerment models of health promotion (see Chapters 7 and 8).

Aligned to these ideas, the practitioner needs to consider whether they are aiming to

- accept the individual and their health-related decisions
- judge the individual and their health-related decisions
- foster autonomy, e.g. encouraging individuals to make their own informed decisions
- foster dependence, e.g. discouraging individuals from making their own decisions because others know better than them

Types of health communication

There are many ways to categorise health communication. For example,

- intrapersonal communication is how we communicate within ourselves
- interpersonal communication is how we communicate with others
- mass communication concerns disseminating information from a single source to a large population through various media

Communication may be verbal, non-verbal or both.

Verbal communication

Verbal communication concerns language, that is: words, the meaning of words and the way their meanings are organised. It includes spoken words and written words. Speech is based on units of sound, takes place in real time and cannot be 'reviewed'. It is a conscious way of communicating, meaning that it is usually under voluntary control and we can be aware of what and how we speak (Berry, 2007). We promote health using speech in one-way communication such as a lecture, talk, or a radio, television or internet programme; and in two-way communication such as during one-to-one counselling, group work or a media event with audience participation. In two-way communication, we may use the skills of listening, summarising and paraphrasing to ensure we have properly understood what is said and to reflect that back to the speaker.

The written word is usually a more precise way of using language in terms of structure and grammar. Unlike speech, there is often a greater need for it to be clearly understood because there is less opportunity to clarify a meaning. Texts and some e-mails tend to be more spontaneous and less grammatically precise. Braille, developed for visually impaired people, is a way of reading by feeling patterns of raised dots on the page. Each pattern represents a word or number. We promote health through written one-way communications in the form of websites; leaflets; books; handouts; stories; posters; lists of contents/ingredients; directions for use; sell-by/use-by dates; learning materials; reports; research papers and through writing diaries to record symptoms and actions or as a means of personal catharsis and reflection (Box 6.2). Written two-way communications include a website with opportunities to ask questions and receive answers, or to engage in live written interactions.

Box 6.2 Writing to express the experience of cancer

"9th May

Cancer and jam, cancer and anger.
The anger keeps oozing out like pus, breaking out like a rash.
I'm angry if I drop something.
I'm angry because I keep losing my glasses.
I'm angry because the skin of my fingers is sore from chemotherapy.
I'm angry because my life's been interrupted.
I'm angry because I'm pushed on one side.
I'm angry because I can't do what I want to.
I'm angry because my body's been invaded by treatments.
I'm angry with the nurses, the specialist, everyone at the clinic even
though I know their intention is to help me.
I'm angry because the drugs make me feel queasy and weak-legged.
I'm angry because I'm unable to eat much at a time. I'm angry because I
can't do much at a time.
I'm angry because I'm afraid I'll never have a full life again.
I'm angry because I wake up four times every night.
I'm angry because the overpowering sickly sweet smell of the air-
freshener in the loo at the clinic makes me feel nauseated.
I'm angry because I'm missing out.
I'm angry because the treatment goes on over so many months.
I'm angry because I'm hot.
I'm angry because I'm cold.
I'm angry because I have to keep considering other people's anxieties.
I'm angry because some people's help is misplaced and unhelpful.
I'm angry because other awful things have happened.

Notes for 'Angry' poem
   What does it feel like, this anger? What does it smell of? What does it sound
like? It is bubbling in my body like a mob of prisoners. I want to throw it out,
slap it like the sea on the shore. I shall shove it out like a bin of rubbish. I want
to hit it into faces, wave it from steeples, dangle it in red flags from the thousand
windows of a great glass building. Crash! I'll crash it against walls kick it along
pavements, throw out its slops. I am going to make a great scene about it, a
drama that will shock audiences into silence, scribble it in furious red across the
clean page of the sky, smash bottlefuls of it on the pavement by Warren Street
tube station …
   … Writing all this has been a breakthrough. It feels as if – well I am – taking
energetic action with my anger and it's incredibly releasing, exciting, fun!"

(Source: Schneider, 2003, pp. 85–86)

Non-verbal communication

Non-verbal communication comprises that which does not rely exclusively on words. Examples include British Sign Language (BSL), images, facial expressions, eye contact, the sound and tone of the voice, gestures, appearance/clothes, symbols, touch and body movement. It also includes the context in which communication takes place such as the physical and social environment, the space between people who are communicating, how they take turns and whether one interrupts or dominates the other. In the context of promoting health, we use the voice, the body, images and the environment to convey messages. Often, the non-verbal cues communicate emotions of encouragement, acceptance, disapproval, urgency, concern or control. For example, when promoting health, we might use a strong image which will communicate danger; we may ensure we sit at the same level as an individual to suggest equality; we may use gestures to emphasise a point and we may use observation to pick up on important non-verbal cues from a communicator.

Both verbal and non-verbal communication

Most communications use both verbal and non-verbal communications together. One may complement or reinforce the other or, if they contradict, the communication might invite scepticism or distrust.

Thinking point:

> Consider what message is being conveyed when
>
> - we invite someone into a private room for a chat and then sit on a high stool while inviting an individual to sit in a very low chair
> - we look out of the window while listening to a recently bereaved individual
> - a poster instructs handwashing and the basins are unclean
> - a notice at the entrance to a leisure centre shows two people standing at a two-metre distance with the caption 'keep your distance', while six members of staff huddle together in a group
> - a campaign claims to be aimed at everyone and all the images are able-bodied

Advice about communication in the context of therapeutic, person-centred communication is shown in Table 6.1.

Communicating with people

One-to-one

One-to-one communication allows communication to be tailor-made for the individual. If this is to be a non-therapeutic, educational, two-way communication, it would ideally include

- establishing trust and a rapport
- demonstrating that the person is unique with their own needs, assets and personality (person-centred)
- asking open questions

Table 6.1 Verbal and non-verbal communication in therapeutic, person-centred, one-to-one communication

	Do	*Don't*
Attributes	Be congruent/genuine. Be accepting, open and convey warmth. Be empathic and try to develop a deep, holistic understanding.	Present a façade, pretend or be closed. Be judgemental, uncaring or cold. Assume an understanding of the individual's frame of reference.
Non-verbal body language	Sit squarely in front of the individual to give them your full attention. Be open in your posture, avoid rigidly crossing your arms and legs. Lean slightly towards the individual. Establish eye contact, but don't stare. Adopt a natural, relaxed posture. Be calm and still.	Use excessive gestures. Make physical contact as this is not an essential part of communication, though the touch of a practitioner in a care setting may be perceived as appropriate and helpful. Be aware of cultural norms e.g. in some cultures, eye contact can be perceived as aggressive.
Listening	Tune in to where the individual is emotionally as well as listening to what they say.	Be thinking about a response instead of listening. Be judgemental because it interferes with listening. Be solving the problem instead of listening.
Verbal	Greet and ask an open question. Paraphrase. Summarise. Reflect. Ask open questions. Ask probing questions e.g. encourage the individual to elaborate or explain what happened next. Ask focusing questions e.g. ask for more detail or focus down on an issue.	Interrupt. Seek out the facts at the expense of hearing the whole of what the individual wants to say. Ask multiple questions in one sentence. Ask leading questions to direct the individual in a particular direction. Ask rhetorical questions, which have no answer.

Source: Hough (2021).

- using active listening skills such as reflection, summary and paraphrasing
- building the individual's confidence
- confidentiality
- providing the necessary information
- helping the individual to make decisions, e.g. agreeing the pros and cons
- helping the individual to make realistic, achievable goals

(Hubley and Copeman, 2008, p. 118)

Motivational interviewing is based on the work of Carl Rogers, person-centredness and the empowerment model of health education/health promotion (see Chapters 1 and 7). Motivational interviewing is a one-to-one communication based on the concept that individuals have within them the resources to change (Miller and Rollnick, 2013). It aims to increase an individual's own confidence and capacities. The process includes building a trusting relationship of two equals, negotiating the focus for their discussions, exploring the individual's thoughts and motivations (e.g. "Why would you want to make this change?" and, "What are the three best reasons for you to do it?"), and then jointly planning how to change when the individual is ready. During the interviews, the communicator/counsellor/educator/health practitioner uses open questions; affirms the individual's strengths and their effort; summarises and reflects back what they hear from the individual to confirm it has been correctly understood and to demonstrate empathy; and takes note of the individual's language such as when they change subject.

Group work

Group work may include

- group meetings, for problem solving or completing a task, e.g. raising awareness of housing standards in the community, fundraising for a hospice or making a plan for supporting local rough sleepers or for a vulnerable individual
- self-help or self-care groups, where participants help one another to understand and cope with a common health concern, e.g. drug dependency or parenting. These include groups of people living with long-term conditions who are trying to help themselves to become more independent. Sometimes they have an agreed common aim, such as abstinence or independence, and sometimes they do not
- a group that comes together for the purpose of formal or informal learning, e.g. to attain a qualification or to learn about nutrition and develop cooking skills
- a group that meets for social or spiritual exchange and to foster relationships

A group may or may not have a leader. Different groups of people may prefer different communication styles from their leader at different points. How the leader communicates influences the participants.

- An authoritarian leader is directive. They hold the power; it resides in their status, qualifications and expertise. Participants may feel secure following their advice, especially in an emergency; but it encourages dependence, does little to encourage them to question, to take responsibility for their own health or to build up their own abilities
- A participative leader shares the power between themselves and the participants who each have knowledge and skills to contribute. The leader acts as a facilitator, encouraging participation, providing encouragement and demonstrating tolerance and impartiality. To do this well, skills of problemsolving and conflict resolution are sometimes needed. Participants learn to trust their own judgements and appreciate the contributions of others. However, the style might not suit those who prefer to be directed by an 'expert', and find the lack of this stressful
- A permissive leader is one who seeks to give power to others. They allow participants to arrive at their own conclusions in their own way. Keeping everyone happy, helping them to enjoy the experience and avoiding conflict is the aim. While some participants may feel nurtured, others may feel insecure with no clear direction, and problems may not be addressed

(Scriven, 2017)

Some groups may come together to discuss personal or sensitive health issues. The setting, meaning the location, privacy and how chairs are positioned, needs careful thought.

To operate within a safe psychological space, it is recommended the group agree their ground rules at the start. These might include:

- what is to be kept confidential to the group
- start on time
- the importance of listening
- no interrupting
- turn taking
- being respectful and sensitive towards others

Groups whose explicit aim is to support health-related learning may adopt participatory/ active learning methods. In contrast to sitting, listening, reading and looking; active learning encourages participants to develop their own communication skills and often their confidence. In addition to learning about the content of a health issue, they are developing the communication skills needed to support their own health and others. These include the skills of listening, clarifying their own values, making health-related decisions, asking for what they need, discussing health issues with others and being able to empathise with the health decisions others make. Active learning includes

- ice breakers, which are often used at the start of a group or even every session. They are simple, fun games that enable participants to get to know one another and create a relaxed atmosphere
- group discussions/buzz groups, which start by giving a group a trigger/theme/issue to discuss, e.g. an ethical dilemma
- problem-solving groups, where a group is given a problem to discuss or a decision to make
- using a case study, an in-depth account of a situation or event which can be discussed
- role plays are excellent for developing empathy for individuals and their situations
- using a trigger video/film as a prompt for discussing a situation or an issue; participants can speak about characters rather than themselves

Mass communication

Mass communication refers to how we disseminate information to 'reach the masses'. Mass media is the medium through which we do this. Mass media includes:

- print media, e.g. books, academic journals, newspapers, magazines and flyers
- broadcast media, e.g. television, radio and films
- outdoor media, e.g. posters, banners, billboards, signs and posters on buses and trains
- digital media, e.g. websites, social media, the metaverse, mobile apps, e-books, podcasts, video platforms and online radio

It used to be thought that mass media would have a direct effect on a population either by acting like an aerosol, spraying information out to many individuals, or a hypodermic syringe where messages could be injected into a population who may, or may not, act on them. In the context of health, much effort went into trying to make media messages more persuasive, but research confirmed that raising awareness and providing knowledge, especially when only one-way communication is used, have little impact

Box 6.3 Mass communication and COVID-19 coronavirus in the UK

Mass communication was used in the UK during 2020 and 2021 during the COVID-19 coronavirus pandemic. The UK and devolved governments, along with public health organisations, used mass communications to raise awareness about: the virus and its spread; infection and death rates; symptoms of the virus, recommended and legislated preventative measures such as 'lock downs', testing and self-isolation; and vaccination development and its rollout. At the same time, many others were adding to the mass communication about the virus. In September 2021, the Office of Communications (Ofcom) carried out a survey with 2,000 people across the UK. It found:

- 73% had accessed news about the virus at least once a day
- 82% gained information from traditional media
- of those that used social media, 79% had seen pop-ups, banners or notices about the virus from official sources such as the Government
- two-thirds of people shared news and information about the virus. This was by talking with friends, family and colleagues (55%), closed messenger groups such as WhatsApp and Zoom (11%), posts on social media (7%) and video calls or other messenger groups (7%)

False or misleading information

- A quarter (24%) had seen what they considered to be false or misleading information. A third of these were under 35 years old
- The most common false/misleading claims were that face coverings offered no protection (22%), the flu was causing more deaths than the virus (19%), the number of deaths from the virus was lower than was reported (17%), the vaccine was a plan to implant trackable microchips in people (15%), the vaccine might reduce fertility (15%) and the virus did not exist or it had been genetically engineered (15%)
- Of those who saw the false/misleading claims, 27% said it had made them think twice about the issue
- 60% of respondents were concerned about the amount of misinformation around
- Those under 35 years old were more likely to report that their friends and families tended to believe the misinformation
- 80% thought that 'untrue' stories should not be posted or shared on social media, while 21% thought it was acceptable provided they were flagged as 'potentially untrustworthy'
- 58% of social media users reported seeing warnings that information might be untrustworthy in the last month

(Source: Ofcom, 2021)

Box 6.4 UK COVID-19 coronavirus media campaign

In February 2022, the England COVID-19 media campaign resources included posters, digital screens, social media (Twitter, Facebook, Instagram and LinkedIn), e-mail signatures, radio resources, web banners, leaflets, artwork, television adverts, and alternative formats and toolkits of resources for hospitals and other employers. There were six groups of resources, and many were presented in several languages.

- COVID-19 Response, e.g. "Wear a face covering in crowded and enclosed settings where you come into contact with people you do not normally meet" and "Here's how fresh air helps stop the spread of COVID-19"
- COVID-19 Vaccine, e.g. "We've been boosted. Join us. Let's get protected"
- Community Testing, e.g. "Keep telling us your test results and help beat COVID-19"
- Pharmacy Collect: notices for pharmacies to indicate whether they had COVID-19 lateral flow tests in stock
- NHS Resources, e.g. useful notices/posters for use in NHS settings
- Antivirals Recruitment, e.g. seeking people to volunteer for a clinical drugs trial for COVID-19

(Source: Public Health England, 2022)

---

on people's health-related behaviour (e.g. Kelly and Barker, 2016). For example, Stead and colleagues (2019) defined a mass media campaign as,

> "The intentional use of any media channel(s) of communication by local, regional and national organisations to influence lifestyle behaviour through largely passive or incidental exposure to media [as opposed to active health seeking]."
>
> (Stead *et al.*, 2019, p. 89)

They carried out a detailed examination of 36 systematic reviews of multiple pieces of international research into mass media campaigns aimed at changing health-related behaviour between 2000 and 2016. This included 3,893 records. They concluded the evidence was very mixed. There was

- no published review of any research into those mass media campaigns focused only on diet or alcohol
- low/weak evidence that mass media campaigns about more than one health-related behaviour had a positive impact on diet
- moderate evidence that mass media campaigns had contributed to a reduction in sedentary behaviour and improved sexual health
- mixed evidence about the impact of mass media campaigns which aimed to increase physical activity or reduce tobacco use. This included some low/weak evidence of a positive impact
- no evidence that mass media campaigns had affected illicit drug use

Mass media can promote awareness and debate about a health issue. It can influence social norms and give credibility to a message, but, without additional interpersonal communication such as further opportunities for reflection and deeper learning, it has very limited impact on people's feelings, beliefs and sustained attitudes. It cannot develop the skills which are a vital prerequisite to changing health-related behaviour. Mass media is best used for

- disseminating health-related information to large numbers of people, and if necessary, quickly
- influencing social and cultural norms which may make an aspect of health more acceptable
- contributing to a focussed health-related campaign
- countering marketing and advertising related to 'unhealthy' products and activities
- advocating for changes in policy

(Green *et al.*, 2019)

To maximise the health impact of using mass media to promote health we need to

- ensure the information presented is relevant, new and placed in an appropriate context
- be clear that its aim is to raise awareness of a health issue or to reinforce information about support for healthy behaviours, e.g. the message that quitting smoking can be made easier with the help of a local smoking cessation service
- use it as part of a wider overall health promotion strategy which addresses related social and environmental factors, and opportunities for learning and face-to-face communication

(Scriven, 2017)

Digital communication

Digital communication means using electronic or online communication to promote health. Unlike most mass media, one of its strengths is its ability to incorporate two-way communication. It can include

- health information alongside 'contact us' buttons, chat lines and online help-lines
- learning about health and/or developing health-related skills through games, films or interactive websites and apps
- accessing or using the arts to improve health, e.g. listening to calming music or creating digital art to communicate a message
- communication between people with common health concerns
- immersive environments in the metaverse which are set up to facilitate health-related communication or to simulate how a population may respond to an epidemic

Digital communication is helping to facilitate patient education within healthcare, particularly in countries with very limited healthcare and vast rural areas. In the UK National Health Service (NHS) digital communication enables communication between healthcare and social care practitioners and individuals. For the public, it includes

- the NHS 111 online service
- booking appointments with General Practices
- e-referral service appointments with medical specialists
- patient portals that give individuals access to their medical records including test results, correspondence and notes

- online/video medical consultations
- NHS facing information via nhs.uk and the NHS App
- an electronic prescribing service

Within the nhs.uk website and App are:

- Health A to Z, which provides succinct information on common health problems
- Medicines A to Z for information about medicines and side effects
- Live well, which provides health education about mental wellbeing, weight, exercise, sleep, alcohol, smoking and sexual health
- Mental health, which provides health education about mental health disorders, mental distress, self-help advice, where to find advice for stressful life situations including being a carer, information about types of therapies and treatments, how to access mental health services and information about dementia, insomnia, substance dependency and autism. It also includes the Every Mind Matters pages which provide information about how to look after mental health and how to deal with common concerns. It includes the opportunity to self-assess one's mental health and suggests appropriate actions
- Social care and support, a guide for those needing social care and carers
- Pregnancy-related education
- Information about the NHS and related healthcare services, such as pharmacies

Social marketing

Social marketing means using the approaches of commercial advertising for social objectives. The aim is to encourage social, environmental or economic change. It often concerns selling behaviours, as opposed to selling products. It often uses 'nudging'.

> "Nudging is defined as changing the presentation of choice options in a way that makes the desired choice – in our case the healthier option – the easy, automatic and default option, without forbidding any options."
>
> (Velema *et al.*, 2017, p. 2)

Social marketing focuses on people as consumers. It 'segments' the population according to features such as age, gender, ethnicity and particular needs. It utilises exchange theory, which means considering the costs to the individual of choosing the healthy option. Costs can include money, time, effort and so forth. The aim of social marketing is to make the costs worth paying. It fits within the social change model of health promotion which is about making healthier choices easier choices (see Chapter 8). For example, to promote healthy eating in a canteen, Velema and colleagues (2017) considered:

- product – what is being promoted and how to present it so that it is attractive to the consumer, e.g. offering ready-to-eat fruit and vegetables, providing water and increasing the proportion of 'healthier' items offered
- price – these are the costs in time, convenience, money or effort, e.g. making the price of a healthier meal slightly cheaper than a less healthy alternative
- promotion – using a range of communication methods to sell the product, including mass media, e.g. positioning promotions for 'healthier' options in a recognisable

permanent spot in the canteen, listing the healthier options first on the menu and using short campaigns to promote healthier options

- place – choose the setting where the product is to be promoted including how to make it accessible, convenient and close to other products or services related to the product, e.g. placing healthier options at the beginning of the route and putting fruit and vegetables at eye level

Communicating is central to promoting health. We need to select the most appropriate communication methods to meet the aim. Communication methods are often informed by the broader health promotion model within which we are working.

World Health Organization's Strategic Communications Framework

The World Health Organization (WHO) (2017) believes effective communication is central to reducing health inequalities and enabling individuals to take control over and make decisions about their own health. It has published its own *Strategic Communications Framework* to support its aim,

"To provide information, advice, and guidance to decision-makers (key audiences) to prompt action that will protect the health of individuals, families, communities and nations."

(WHO, 2017, p. 2)

The WHO communicates with anyone concerned with health including individuals, policy-makers, health practitioners, communities, international organizations and their own staff. The WHO's own communications include

- its own internal communications
- building the communication skills of its workforce
- brand and corporate identity communications such as explaining what the WHO does
- developing its own communications strategy to ensure its work reaches a global audience
- audio visual services, such as creating images and timelines to complement and better communicate text to their audience
- emergency communications, e.g. ensuring people have the correct information to best protect their health and safety
- leading on world campaigns, e.g. World Malaria Day and World AIDS Day
- communicating in many languages
- engaging with digital and traditional news-related mass media
- working with social media, e.g. Twitter, Facebook, Google, YouTube, Instagram etc.
- the WHO website

It has developed six principles which lie at the core of all its communication activities. Communications must be

- accessible – they must use the most appropriate communication channels including mass media, those within communities and organisations, and interpersonal communications such as one-to-one conversations. They should consider how audiences approach the information and make it logical and accessible for all

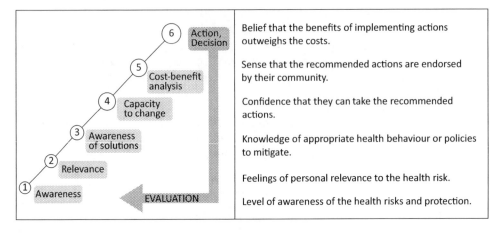

Figure 6.1 The communications continuum: moving audiences towards health action

Source: World Health Organization, 2017, p. 10. Reproduced with permission from the World Health Organization

- actionable – communications must meet the needs and characteristics of the target audience. They begin by raising awareness about a health issue; explaining the risks are real; providing knowledge, answering questions and providing solutions; instilling confidence, capacity to change and self-empowerment including the teaching of skills; encouraging the healthy action to become the social norm to increase its acceptability; addressing barriers, emphasising benefits and providing encouragement for the healthy steps to be taken; and finally the communications are evaluated
- credible and trusted – communications must be accurate and consistent; open and honest including online questions and answers; be dependable and demonstrate commitment and care
- relevant – they must be relevant to the audience; be responsive to the audience and tailored to them; based on listening to many stakeholders and using many channels; and then the messages need to be tailored in ways to build confidence and motivate this audience
- timely – information and guidance need to be timed so audiences have what they need, when they need it
- understandable – information needs to be tailored to its audience; some may have more technical knowledge than others. It needs to use clear, plain, familiar language and include real stories and visual images. Where needed, it should capture the attention of the public or journalists

The sequence of communication steps that aim to move populations towards health-related action are illustrated in the WHO's communications continuum (Figure 6.1).

The World Health Organization aims to model effective health-related communication to the world.

Health communication theories

Very many theories contribute to understanding health-related communication. Here we summarise three theories of behaviour change, two communication theories and the concept of self-efficacy.

Theories of behaviour change

Psychological theories, or models, can help us to understand and predict whether an individual is likely to adopt a health-related behaviour. They illuminate the factors which influence people's decision making, and therefore can provide guidance about the most pertinent type of health communication. These are discussed more fully in Chapter 5, but here we provide three illustrative examples.

Health belief model

Becker's health belief model (Becker, 1974) helps to explain how individuals weigh up their beliefs about their risks of contracting disease and its severity against their beliefs about adopting a health-related behaviour such as having a vaccination or attending for screening. They weigh up the costs and benefits. Listening to their beliefs can provide guidance about any factual misinformation which could be corrected and any fears that require empathic communication. The communication could be tailored to help them to make their own decision.

Theory of planned behaviour

The theory of planned behaviour (Ajzen, 1991) suggests people's intentions to perform a behaviour can be predicted from their attitudes towards the behaviour, their perceptions of what is 'the norm' and their perceptions about how easy or difficult it would be to perform the behaviour. Health communication can be tailored to influence these perceptions. For example, it could explore a person's strengths, past experiences or abilities; check how much their understanding of the health issue is based on the best evidence to date and it may include discussing how they assess what is 'normal' for other people.

Transtheoretical model

The transtheoretical model, or 'stages of change', can be used to assess where an individual thinks they are along a process of changing health-related behaviour, from giving it no thought (precontemplation), to thinking about it (contemplation), to making a decision and being ready to change (commitment), to action, to maintenance and possible relapse (Prochaska *et al.*, 1992). Through communication, we can identify where an individual is in the process and we can tailor the aims of the communication appropriately to move the individual along to the next stage towards their goal. At

- precontemplation – we need to communicate to raise awareness of a health issue or behaviour; this includes the personal health risks of no change and the benefits of making a change
- contemplation – we need to self-empower someone with the knowledge they need to make a change; enable them to develop the necessary skills; raise their confidence

and help them with the process of making their own decision. This includes exploring potential personal, social/financial and environmental barriers to making a change and considering who, such as friends or family, can provide support

- preparation – we communicate to enable them to put their decision into a realistic plan of action that will fit in with their lives. We help them to believe they can do it (self-efficacy) and identify rewards
- action – we communicate to encourage and motivate the start of the new health-related behaviour
- maintenance – we communicate to sustain motivation, the 'new norm', identify health benefits and possibly set further goals
- relapse – we use communication to help individuals to reflect and learn from the experience, and consider the next step

(Scriven, 2017)

Communication models and theories

Communication theories are concerned with how people process communication and they can provide guidance about how to manipulate communication towards different outcomes (Zhao, 2020).

Elaboration likelihood model

The elaboration likelihood model (Petty and Cacioppo, 1986) suggests people can be persuaded via one of two processes, the one that is selected depends on how much a person thinks about, 'elaborates' on, the issues raised. The two processes are

- there may be a great deal of thinking about a health-related message and this will inform the decision that is made, e.g. after having a one-to-one discussion with a healthcare practitioner about preventing a serious health problem
- there may be very little thinking and a decision is made according to relatively peripheral factors such as who is providing the health message or how attractively it is presented, e.g. a Public Health Wales mass media campaign with a very simple message might be quickly trusted compared to a commercial advert

Which process is followed depends on many factors such as the individual's own motivation, their personal involvement with the health issue and how much time and energy a person has to devote to considering the health issue. Berry (2007) notes that there is no reason why health communication cannot target both processes by being well-argued, credible and attractively presented.

Heuristic-systematic model

The heuristic-systematic model of information processing (Boohner *et al.*, 1995) also suggests people process information in two ways which they call systematic and heuristic.

- Systematic processing is where people are motivated to put effort into reading, examining, searching and comparing information in order to make a judgement
- Heuristic processing is more superficial. It is where people use 'short cuts' to make a judgement such as putting faith in the author, the journal, the number of references, or the established credibility of a broadcaster or brand

An individual who uses systematic processing may also use heuristic processing, but one who uses heuristic processing will not be using systematic processing. Individuals will be influenced by what motivates them for example caring about accuracy and evidence; the need to defend a conclusion which matches their own self-concept; or the desire to maintain existing beliefs, attitudes and actions, or an existing self-image, because it suits the individual's social situation.

Thinking point:

> In the context of a health communication about cannabis, how might these five people process the information from a media campaign, led by the Royal College of Psychiatrists, suggesting cannabis may be harmful to health.
>
> - A director of public health
> - An individual who uses cannabis regularly for muscle spasms
> - An individual who regularly smokes cannabis with their friends
> - A medical student
> - An individual whose partner is leading the campaign

Self-efficacy

Self-efficacy (Bandura, 1977) concerns how an individual appraises their ability to carry out an action, for example a healthier behaviour. They may believe it to be worthwhile, but their thoughts and feelings are assessing whether they have enough knowledge and the right skills to be successful. If they assess that they have a good chance of being successful, they may attempt to make the change; if they do not, they may avoid it or refuse to try. Communication/education aimed at enabling an individual to realistically appraise their capabilities includes examining their emotions about the health issue and proposed new behaviour, for example their anxieties; discussing the wider influences on their thinking such as what they think others do and think, and their previous experience of attempting a health-related change. With this understanding, we can 'start from where they are'. The aim may be to

- increase their knowledge and provide support to develop their personal skills, e.g. assertiveness or problem-solving skills
- influence their beliefs, e.g. challenge misinformation
- develop their knowledge and skills to address and remove the social and environmental barriers to making healthier changes

(Green *et al.*, 2019)

There are many psychological theories which can inform how we approach communication in the context of promoting health.

Health literacy

We may summarise health literacy as the ability to understand, evaluate and act on health-related information. It supports decision-making and the ability to express personal and social health needs. Health literacy is not the sole responsibility of individuals, but of all those who provide information such as the media, governments and public services. One definition of health literacy is,

> "Health literacy represents the personal knowledge and competencies that accumulate through daily activities, social interactions and across generations. Personal knowledge and competencies are mediated by the organizational structures and availability of resources that enable people to access, understand, appraise and use information and services in ways that promote and maintain good health and well-being for themselves and those around them."
>
> (WHO, 2021, p. 6. Reproduced with permission from the World Health Organization)

In the UK, it is thought between 15 and 21 million people might not have sufficient health literacy skills to lead a healthy life. In England, among 16 to 65 year olds, about

- 42% cannot understand and make use of health-related information
- 61% cannot understand numerical health information
- 43% struggle to understand the childhood dose of paracetamol

(PHE/UCL IHE, 2015)

In 2018, 2,309 people across Great Britain participated in a survey about health literacy (Simpson *et al.*, 2020). Face-to-face interviews, based on a questionnaire, were completed. The researchers found

- 19.4% had some difficulties with reading and understanding written health information
- 23.2% reported problems discussing health concerns with healthcare providers
- those who struggled most were more likely to be living in socio-economically deprived circumstances, have a long-term disability or chronic illness and/or have no educational qualifications

Within healthcare, concerns about health literacy relate to patients being unable to follow instructions which can exacerbate health problems and waste limited healthcare finances (Palumbo, 2017; Protheroe *et al.*, 2009). Poor health literacy has also been linked to

- poor health-related behaviours, e.g. poor diet, little physical activity and smoking
- greater use of emergency services
- poor management of long-term health conditions
- increased illness and premature death

(PHE/UCL IHE, 2015)

Health literacy is an outcome of health education. The skills of health literacy are both cognitive and social. They include the general literacy skills of reading, writing, listening, numeracy and speaking which are used to develop an understanding of health-related communication; to appraise and synthesise it; to apply it and to communicate it to others (Liu *et al.*, 2020). It also includes understanding non-verbal and visual information as well as having access to and using digital resources. Health literacy contributes to empowerment, discussed in Chapter 7, because having the tools of health literacy enables people to better understand their health, to communicate their health needs, to question health-related advice, to give them a sense of control over their health and to develop their health potential. In this way, health literacy makes an important contribution to reducing health inequalities (PHE/UCL IHE, 2015; WHO, 2021).

Accessible Information Standard

In the UK, all organisations that provide healthcare or social care are legally required to follow the Accessible Information Standard which sets out,

> "… a specific, consistent approach to identifying, recording, flagging, sharing and meeting the information and communication support needs of patients, service users, carers and parents with a disability, impairment or sensory loss."
>
> (nhs.uk, 2022)

The organisation must:

- ask people if they have any communication or information needs, and find out how to meet their needs
- record these needs clearly, using a set format
- insert a flag on the individual's notes/file to show the individual has communication needs and how to meet them
- with the individual's permission, share the individual's communication needs with other providers of healthcare and social care
- act to ensure individuals will receive information in a way that they can understand it, including providing communication support if needed

(nhs.uk, 2022)

Within the National Health Service (NHS), an online e-learning resource called the Health Literacy Toolkit has been developed to provide practitioners with the knowledge, understanding and skills to support individuals to participate in person-centred care and to navigate the healthcare and social care systems (HEE, 2022). The NHS has trained those working in the NHS library and knowledge services, such as librarians, to cascade the knowledge and skills to others. Examples include:

- Leeds Libraries for Health held an Away Day in 2019 to improve the health and wellbeing of the citizens of Leeds, including strengthening links between NHS and public libraries. It included sessions about the impact of health literacy on health, how to develop the public's digital and health literacy skills and how healthcare staff and NHS librarians could work together
- an NHS librarian ran a session about 'jargon busting' for junior doctors in 2019. It included a 'Dr Jargon' game where doctors had to describe a health term without using jargon and 'Crack a code' which helped the doctors to empathise with how it feels to not understand information. The doctors learnt to avoid assuming patients understand, to check understanding with their patients, to tailor information to each individual and to reduce their jargon

(Naughton *et al.*, 2021)

Mental capacity

One impediment to health literacy may be mental capacity. The UK Mental Capacity Act (2005) seeks to protect all people over 16 years old to make their own decisions wherever possible (Legislation.gov.UK, 2005). It states that clear, concise information must be provided to the individual. All parties involved need to feel confident that the individual is competent to make the decision. This means assuming an individual *does* have the capacity and then checking they are able to

- understand the information relevant to a decision
- retain the information
- use, or weigh up, that information as part of the process of making the decision
- communicate the decision

Wherever possible, an individual should be supported to make their own decisions. The charity Mencap, which champions people with learning disabilities, suggests we should

- provide all the relevant information, including information about any alternatives
- communicate in an appropriate way, e.g. using simple language, visual images, non-verbal communication and inviting others such as a family member, advocate or speech and language therapist to help
- put the individual at ease, e.g. consider where and when are best for the individual to take in the information
- support the individual and consider who else might be able to provide support or express a view

If it is concluded an individual does not have the mental capacity to make *this* decision, decisions must always be made in the individual's best interests.

(Mencap, 2022)

Health literacy is an important asset when making informed health-related decisions. We can support people's health literacy through education, and we can ensure all health communication meets the needs of those who may have low health literacy.

Summary

This chapter has

- defined the aims, scope, purpose and characteristics of health communication
- explored different types of health-related communication and how the process of communication influences outcomes
- provided guidelines for best practice in health communication
- described how the World Health Organization aims to communicate with the world
- outlined examples of health communication theories and models
- described the importance of health literacy to understanding and creating health communications

Further reading

Green, J., Cross, R., Woodall, J. and Tones, K. (2019) *Health promotion: planning and strategies.* 4th edn. London: Sage

Scriven, A. (2017) *Promoting health. A practical guide.* 7th edn. London: Elsevier

Useful websites

Communications. Available at: https://www.publichealth.hscni.net/directorate-operations/communication-and-knowledge-management/communications

Health communication and public health messaging. Available at: https://www.nihr.ac.uk/documents/health-communication-and-public-health-messaging-commissioning-brief/30239

Health literacy UK. Available at: https://www.healthliteracy.org.uk

References

Ajzen, I. (1991) 'The theory of planned behaviour', *Organizational Behavior and Human Decision Processes,* 50(2), pp. 179–211

Bandura, A. (1977) 'Self-efficacy toward a unifying theory of behavioural change', *Psychological Review,* 64(2), pp. 191–225

Becker, M.H. (1974) 'The health belief model and sick role behavior', *Health Education Monographs,* 2(4), pp. 409–419

Berry, D. (2007) *Health communication. Theory and practice.* Maidenhead: McGraw-Hill

Bohner, G., Moskowitz, G.B. and Chaiken, S. (1995) 'The interplay of heuristic and systematic processing of social information', *European Review of Social Psychology,* 6(1), pp. 34–68

Green, J., Cross, R., Woodall, J. and Tones, K. (2019) *Health promotion. Planning and strategies.* 4th edn. London: Sage

Health Education England (2022) *Educating and training the workforce.* Accessible at: https://www.hee.nhs.uk/our-work/population-health/training-educational-resources (Accessed 28th February 2022)

Hough, M. (2021) *Counselling skills and theory.* 5th edn. London: Hodder Education

Hubley, J. and Copeman, J. (2008) *Practical health promotion.* Cambridge: Polity Press

Ishikawa, H. and Kiuchi, T. (2010) 'Health literacy and health communication', *BioPsychoSocial Medicine,* 4(1) doi:10.1186/1751-0759-4-18

Kelly, M.P. and Barker, M. (2016) 'Why is changing health-related behaviour so difficult?', *Public Health,* 136, pp. 109–116

Legislation.gov.UK (2005) *Mental capacity act 2005.* Available at: www.legislation.gov.uk/ukpga/2005/9/contents (Accessed 24th February 2022)

Liu, C., Wang, D., Liu, C., Jiang, J., Wang, X., Chen, H., Ju, X. and Zhang, X. (2020) 'What is the meaning of health literacy? A systematic review and qualitative synthesis', *Family Medicine and Community Health,* 8 doi:10.1136/fmch-2020-000351

Mencap (2022) *The mental capacity act.* Available at: https://www.mencap.org.uk/advice-and-support/mental-capacity-act (Accessed 24th February 2022)

Miller, W.R. and Rollnick, S. (2013) *Motivational interviewing: helping people to change.* 3rd edn. New York: Guildford Press

Naughton, J., Booth, J., Elliott, P., Evans, M., Simões, M. and Wilson, S. (2021) 'Health literacy: the role of NHS library and knowledge services', *Health Information and Libraries Journal,* 38(2), pp. 150–154

nhs.uk (2022) *Accessible information standard.* Available at: https://www.england.nhs.uk/ourwork/accessibleinfo (Accessed 28th February 2022)

Office of Communications (Ofcom) (2021) *Covid-19 news and information: consumption and attitudes.* Available at: https://www.ofcom.org.uk/research-and-data/tv-radio-and-on-demand/news-media/coronavirus-news-consumption-attitudes-behaviour (Accessed 23rd February 2022)

Palumbo, R. (2017) 'Examining the impacts of health literacy on healthcare costs. An evidence synthesis', *Health Services Management Research*, 30(4) doi:10.1177/0951484817733366

Petty, R.E. and Cacioppo, J.T. (1986) *Communication and persuasion: central and peripheral routes to attitude change*. New York: Springer

Prochaska, J.O., DiClemente, C.C. and Norcross, J.C. (1992) 'In search of how people change: applications to addictive behaviours', *American Psychologist*, 47(9), pp. 1102–1114

Protheroe, J., Nutbeam, D. and Rowlands, G. (2009) 'Health literacy: a necessity for increasing participation in health care', *British Journal of General Practice*, 59(567), pp. 721–723

Public Health England (2022) *Coronavirus (COVID-19) Resource Centre*. Available at: https:// campaignresources.phe.gov.uk/resources/campaigns (Accessed 26th February 2022)

Public Health England/UCL Institute of Health Equity (2015) *Local action on health inequalities. Improving health literacy to reduce health inequalities*. Available at: https://assets.publishing. service.gov.uk/government/uploads/system/uploads/attachment_data/file/460710/4b_Health_ Literacy-Briefing.pdf (Accessed 28th February 2022

Readable (2022) *About readability*. Available at: https://readable.com/readability/smog-index (Accessed 24th February 2022)

Schneider, M. (2003) *Writing my way through cancer*. London: Jessica Kingsley

Scriven, A. (2017) *Promoting health. A practical guide*. 7th edn. London: Elsevier

Simpson, R.M., Knowles, E. and O'Cathain, A. (2020) 'Health literacy levels of British adults: a cross-sectional survey using two domains of the Health Literacy Questionnaire (HLQ)', *BMC Public Health*, 20 doi:10.1186/s12889-020-09727-w

Stead, M., Angus, K., Langley, T., Katikireddi, S.V., Hilton, S., Lewis, S., Thomas, J., Campbell, M., Young, B. and Bauld, L. (2019) 'Mass media to communicate public health messages in six health topic areas: a systematic review and other reviews of evidence', *Public Health Research*, 7(8) doi:10.3310/phr07080

Velema, E., Vyth, E.L. and Steenhuis, H.M. (2017) 'Using nudging and social marketing techniques to create healthy worksite cafeterias in the Netherlands: intervention development and study design', *BMC Public Health*, 17(63) doi:10.1186/s12889-016-3927-7

World Health Organization (2017) *WHO strategic communications framework for effective communications*. Available at: www.who.int/mediacentre/communication-framework.pdf (Accessed 23rd February 2022)

World Health Organization (2021) *Health promotion glossary of terms 2021*. Geneva: World Health Organization

Zhao, X. (2020) 'Health communication campaigns: a brief introduction and call for dialogue', *International Journal of Nursing Sciences*, 7 doi:10.1016/j.ijnss.2020.04.009

7 Health education

Sally Robinson

Key points

- Introduction
- The beginnings of UK mass health education: 1848 to 1930
- Health education
- Preventive model
- Educational model
- Empowerment model
- Social change model: health education becomes health promotion
- Summary

Introduction

For centuries, health was perceived as a private matter to be managed at home. Knowledge was gained from experience and passed by word of mouth through generations of family, friends, healers, physicians and midwives. The knowledge and skills associated with preventing illness or death are as precious as life and those who are deemed to have them gain influence and then a prestige and power they fiercely protect. This includes limiting who is given the knowledge and skills, then controlling their practice by law, procedures, exams and professional registration while denigrating anyone who presents alternative knowledge and skills as worthless, heretical, unscientific, dangerous or 'mad'. In Europe, in the Middle Ages, the Church, encouraged by male physicians, asserted control over women-healers by declaring them witches (Minkowski, 1992; Ussher, 1991). In the 20th century the medicalisation of childbirth, led by male obstetricians, undermined the traditional partnership of women and midwives (Oakley, 1980). History shows countless examples of the Church having power over people's souls, men having power over women, the rich having power over the poor and the educated having power over the uneducated. The words and actions of the powerful have always held higher status and influence than those of the powerless, and this continues. In Chapter 1, we discussed how people with influence can shape what people think the word 'health' means. Health education has much to do with power, who has it and whether it is shared, kept, used for self-interest or given away.

DOI: 10.4324/9780367823696-9

Box 7.1 Power

Glenn Laverack draws on the work of philosophy and feminism to summarise three types of hard power.

- 'Power-over' is where one party is made to do what another wishes. It may be negative or positive. It may comprise dominance; exploitation where one party controls another's choices because they have money or knowledge; or hegemonic power which is invisible and so internalised that it is taken for granted. Living within a culture of hegemonic power-over leads people to lose confidence, to believe problems are their own fault, develop low self-esteem and ultimately feel powerless. Hegemonic power is the type of power enjoyed by the medical profession. It is unhealthy because,

"... it shuts down critical thinking, public debate and the possibility of change. One of the subtle ways in which health practitioners participate in hegemonic power-over is when they continually impose their ideas of what are important problems without listening to what others think are important."

(p. 15)

- 'Power-from-within' is personal, psychological power. It is our own inner sense of value, truth, individual mastery or sense of self
- 'Power-with' is where people with 'power-over' deliberately use it to increase people's power-from-within. It starts with listening, and deliberately encouraging a person's self-esteem and confidence. It demands restraint and focus. A sign of success is that the person makes their own choices and decisions

(Source: Laverack, 2013)

The beginnings of mass health education: 1848 to 1930

'Health education' is a phrase which has been applied to coercion, propaganda, indoctrination, instruction, training, education, facilitation, enablement and empowerment.

- *Coercion* means persuasion by using threats, promises or force
- *Propaganda* means spreading information, or a message, in support of a cause. The information may be true or false
- *Indoctrination* means to instruct, to teach an idea or opinion, to imbue with a doctrine to persuade someone into thinking or behaving in a certain way
- *Instruction* means telling someone, or providing information that tells someone, what to do. Like indoctrination, it is concerned with 'what to think' not 'how' to think

Across Europe, for centuries, the only measure designed to protect the health of populations was coercion. Mayors, aldermen and justices of the peace imposed quarantine, or 'lockdown', on the infected people of a parish during epidemics such as plague.

In the UK, the era of the first public health movement in the 19th century marked the beginning of greater state involvement in the public's health. It comprised

- health protection, e.g. environmental changes to introduce clean water and sanitation
- disease prevention, e.g. the smallpox vaccine and identifying harmful bacteria in unclean water
- health propaganda, e.g. communicating the causes of a disease and how to avoid it

It saw coercive legal requirements being used alongside widespread health-related propaganda, indoctrination and instruction for the first time. The aim was to ensure every person was informed about what they were expected to do, and to do it. These three examples, namely, propaganda for the population, instructing mothers and coercion to vaccinate, reveal the tensions that arose in the UK prior to it becoming a full democracy in 1928. They show what happens when an authoritarian approach meets individuals' desire for autonomy, liberty and freedom of expression.

Propaganda for the population

The Industrial Revolution created the need for a large labour force to work in the new factories. Workers lived in overcrowded housing with poor nutrition and river water for drinking. The streets were filled with dirt, excrement and refuse because of the lack of water supplies, drainage and sewers. Information about deaths, beginning to be collected by local registrars, showed that epidemics of infectious diseases such as cholera, smallpox and measles were rampant killers. Between 1839 and 1842 the Poor Law Commission, led by Edwin Chadwick, confirmed the links between the poor environment and the poor health of the workers across England, Wales and Scotland. They thought diseases were caused by miasma, invisible particles, hanging in the foul air. Chadwick's report to Parliament concluded that it was not only more humane to improve sanitation to 'clean the air' and prevent deaths, but also economically expedient as the costs associated with lost productivity and burials were greater (Fee and Brown, 2005). Edwin Chadwick was described as,

> "... tenacious in pushing a reform by all means until action was taken, but he was overbearing and unresponsive to the views of others. He did not negotiate or converse but lectured people, again and again, until they acted."
>
> (Hamlin and Sheard, 1998, p. 588)

The 1848 Public Health Act established a General Board of Health (Figure 7.1) and local districts in England and Wales which had the authority to deal with sewerage, water supplies, the quality of food, street paving, the removal of waste and other sanitary measures. They could appoint a medical officer of health and an inspector of nuisances, forerunner of the sanitary inspectors and later environmental health officers. The Act recognised that disease in the population could not be prevented by central government alone. It could enforce standards through the law, finance and technology and it could issue instructions, but the government needed local communities to carry the message to individuals. The Metropolitan Health of Towns Association aimed to disseminate the valuable information about sanitation among

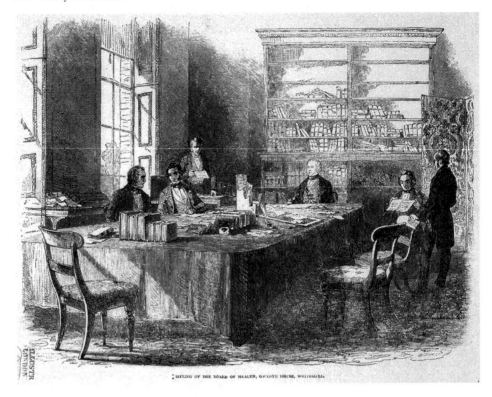

Figure 7.1 The General Board of Health, 1846

Source: Sitting of General Board of Health published in the Illustrated London News, October 6th 1846
Wellcome collection made available under a CC BY 4.0 licence

the population (Sutherland, 1987) (Figure 7.2). The Association for Promoting
Cleanliness among the Poor became responsible for the new public wash houses,
which often combined bathing and laundry facilities. Members taught the poor about
hygiene using the Methodist mantra 'cleanliness is next to Godliness', reinforcing the
belief that being in a poor physical state was related to being in a poor moral state.
Poverty was widely believed to be the result of criminality, alcoholism and degenerative
behaviour, while disease was the result of ignorance.

The backlash

By 1853, there were signs that the health of the population was slowly improving due
to a combination of the engineering skills which had improved the water supplies and
sanitation for about two million people, alongside social and behavioural changes
resulting from written, spoken and persuasive propaganda (Sutherland, 1987). In the
same year, violent riots broke out in several towns and in 1858, the General Board
of Health was terminated due to it being politically unpopular. Its work challenged
'vested interests', meaning those who gained personally or financially from the unsan-
itary status quo, and it was accused of threatening human freedoms through its propagandism and bullying. The Times newspaper commented that people would rather
take their chance with cholera than be bullied into health (Sutherland, 1987).

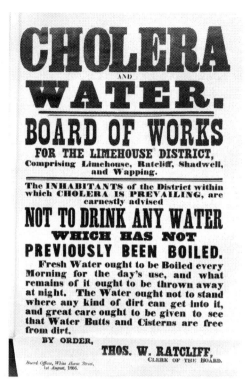

Figure 7.2 Broadsheet: cholera and water, 1866

Source: Wellcome collection made available under a CC BY 4.0 licence https://creativecommons.org/licenses/by/4.0

Indoctrination and instruction for mothers

Although women worked as sanitary inspectors, they were not welcomed by the male-led Sanitary Inspectors Association. In response, and as part of the wider Victorian women's movement, sanitary associations were formed around the UK (Haynes, 2006). They disseminated a blend of religious tracts and sanitary advice. Written materials included *Household Verses on Sanitary and Other Subjects*, where topics included the importance of fresh air, cleaning, cooking, childcare and tidiness (Box 7.3).

Box 7.2 Kitty Wilkinson, the 'saint of the slums'

Mrs Kitty Wilkinson, a mother of two children, was fortunate to have a boiler and a mangle in her Liverpool home where she earned a living as a laundress. In 1832, during a cholera epidemic, Kitty allowed local people to come and wash their clothes and bed linen at her house. She showed them how to use bleach in the washing. She and others noticed how this cleanliness helped to protect against cholera, and she began to campaign for public wash houses to be provided for the local people. The first public wash house in the world was opened in Frederick Street, Liverpool, in 1842.

Box 7.3 Fresh air

> Do you wish to be healthy? –
> Then keep the house sweet;
> As soon as you're up
> Shake each blanket and sheet.
>
> Leave the beds to get fresh
> On the close crowded floor;
> Let the wind sweep right through –
> Open window and door.
>
> The bad air will rush out
> As the good air comes in,
> Just as goodness is stronger
> And better than sin ...

> (Source: Ladies Sanitary Association 1850, p. 35. Wellcome
> collection made available under a CC BY 4.0 licence)

Recognising many of the poor were illiterate, the sanitary associations organised volunteers, known as home missionaries or lady health missioners, to teach the poor at mothers' meetings. In 1861, the Ladies Auxiliary of the Manchester and Salford Sanitary Association was formed. It sent out intelligent, trained, working-class women to live in the poorest districts, where they carried out home visits under the guidance of a supervisor. Their job was to visit the poor and give them practical instruction about sanitation in the home (Figure 7.3), alongside practical help such as helping

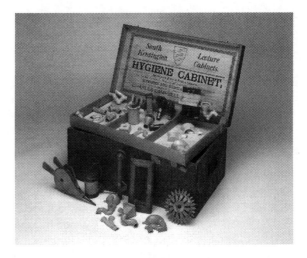

Figure 7.3 Hygiene demonstration cabinet, 1895

Source: Charles Campbell, 1895 Science Museum Group Collection made available under a CC BY 4.0 licence
https://creativecommons.org/licenses/by/4.0

with babies, cleaning and washing. They provided brushes and cleaning products and encouraged mothers to send children to school and adults to church. The success of these women owed much to living in the same local area as the families they visited and having a similar social position to the mothers they supported. These forerunners of health visitors were of interest to the increasingly powerful male medical officers of health, who later employed them within the local districts. The medical officers believed,

> "... there were too many incompetent mothers who, through ignorance and carelessness, jeopardised the lives of their children ... The cheapest and simplest solution seemed to be to educate women in hygiene, encourage them to breastfeed their young and keep their houses cleaner, particularly by getting rid of flies ... In fact, sub-standard sanitation caused many of the problems ... but improved sanitation was a long-term and far more costly project than teaching women how to be better mothers. Motherhood was ... not just a personal duty but a national one. Women were expected to take pride in being mothers of the race and they had to do the job properly."

> (Holdsworth, 1988, p. 113)

Thinking point:

> Note what Holdsworth says about the cost of teaching people to 'behave better' versus the cost of changing the environment in which they were living.

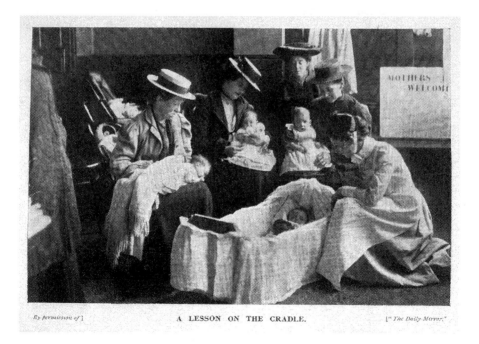

A LESSON ON THE CRADLE.

Figure 7.4 A School for Mothers, 1907

Source: Evelyn Bunting *et al.* (1907). Wellcome collection made available under a CC BY 4.0 licence.

The impetus to teach mothers was driven by a wish to reduce high infant deaths. For socialists it was about improving the conditions of the poor, but for others it was about the necessity of growing the population to support the British Empire (Davin, 1978). Charles Darwin's work on the 'survival of the fittest' fuelled the Eugenics movement which was concerned with improving the quality of the race, which meant the virile, not weaklings and the upper, not lower, classes (Davin, 1978). Attention was paid to the health of children; boys needed to be able to fight to defend the Empire and girls needed to be healthy to produce the next generation. As the 20th century began, the Education Act of 1907 brought health and education together in legislation. Physical education, domestic science and hygiene instruction were introduced into schools, alongside medical inspections and meals. For adults, there was the temperance movement, parenthood education, Schools for Mothers (Figure 7.4) and the refusal of marriage licences to those considered to be 'unfit' (Davin, 1978; Sutherland, 1987).

The backlash

Marie Stopes, a eugenicist who set up the Society for Constructive Birth Control and Racial Progress, provided information on contraception, helped to set up family planning clinics and wrote her scandalous book Married Love in 1918. Stopes is credited as the first health educator in the UK to present information to her readers in a way that encouraged their interest. She based her writing on an understanding of what people wanted to know, rather than what they needed to be told. She dealt with real situations, presented her arguments and did not resort to the propaganda on posters and pamphlets (Blythe, 1987). The birth control movement grew and included many women from the Labour Party and female doctors who were concerned about the appalling health of women worn down by childbearing. Building on the long-established tradition of women supporting women in matters of health through the feminine grapevine, they provided information about contraception despite contravening the obscenity laws and experiencing significant assaults on their own reputations. Holdsworth (1988) summarises,

> "… the combined forces of Medicine, Church and State did their best to slow down the development and spread of contraception."
>
> (Holdsworth, 1988, p. 96)

As for the mothers, Hilda Bates, who worked as a health visitor in the period around 1918 when local authorities started to provide free clinics for married pregnant women and infants, said,

> "They couldn't see why the government should want to register or take any interest in their child. And they wouldn't bring their children to the clinic every month as they were supposed to do. Anyway, the clinic was awful."
>
> (Holdsworth, 1988, p. 92)

Coercion to vaccinate

In 1840, the UK Vaccination Act made the world's first vaccination, against smallpox, freely available in England and Wales. In 1853, the Government passed the Vaccination Act for England and Wales, making the smallpox vaccination compulsory for babies.

Parents would be either fined or imprisoned if their babies were not vaccinated. This marked the first time that the state intervened with individuals' civil liberties in the name of public health. By 1864, the vaccination was available throughout the UK. In 1867, the vaccination became compulsory for those up to 14 years old, with various penalties for non-compliance.

The backlash

The 1853 Act sparked riots in several towns in England and Wales and the 1867 Act prompted the founding of the Anti-Compulsory Vaccination League in London. In an era where people looked to the quality of the air and to sin as causes of disease, people were afraid of the new vaccine. The anti-vaccine propaganda, in the form of pamphlets, described the vaccine as a fearful and destructive monster that could damage people's health (Wolfe and Sharp, 2002). The League argued that it was the duty of Parliament to protect the 'rights of man' which included the right for parents to protect their children from disease, to resist invading their subjects' liberty and their right to good health. A royal commission sat for several years and concluded the vaccine was safe, but there would be no penalties for those who refused it. The Vaccination Act of 1898 introduced the concept of the 'conscientious objector' into English law, meaning that if someone did not believe the vaccine was safe, they could be exempt from having it. This was replicated in Scottish law in 1907. In 1947 all vaccinations simply became optional. The UK continues to have no mandatory vaccines, though some are a requirement of certain occupations and COVID-19 coronavirus vaccination was required for entry to some venues during the pandemic. Figure 7.5 shows protests against the latter in London, and against the legally enforced 'lockdowns', during 2020 and 2021.

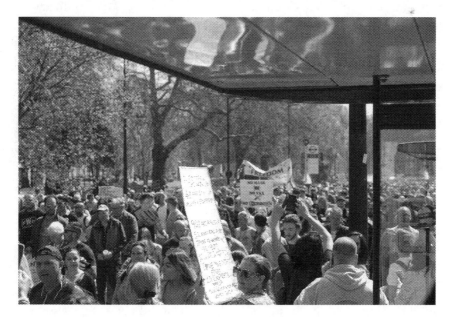

Figure 7.5 Protests against COVID-19 coronavirus regulations in London

Early health education

Early mass health education in the UK

- was characterised by 'top down' communication mostly in the form of propaganda, coercion, indoctrination and instruction with the aim of achieving obedience and compliance
- was an essential ingredient in reducing deaths from disease alongside the creation of a sanitary environment and the smallpox vaccination
- was often linked to national, economic, political, medical or religious agendas set by those who had authority and influence
- was focussed on changing people's attitudes and behaviour while ignoring the social, environmental and economic constraints in which individuals lived
- blamed a homogenous group called 'the poor' for their ill health
- held mothers responsible for the ill health of their children
- was unconcerned about the health of women, only their childbearing potential
- was central to the role of health visitors, medical officers and some social activists and charities
- started to attract the attention of some teachers, dentists and nurses
- revealed tensions between authoritarian communication and people's freedom to make their own health-related choices

Once people's poor health became a political, social and economic problem and not merely a private one, it was added to the list of ways in which the most powerful people and organisations sought to influence the thoughts and actions of the least powerful so that their particular vision of society could emerge. Many ordinary people benefited from the new engineering and environmental improvements while following instructions to adopt hygienic behaviours, to be dutiful mothers and to ensure children were vaccinated against smallpox. We know this because the death rates fell, 'absence of disease' was achieved. It was at a cost. In parallel, some people actively worked together to defend people's right to determine their own health and others recognised that people needed more than propaganda. Note how Kitty Wilkinson (Box 7.2) provided knowledge, skills and then campaigned for public wash houses; how the Manchester and Salford Sanitary Association immersed themselves into the lives of poor women only to find they needed to provide cleaning products alongside knowledge and skills; and how Marie Stopes answered the questions and needs of ordinary people. These women did not yet know they were pioneers for a different kind of health education.

In 1927, the Central Council for Health Education was set up for England and Wales as a lead agency to assist the statutory authorities by encouraging and coordinating health 'propaganda' and 'education' related to the science and art of healthy living, prevention or cure of disease. It comprised representatives from directors of education, medical officers of health and other doctors, dentists, teachers, nurses, voluntary organisations and selected individuals (National Archives, undated). However, health education as a movement did not gain traction beyond enthusiastic individuals. For a range of bureaucratic reasons neither central government, local government nor industry were interested and most argued people's health was their personal affair. Many professions were generally disinterested in health education because

- it was associated with charities and volunteers
- the teachers disliked the propaganda approach which conflicted with the aims of education as well as the inconvenience of adding health-related teaching to their responsibilities
- many of the healthcare professions were focused on developing their specialisms in aspects of treatment, therapies or care
- most doctors were developing their professional strength around curing disease with little interest in disease prevention
- many female health visitors worked under the authority and direction of male medical officers of health who directed their work towards instructing mothers about infant welfare, infectious diseases and domestic hygiene. Health visitors had neither the power nor freedom to educate as they would have wished, and to work for the much-needed social reform that they knew was needed to improve the conditions of the poor

(Blythe, 1987; Haynes, 2006; Sutherland, 1987)

The Central Council deliberately used the phrases 'propaganda' and 'education' in setting out its aims (Sutherland, 1987). It is an important distinction which reflected two different processes, one coming from doctors who considered themselves to be experts in 'health' and one coming from educators, such as teachers, who considered themselves to be experts in 'education.' Health 'education and propaganda' were also part of the duties of the Department of Health for Scotland, established in 1929 (National Records of Scotland, 2020). It is the fault line that goes to the heart of how health education, health promotion and public health are understood and practised today.

Health education between 1848 and 1930 was characterised by authoritarian approaches which encouraged both compliance and resistance. There were early signs of a division between the approach advocated by the male-dominated medical profession and that taken by the education profession and others, including some women.

Health education

Contemporary health education is,

> "… any intentional activity which is designed to achieve health or illness related learning, i.e. some relatively permanent change in an individual's capability or disposition. Effective health education may, thus, produce changes in knowledge and understanding or ways of thinking; it may influence or clarify values; it may bring about some shift in belief or attitude; it may facilitate the acquisition of skills; it may even effect changes in behaviour or lifestyle."

(Tones and Tilford, 1994, p. 11)

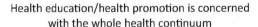

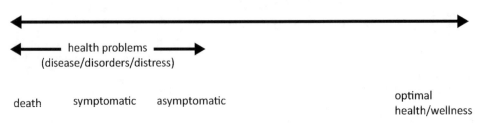

Health education/health promotion is concerned with promoting health at every point along the health continuum. We promote health when people feel well, when they experience health problems and at the end of life. Deterring movement to the left is disease prevention. Encouraging movement to the right is salutogenic.

Figure 7.6 The health continuum

Health education is concerned with health-related learning

- for individuals, families, groups, communities and populations
- at all points across the life course from pre-conception to death
- across the health continuum (Figure 7.6), for those who

    - are experiencing optimal health/wellness
    - have a health problem but are asymptomatic/it is not yet known
    - have a health problem and are symptomatic/it is known
    - are dying or bereaved

- where the *process* of learning and its impact on people's future abilities is a core concern
- pertinent to people's health-related awareness, knowledge, values (see Chapter 1, Table 1.1), attitudes, feelings, motivations, decisions, skills and behaviours
- where the concept of health may vary according to who defines it, e.g.

    - an expert who may think health means absence of disease
    - an educated person who may think health is a holistic and personal concept
    - a client who may think health is about developing coping skills, resilience and enablement
    - individuals, families, groups or populations who may think health is about the society in which they live and the decisions made by those with influence and power

- towards a range of outcomes that include disease prevention, optimal health and autonomous health-related choices and actions
- that is disease-centred, aiming to prevent disease (pathogenic), but it is also person-centred and salutogenic, aiming to enhance a person's health and their capacity to take control and change their own and others' health (Table 7.1, Boxes 7.4 and 7.6 on p.181).

Table 7.1 Disease prevention versus health education

	Disease prevention	*Health education*
Primary	Preventing the development of disease by reducing risks and enhancing protection	Learning how to prevent disease and optimise health e.g. be aware of media bias and vested interests; to know how to prevent accidents, keep safe and keep active; developing the knowledge and skills for healthy eating; to understand how to build resilience and practice life skills
Secondary	Early detection of disease to reverse or limit its progression	Learning how to identify signs and symptoms of potential disease and to optimise health e.g. to understand screening procedures such as blood pressure checks; to know how to reduce excess weight, to stop smoking and to provide first aid; to identify when emotional or spiritual support is needed and know how to find it; and to use life skills to support self and others
Tertiary	To prevent deterioration of existing disease, to maximise potential for healthy living	Learning how to manage and prevent deterioration and optimise health e.g. to measure blood glucose levels for those with diabetes; to understand the pros and cons of treatments; to carry out daily living activities independently; to identify emotional, spiritual and practical needs and know how to find support; to use life skills to improve quality of life at the end of life; and to understand loss and bereavement

---

Box 7.4 Salutogenesis

Aaron Antonovsky's development of his salutogenic model originated with his research into women and ageing. He found that 29% of those women who had survived Nazi concentration camps had positive emotional health; they were *not* emotionally impaired by the experience. He set out to understand more about their resilience and coping skills. He found when people have, what he called, 'a sense of coherence', they find the world is understandable, meaningful and manageable.

Salutogenesis is concerned with what causes health, in contrast to pathogenesis, meaning what causes disease. Both are needed.

Salutogenesis is a constant learning process that supports a person's movement towards their concept of optimal health/wellness. Learning is itself a health promoting activity.

Salutogenic learning includes learning to improve wellbeing, quality of life, inner strength, resilience, health literacy, self-efficacy, social and emotional learning, mindfulness/contemplative learning, connectedness, humour and flourishing.

(Source: Antonovsky, 1987; Eriksson, 2017; Jensen *et al.*, 2017; Weare, 2019)

Process of learning

A health education model, or an approach, describes a communication process designed for learning (see the end of this chapter to see why we call this a health promotion model today). It determines whether the educator keeps or gives away power to the learner. It comprises

- who sets the agenda for the communication, e.g. the educator or the person/people
- the direction of communication, e.g. top-down/authoritative, bottom-up/person-led or side-to-side/equal discussion
- the role that is played by the educator and the person/people, e.g. passive or active
- desired outcome of the communication, e.g. compliance to prevent disease, informed choice or empowerment

The 'educator' denotes a person whose communication aims to achieve a person or population's learning. They can be anyone including a nurse, a broadcaster, an educational professional, therapist, social influencer, artist, activist, neighbour or friend. Communication can be verbal or non-verbal (see Chapter 6). We will examine three models (Table 7.2).

- Preventive model, which includes the medical approach and the behaviour change approach
- Educational model
- Empowerment model

Table 7.2 Preventive, educational and empowerment models

	Preventive model	*Educational model*	*Empowerment model*
Direction of communication	Top-down, one-way, expert leads	Side to side, two-way, educator leads	Bottom-up, two-way, learner leads
Role of educator	An expert in the causes of disease who draws upon medical research and epidemiology to persuade	An educated person who draws upon a wide range of health-related knowledge and applies core principles of education	A facilitator who practices congruence, acceptance, empathy and participatory/active learning methods
Agenda	Educator decides what a person needs to learn and sets the agenda	Educator normally decides what a person needs to learn and sets the agenda, but there may be some room for negotiation	Learner decides what they need to learn and sets the agenda but may work with the educator as an equal to agree detail
Focus of communication	Causes and risk factors for disease, or health-related behaviours that contribute to disease	Any aspect of health e.g. physical, mental, emotional, spiritual, social, societal, sexual	Personal insights, knowledge and skills relating to any aspect of health e.g. physical, mental, emotional, spiritual, social, societal, sexual

(Continued)

Table 7.2 Preventive, educational and empowerment models *(Continued)*

	Preventive model	*Educational model*	*Empowerment model*
Content	Presents information about body malfunctions and persuades compliance with medical solutions or healthier behaviours	Provides access to health-related knowledge and skills; fosters thinking, reasoning, exploration of values, attitudes and motivations; encourages rational decision making	Provides opportunities to explore health-related personal and social experiences; to think, feel and share; to practice and apply transferable life skills; to understand power imbalances and develop one's own potential
Types of communication	Instruction Training Demonstration	Education Facilitation Enablement	Facilitation Enablement Empowerment
Learning domains	Cognitive, psychomotor	Cognitive, affective, conative, psychomotor	Cognitive, affective, conative, psychomotor
Role of client	Compliance	Active, questioning, personal reflection, decision-making	Active, questioning, personal reflection, decision-making, action
Aim and criteria for success	Absence of disease due to compliance with screening, treatment or adopting healthier behaviours	Autonomy, person makes informed choices about their health	Autonomy and empowerment, person has knowledge and skills to take control of their health and to reach their full potential
Desired outcome	The progression of disease is halted or reversed	The person is changed by the learning experience. They own the health-related choices they make and are equipped to make informed choices in the future	The person is changed by the learning experience. They are empowered to navigate, negotiate and act on their health-related choices

Preventive model

The aim of the preventive model is to prevent disease either by complying with medical advice or by changing health-related behaviours (Table 7.3). Disease is defined as,

"Any impairment of normal physiological function affecting all or part of an organism … a specific pathological change caused by infection, stress etc. producing characteristic symptoms; illness or sickness in general."

(Collins dictionary, 2021)

Medical approach

As we progressed through the 20th century, the death rates from infectious diseases were much reduced and the political incentive to interfere with people's health diminished, but the advances in science and the power of the medical profession ascended.

Table 7.3 The preventive model

	Preventive model	
	Medical approach	*Behaviour change approach*
Direction of communication	Top-down, one-way	
Role of educator	Expert in causes of disease who draws upon medical research and epidemiology to persuade	
Agenda	Educator decides what the person needs to know and sets the agenda	
Focus of communication	Disease	Health-related behaviours which contribute to disease
Underpinning content	Presents information about body malfunctions and persuades compliance with medical solutions	Presents information about body malfunctions caused by unhealthy behaviours and persuades compliance with healthier behaviours
Types of communication	Instruction Training Demonstration	
Learning domains	Cognitive, Psychomotor	
Role of client	Compliance	
Aim and criteria for success	Absence of disease due to compliance with screening or treatment	Absence of disease due to adopting healthier behaviours
Desired outcome	The progression of disease is halted or reversed; this can be objectively measured	
Examples	Instructions to have vaccinations, to attend screening services, to take medicine prior to an operation or to comply with medical tests	Instructions to avoid taking recreational drugs, to stick to low-risk drinking guidelines, to give up smoking, to lose weight, to attend cardiac rehabilitation classes or to adopt a 'healthier lifestyle'

The medical profession's work was, and still is to a great extent, characterised by the medical model of health and illness (Robinson, 2021). This means their thinking and practice was guided by viewing the body as a machine which needed to be fixed by an expert to prevent or cure disease. Medical officers and other doctors took the same approach when communicating with the population (Figure 7.7). Sutherland (1987) explains this as,

> "… an engineering model: since the human body can be thought of as a machine it can also be thought to run better if the right things are done to it. It was consistent with this model to give a mother a pamphlet with some instructions on it,

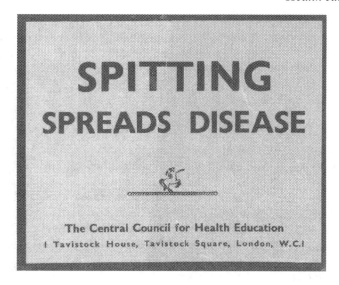

Figure 7.7 A sticker illustrates the preventive model/medical approach, dated between 1950 and 1970

Source: Central Council for Health Education, Science Museum Group Collection made available under a CC BY 4.0 licence.

Box 7.5 Be Clear on Cancer

The Be Clear on Cancer campaign, for England and Wales, began in January 2011. Its aim to was to raise the public's awareness about the signs and symptoms of cancer and to visit their GP. It was an example of secondary disease prevention/health education, the preventive model: medical approach and instruction. The campaign included several sub-campaigns such as skin cancer, ovarian cancer, lung cancer and bowel cancer. Each had a key message such as

- have you had a cough for more than 3 weeks? Then it is time to tell your doctor
- see your doctor straight away if, for the last three weeks, you've had blood in your poo or looser poo
- feeling bloated, most days, for three weeks or more could be a sign of ovarian cancer. Tell your doctor
- having heartburn, most days, for 3 weeks or more could be a sign of cancer – tell your doctor

The campaign utilised one-way communication via TV and radio advertising, posters, leaflets and briefing materials for health professionals. Some of the results from the evaluation of the campaign, in England in 2013, showed a statistically significant increase in people's awareness of key symptoms of bowel cancer, kidney/bladder cancer and ovarian cancer after the campaigns.

(Source: Cancer Research UK, 2014, 2021)

expecting her to accept the instructions and to behave accordingly. To instruct by means of a pamphlet was like adjusting a machine; the adjustment would produce a beneficial effect … It was from that time onwards a small step to change a tract or a pamphlet into a poster, a leaflet, an exhibition, or a lecture and so to expect the required lesson to be learnt. These became the traditional tools of health propagandism, and are consistent with the model of doctors as engineers."

(p. 12)

Today's persuasive one-way communication, in the form of leaflets, lectures, advertising; and social, broadcast, visual and print media continues to instruct people in the workings of the body, to be hygienic, have vaccinations, comply with treatment and follow doctors' orders. The success of this medical approach is measured in terms of its outcome, an absence of disease, either within an individual or within a population. It is disease-centred, detached from the messiness of human values or concerns about what health might mean to any individual and their emotional or social life, and importantly it is divorced from politics. It continues to contribute to the decline in many diseases by giving people clear instructions to save someone's life or prevent known disease (Box 7.5). We note that this approach focuses on disease, not the whole of health, and it comprises persuasive instruction, which is not education. To call it health education sounds like a misnomer, but it meets the definition, "… any intentional activity which is designed to achieve health or illness related learning" (Tones and Tilford, 1994, p. 11).

Behaviour change approach

By the 1970s, as we learnt more about the causes of cardiovascular disease and cancer, people were instructed to take responsibility and change their health-related behaviour such as to eat less saturated fat, be more physically active and practice safe sex (Figure 7.8). Like the instruction to boil water to avoid cholera in Victorian times, the assumption was that if experts provided health-related information then people would change their behaviours to avoid disease and early death. Simultaneously, advertisers were paid by industries to encourage people to buy and consume high-fat food, smoke cigarettes and drink alcohol, wrapped up in an attractive, glossy lifestyle. They were selling products as life-enhancers. From this propaganda and advertising, health educators learnt they needed to engage with people's emotions and sometimes resorted to shock tactics, that is, using images, stories and messages that aim to scare people into changing behaviour. Such images are sometimes printed on cigarette packets today. They may raise awareness but, unless they are complemented by other types of education, this approach has been found to be ineffective at changing behaviour and probably unethical (Green *et al.*, 2019; Scriven, 2017).

Pros and cons of the preventive model

There are times, particularly when we are in great pain, incapacitated or feeling very vulnerable, when we might be grateful to hand over to an expert to tell us what to do. This quick and efficient transmission of knowledge, with its credentials of being evidence-based, safe, 'proven' or risk-reducing, can occur in flexible spaces and represents value for money. Managers are happy, and experts may go unchallenged. However, if the person does not choose to comply or is unable to comply due to lack

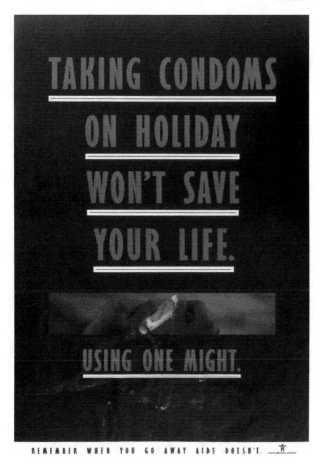

Figure 7.8 A poster illustrates the preventive model/behaviour change approach, 1988

Source: Health Education Authority, Science Museum Group Collection made available under a CC BY 4.0 licence. In 1988, HIV/AIDS was always fatal.

of time, skills, understanding, social pressure or money, it is a failure that becomes their fault. Sometimes health-damaging behaviours are called 'lifestyle' and, although behaviour is influenced by a range of factors, 'lifestyle' has more than a hint of blaming the lives that people lead as if these are always based on free choices. Victim blaming means blaming the victim of the problem for the problem. The problem may be a social or economic difficulty over which the person is powerless. Used over a long time, a preventive model of health education may induce dependency on experts or rebellion against 'being told what to do'. Persuasion may be considered unethical when it becomes disempowering. For a democratic, evolving society, neither passive dependence nor active rebellion are desirable population characteristics.

> *The preventive model is an authoritarian approach where the educator seeks to persuade people to comply with instructions to prevent disease based on medical science and epidemiological evidence.*

Educational model

At the same time the Victorians were introducing public health measures, they were also introducing universal education. The history of education influenced health education just as much as the history of health. Both occurred as the UK was becoming a country where ordinary men and, later, women could vote and have a say in the running of the country. As the 20th century began, teachers were uncomfortable with being asked to introduce health propaganda into schools beyond physical training. Education, as inherited from the ancient Greeks, was, and is, about teaching someone 'how' to think, not 'what' to think. It is about facilitating their learning and enabling them to develop the critical thinking skills which can be used throughout their whole life. Education supports people's ability to make informed decisions for themselves, quite the opposite of coercion or propaganda, and not the same as training, though both education and training are often present in education institutions.

- *Training* is close to indoctrination and instruction. It is the imparting of a single set of ideas, habits, behaviours and values with a view to these being perfectly replicated by the trainee
- *Education* is about autonomy. Autonomy means being able to make one's own decisions. It is,

    "... to be free, in control of one's own life, able to think rationally and logically and make decisions without coercion or fear... It is not about persuading a person to do what others think they should."

    (Weare, 1992, p. 66)

Katherine Weare (1992) summarises one of the oldest debates about the purpose of education. At its heart is the idea that human nature is either naturally good or naturally evil. Rousseau, a philosopher writing in the 18th century, argued that education is about enabling a person to develop their intrinsically good self. If we remove constraints such as the curriculum, educational structures and social prejudices; create learning opportunities and give the person freedom to choose; they will naturally want to learn, to discover and flourish at a pace that suits them. Their whole being, their mental, physical, emotional and moral capacities, will thrive and be free. Education has the power to shape the type of society in which we live, and here the thinking is that a fair and just society, where people are respectful of others, will naturally emerge. In summary, to be healthy we need to give people the freedom and resources to learn and foster their confidence so that they can make autonomous decisions about their health.

Thinking point:

    Consider something that you have learnt, perhaps a hobby, which you largely taught yourself. Think about how you felt when you were learning. Compare this experience to something you had to learn at school to achieve a qualification.

The alternate view, which starts from the position that human nature is evil, bad or at least naive, was held by philosophers such as John Locke writing in the 17th century who argued people needed strict, active guidance from an educator. Educators needed to recognise that people can be drawn to evil, perhaps caught up in the harmful indoctrination and propaganda of others. Locke took the idea of Aristotle that a person's mind was a 'blank slate' onto which useful knowledge needed to be imprinted. Recently there has been a much greater attention paid to understanding how people learn and then adapting styles of teaching accordingly. The aim is to help the learner acquire the knowledge, attitudes and behaviours which may help them to counter pressure such as peer pressure or advertising, make *informed* choices and protect their own autonomy.

No matter where one stands on the continuum between a naturalist and more directed learning, the educational model respects the person's decision about what is best for their own health. It accepts that their health may not only be about the absence of disease; it accepts that health is a personal and holistic concept, aligned with the many factors that affect people's quality of life. Respecting people's right to make informed choices about their health may resonate with societies who seek to support human rights and democratic rights, but it is significantly more challenging than an authoritarian approach. There is a balance to be struck between the individual's right to health and the rights of others around them. Consider someone who chooses not to have a vaccination for a communicable disease, who chooses to smoke tobacco in an enclosed space or who sings loudly in the middle of the night. Immediately, we ask who decides what is acceptable within a community, and so health becomes a matter for society and highly political.

Holistic health and holistic learning

In education, both 'health' and 'learning' are understood to be holistic and mutually reinforcing concepts, meaning more learning leads to better health and better health enables more learning. Both concern the engagement of the whole person in their environment. Holistic health is captured in six dimensions by Scriven (2017).

- Physical health is concerned with the body and how it functions
- Mental health is being able to think clearly and coherently
- Emotional health is about recognising and expressing feelings appropriately
- Spiritual health is about personal creeds and ways of achieving peace of mind which, for some, may be influenced by a formal religion
- Social health is the ability to make and maintain relationships with others
- Societal health captures the physical and social environment in which people live and includes culture, social and economic inequalities, environmental hazards, political oppression, discrimination and powerful industries

These six dimensions of health are interdependent and may be contested. For example, sexual health may be included as a seventh dimension (Naidoo and Wills, 2009). Emotional health may be defined as people's social and emotional functioning (FLTCEH, 2018). In healthcare, mental health is often used as a catch-all for anything that is not physical. Mental and emotional health together are often called psychological health. Mental health may be understood more broadly to include the continuum of mental disorders, mental health problems and mental wellbeing, which is about feeling good and functioning well (FPH/MHF, 2016). Mental, emotional and social dimensions of health are sometimes collectively called wellbeing (Aked *et al.*, 2008). Wellness means optimal health (Smith *et al.*, 2006). Figure 7.9 illustrates a leaflet produced in the early 1990s. It demonstrates a holistic approach to health and encouragement to take self-control.

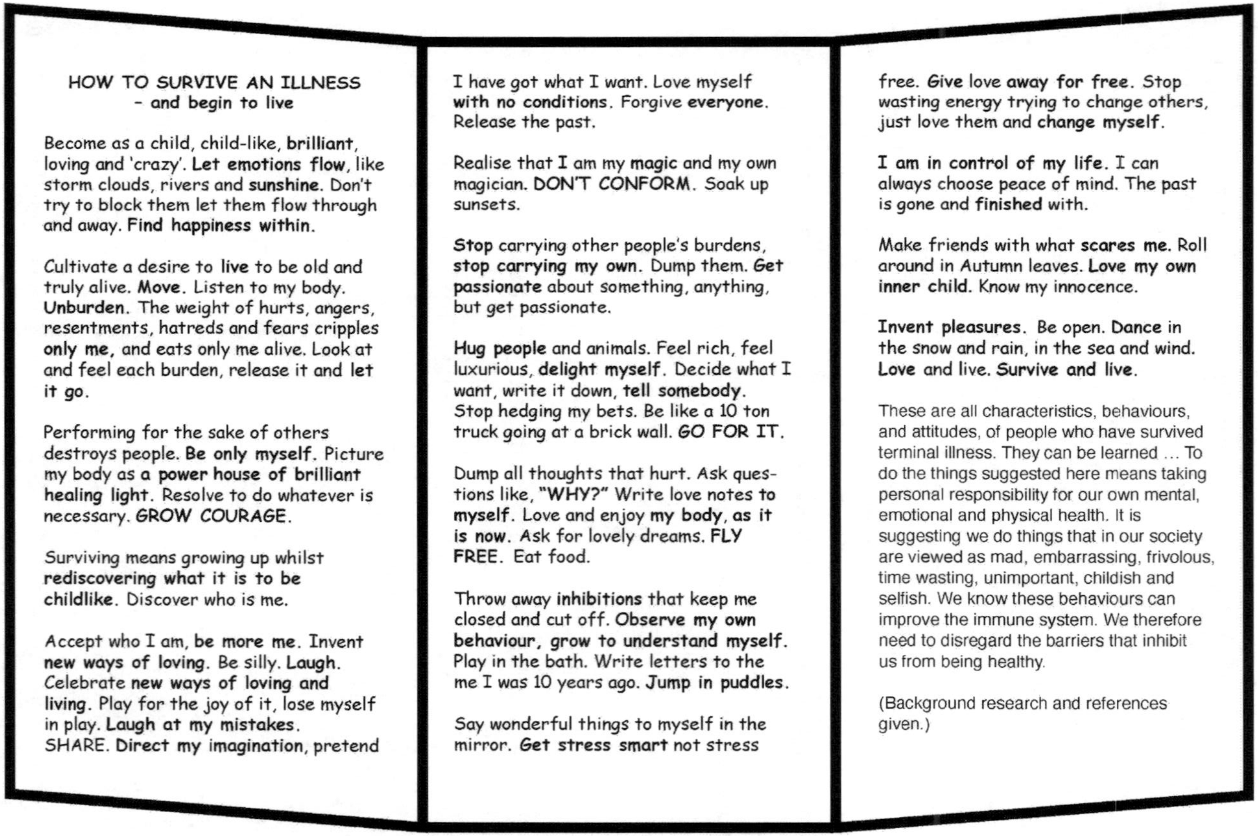

HOW TO SURVIVE AN ILLNESS
– and begin to live

Become as a child, child-like, brilliant, loving and 'crazy'. Let emotions flow, like storm clouds, rivers and sunshine. Don't try to block them let them flow through and away. Find happiness within.

Cultivate a desire to live to be old and truly alive. Move. Listen to my body. Unburden. The weight of hurts, angers, resentments, hatreds and fears cripples only me, and eats only me alive. Look at and feel each burden, release it and let it go.

Performing for the sake of others destroys people. Be only myself. Picture my body as a power house of brilliant healing light. Resolve to do whatever is necessary. GROW COURAGE.

Surviving means growing up whilst rediscovering what it is to be childlike. Discover who is me.

Accept who I am, be more me. Invent new ways of loving. Be silly. Laugh. Celebrate new ways of loving and living. Play for the joy of it, lose myself in play. Laugh at my mistakes. SHARE. Direct my imagination, pretend

I have got what I want. Love myself with no conditions. Forgive everyone. Release the past.

Realise that I am my magic and my own magician. DON'T CONFORM. Soak up sunsets.

Stop carrying other people's burdens, stop carrying my own. Dump them. Get passionate about something, anything, but get passionate.

Hug people and animals. Feel rich, feel luxurious, delight myself. Decide what I want, write it down, tell somebody. Stop hedging my bets. Be like a 10 ton truck going at a brick wall. GO FOR IT.

Dump all thoughts that hurt. Ask questions like, "WHY?" Write love notes to myself. Love and enjoy my body, as it is now. Ask for lovely dreams. FLY FREE. Eat food.

Throw away inhibitions that keep me closed and cut off. Observe my own behaviour, grow to understand myself. Play in the bath. Write letters to the me I was 10 years ago. Jump in puddles.

Say wonderful things to myself in the mirror. Get stress smart not stress

free. Give love away for free. Stop wasting energy trying to change others, just love them and change myself.

I am in control of my life. I can always choose peace of mind. The past is gone and finished with.

Make friends with what scares me. Roll around in Autumn leaves. Love my own inner child. Know my innocence.

Invent pleasures. Be open. Dance in the snow and rain, in the sea and wind. Love and live. Survive and live.

These are all characteristics, behaviours, and attitudes, of people who have survived terminal illness. They can be learned .... To do the things suggested here means taking personal responsibility for our own mental, emotional and physical health. It is suggesting we do things that in our society are viewed as mad, embarrassing, frivolous, time wasting, unimportant, childish and selfish. We know these behaviours can improve the immune system. We therefore need to disregard the barriers that inhibit us from being healthy.

(Background research and references given.)

Figure 7.9 A leaflet demonstrates a holistic approach to health and self-help

Source: Sheila Warne (undated), West Glamorgan Health Authority, Health Promotion Unit, Swansea. Reproduced with permission from Public Health Wales.

Learning is a holistic process. People learn with their minds, hearts and bodies; it is a mental, emotional, spiritual, social and physical process influenced by the wider environment. We learn best from that which is personal to us because it resonates with an emotional need or desire to learn. There are four domains of learning.

- Cognitive learning is about gaining knowledge, understanding, beliefs and ways of thinking. Whereas knowledge is based on a standard of evidence, it is 'true'; beliefs are based on subjectivity, what we think is probably true. Beliefs are a powerful influence on people's behaviour. Cognitive learning is associated with mental health, when defined as clear thinking. Thinking and memory are powerfully influenced by emotional health. For example, in situations of high stress, the body activates its 'fight, flight or freeze' response which overwhelms the brain's ability to think, learn and remember
- Affective learning is about feelings, values and attitudes. It is about processing how we feel about something, whether we are anxious or excited, and how much it has meaning or importance for us. An attitude is the outcome of both feeling and believing. It is a personal judgement. We like or dislike something; we are in favour or against something. Affective learning is associated with emotional and spiritual aspects of health. We are more likely to learn when we care about a subject. All aspects of health are inherently emotional because they are personal. How we feel during learning is influenced by our social health, that is our relationships with the educator or peers. Learning about relationships and the emotions of others is called social, or social and emotional, learning. We cannot learn if we are cold, afraid or do not possess the appropriate resources, and these are influenced by aspects of societal health such as deprivation and discrimination
- Conative learning is about becoming motivated, intentional, striving, persistent, planning and being self-directed towards a goal with the expectation of success. It is central to autonomy. It determines whether what we know (cognitive) and what we feel (affective) is likely to result in behaviour (psychomotor). We may lose momentum if we suffer from poor physical health or gain momentum when we feel strong. Similarly, conative learning is associated with mental, emotional and spiritual health and is influenced by social and societal health
- Psychomotor/behavioural learning is about doing; developing practical, social and physical skills. Skills require the application of cognitive, affective and social learning and are influenced by all dimensions of health

Thinking point:

> Consider the knowledge, feelings, conation and social skills involved in declining the offer of a joint among a group of friends who are all smoking cannabis.

Education for health is cognitive, affective, conative and skills-based. The learner needs to participate with their whole being. The health-related learning needs to be active while the educator facilitates the learning (Table 7.4). Some principles include

- start from where the person is in terms of what they already know, feel or can do
- build on prior learning, gradually introducing what is new or more challenging
- recognise this is only one piece of learning among all the other learning that is going on in their lives via their wider social network

Table 7.4 Methods to meet learning objectives

Domain of learning	Learning objectives		Suitable methods to achieve objective
Cognitive	To raise awareness	"I have heard of new disease X"	A talk/lecture, media, posters, exhibitions, campaigns, group teaching/discussion
	To gain knowledge and understanding	"I understand how people develop disease X and I know what I need to do to keep myself healthy"	Media, posters, leaflets, exhibitions, campaigns, lectures/talks, group discussion. Better, if complemented by opportunities to ask questions
Affective	To increase self-awareness	"I feel concerned that I could develop disease X"	Opportunities for discussions with people who have experienced disease X, role play, one-to-one discussion, counselling/therapy, reflective diary
	To raise self-esteem	"I am worth this, I feel OK"	Group or one-to-one activities and discussion, confidence building exercises, self-care skills, counselling/therapy
	To clarify values	"I realise that this is more important to me than that"	Values continuum, ranking, group activities and discussions, counselling/therapy
	To clarify attitudes	"I agree with this. I disagree with that"	Use polarised arguments, group activities, quizzes and discussions
Conative	To clarify motivations and intentions	"I know I want to do this because I feel this"	Discussions using challenging questions about beliefs, values and consequences
	To encourage self-direction	"I'm going to take this forward"	Group work, self-esteem exercises, practice social skills, setting personal targets or rewards
	To make decisions	"I've decided to do this"	Clarify desired outcome, then write or discuss the costs and benefits, consider alternatives and consequences, "What would happen if?" questions
Psychomotor	To develop a new skill	"I can do this"	Demonstration, break down skill into its components, observe, listen, practice, repeat, build components into whole skill, apply to something real or meaningful
	To change behaviour	"I have changed behaviour"	Social and practical support, plan, application of skills to real situations, set realistic targets, reward, self-monitoring diary
	To maintain behaviour	"I have continued with my new behaviour"	Coping skills such as problem-solving, peer support network, refresh motivations

- encourage multi-sensory learning incorporating speaking, seeing, listening, doing, sharing, interacting and simulation. It can be creative, dynamic and playful, with a view to encouraging the development of social and practical skills
- encourage personal reflection, recognition of learning and the transfer of learning to new situations

- take a positive approach, such as encouraging decisions to keep safe and gain enjoyment rather than negative approaches which communicate fear, criticism or promote guilt
- keep information realistic and relevant, where possible it should reinforce positive social norms
- keep the learning environment a safe, secure, nurturing place
- encourage the learner and support them to feel heard and valued

(adapted from PSHE Association, 2014)

Examples of the educational model

The educational model is commonly found in educational settings and in many others such as in citizen's advice services and commercial weight loss groups. It is likely to have been the approach taken by Mrs Kitty Wilkinson when talking with her neighbours about using bleach in the wash (Box 7.2). In healthcare, we see the educational model described as 'patient education', for no other reason than the recipient is a 'patient.' It is where a health professional explains why an intervention, such as a hearing aid or an injection, may help the patient. The patient may ask questions, there is a two-way discussion, the patient reaches a point when they have a good understanding, and then the patient decides whether they would like to have the intervention. Examples of the educational model are shown in Boxes 7.6 and 7.7. Note how Five Ways to Wellbeing takes a salutogenic approach.

Box 7.6 Five Ways to Wellbeing

There are five evidence-based actions that can improve personal wellbeing.

"*Connect*
Connect with the people around you. With family, friends, colleagues and neighbours. At home, school or in your local community. Think of these as the cornerstones of your life and invest time in developing them. Building these connections will support and enrich you every day.

Be active
Go for a walk or run. Step outside. Cycle. Play a game. Garden. Dance. Exercising makes you feel good. Most importantly, discover a physical activity you enjoy and that suits your level of mobility and fitness.

Take notice
Be curious. Catch sight of the beautiful. Remark on the unusual. Notice the changing seasons. Savour the moment, whether you are walking to work, eating lunch or talking to friends. Be aware of the world around you and what you are feeling. Reflecting on your experiences will help you appreciate what matters to you.

Keep learning
Try something new. Rediscover an old interest. Sign up for that course. Take on a different responsibility at work. Fix a bike. Learn to play an instrument or how to cook your favourite food. Set a challenge you will enjoy achieving. Learning new things will make you more confident as well as being fun.

Give

Do something nice for a friend, or a stranger. Thank someone. Smile. Volunteer your time. Join a community group. Look out, as well as in. Seeing yourself, and your happiness, linked to the wider community can be incredibly rewarding and creates connections with the people around you."

(Source: Aked *et al.*, 2008, p. ii. Reproduced with permission from New Economics Foundation)

Box 7.7 Becoming a good listener

You are speaking and someone is listening. Tick the behaviours which you would find rewarding or encouraging in your listener. Put a cross next to the ones you would find off-putting or discouraging.

> Fiddles with papers
> Calm manner
> Sits on same level as you
> Bounces a leg
> Waves arms
> Voice is easy to hear
> Leans far back
> Their head is very close to yours
> Stares at you
> Tugs at their ear
> Looks towards you
> Looks clean
> Speaks at a comfortable pace
> Has a high-pitched voice
> Looks out of the window
> Relaxed seating position
> Slouches
> Body posture is open to you
> Shuffles about
> Raises an eyebrow
> Looks alert
> Sits higher than you
> Whispers
> Looks anxious
> Shuts eyes
> Leans slightly towards you
> Has vacant look
> Has warmth in voice

Consider whether you think you have behaviours which may discourage others from talking to you. Discuss the exercise with others.

(Source: Adapted from Nelson-Jones, 1986, p. 149)

Pros and cons of the educational model

The educational model engages people with a variety of methods, or personalised methods, to foster the effective and deep learning needed for true comprehension, reflection and the ability to prioritise and choose. It encourages the learner to practice thinking and communication skills so they can critically evaluate what is right for their health, to communicate it and be autonomous. These skills can be transferred to other aspects of their life and to wider society. A democratic, evolving society welcomes independent thinking and rational critique. However, learning is more time consuming than simple instruction and a manager may not pay for such time. The educator may struggle to fully accept a person's free and informed choice as different from the one they would advocate based on their own knowledge, experience and values. Fully accepting another person's own decision is an act of humility not all can achieve. It may conflict with the desired outcomes of those who fund the education. It may be tempting, and not uncommon, for the educator to slip into the preventive model of health education.

> *The educational model is where the educator understands that the 'process of learning' and 'health' are both holistic and mutually reinforcing concepts. The aim is to enable people to make free and fully informed choices by facilitating their learning.*

Empowerment model

Empowerment is a form of learning where the educator facilitates learning in a way that gives more power to the learner, moving beyond making choices to having the confidence and abilities to make changes.

- *Facilitation* means providing a suitable, safe, nurturing, well-resourced, learning environment which includes resources and then supporting a person's choices about their learning, e.g. what they learn, how they learn and what successful learning means to them
- *Enablement* means providing a person with the power, opportunities, knowledge, confidence, resources and/or abilities to achieve something
- *Self-empowerment* is where an individual has a genuine potential to make their own choices because they have a relatively high degree of actual power, realistically-based good self-esteem and a range of life skills

(Green *et al.*, 2019)

It is summed up in a variation of the proverb:

> If you give someone a fish, they will eat for one day. If you teach someone to fish they will eat for a lifetime (enablement). If, in addition, someone has negotiated and gained permanent rights to fishing in an area, they can confidently feed themselves and others for a lifetime (empowerment)

- *Community empowerment* comprises a series of organized, community-led social and political actions to challenge social injustice and to redistribute power and resources

(Green *et al.*, 2019)

The naturalist view of education, based on the assumption that human nature is naturally good, gained popularity in the late 1960s and 1970s amid concerns about professional power, both in medicine and in education. Ivan Illich (1971;1976) argued professional institutions and mantras about what should be learnt and how people should behave seemed to be eroding people's rights to feel free to learn and to direct their own health journeys. Illich was not alone. The international community endorsed the *Declaration of Alma Ata* (WHO, 1978) which stated that people had a right and a duty to participate in their healthcare, the world united behind the *Health for All* movement (WHO, 1981), and Carl Rogers argued the case for his person-centred counselling and wrote about 'freedom to learn' within a person-centred approach to education (Rogers, 1983).

In 1957, Carl Rogers proposed the necessary conditions that enable a person to reach their full potential, their true self. This humanistic concept of health is discussed in Chapter 1. There are three core conditions of person-centred counselling and person-centred education and health education.

- Congruence means that the educator is authentic, genuine and sincere in believing in the person, their ability to become self-directing, gain insight and make progress towards their concept of fulfilment. It means respecting, valuing and giving power to the person
- Acceptance means having an unconditional, positive, non-judgemental attitude towards the person. This allows the person to drop their natural defensiveness and be who they really are, to express their true self and allow it to be strengthened, and then to be able to make the choices that are right for them
- Empathy means stepping into the person's shoes, seeing the world from their perspective and reflecting this back to them. This validates the person's thoughts, feelings and experiences. It helps them to feel safe, fully understood and accepted

In practice, a person-centred, empowering approach to health education means that the learner is encouraged to lead, to be active and to fully participate in this joint endeavour of learning. The educator facilitates the learning process by

- creating a supportive environment which includes access to resources
- creating a non-hierarchical, equal relationship between the educator and learner
- co-creating some ground rules, or a contract, which may include the frequency and times for learning and confidentiality boundaries
- allowing the learner to identify the issue they want to examine; it is often something that is meaningful to them at that moment, a need or an aspiration
- asking open questions that encourage thinking and reflection
- following where the learner's thoughts take them
- summarising to see if both agree on what has been discovered or where they are on the journey
- supporting the learner's ability to learn, to find out, to master an idea or a skill and to accomplish. If asked, this may include guidance about how to get started
- always believing that the learner has the capacity and capability to succeed

---

Box 7.8 Learning to recognise we have choices

Write down five things that you think you should be or should do e.g. 'I should be more active' or 'I should be tidy'.

Working with a partner, read out each statement emphasising the word 'should' e.g. "I *should* be more active." After each one, your partner says, "No you *shouldn't*," convincingly (even if they don't agree).

Read out the list again, but this time substitute 'could' for 'should' e.g. "I *could* be more active." Your partner will respond, "Yes you *could* …. and you have a *choice,*" e.g. "Yes, you *could* be more active and you have a *choice.*"

When you have read out the list of 'coulds', you may repeat any statements you have difficulty accepting that you do have a choice.

Finally, choose one of the statements and add the words, "… and I choose to," e.g. "I *could* be more active and I *choose* to."

Reflect on the difference that changing 'should' to 'could' made.

(Source: adapted from Townsend, 1985, p. 25)

The educator knows they are working in a person-centred, empowering way when they receive feedback such as,

"… Your sense of humour was cheering … we all felt relaxed because you showed us your human self, not a mechanical teacher image …"

(Rogers, 1983, p. 123)

"… someone we could trust and identify as a 'sharer'. You were so perceptive and sensitive to our thoughts, and this made it all the more 'authentic' for me."

(Rogers, 1983, p. 123)

"I feel important, mature and capable of doing things on my own … I think you see me as a person with real feelings and needs, an individual. What I say and do are significant expressions from me, and you recognize this."

(Rogers, 1983, p. 124)

By facilitating the development of knowledge, insight and skills a person grows and gains more power and control over their lives and therefore their health. Life skills are particularly important for dealing effectively with the challenges of life that can damage health. Many health-related decisions and actions require skills that can be learnt. The World Health Organization (2003) suggests there are ten core life skills, or skills for health:

- self-awareness
- self-management
- critical thinking
- decision-making
- problem-solving
- empathy
- creativity
- communication
- interpersonal relationship skills
- coping with stress

Box 7.9   Being a self-empowered person

- You are able to look at yourself from the outside and believe that you are open to change
- You can use your feelings to recognise discrepancy between what you are and what you would like to be
- You have the skills to change some aspects of yourself
- You have the skills to change some aspects of the world in which you live
- You can identify the specific action steps needed to reach your aspiration
- You can implement your action plans. You can do
- You live each day knowing you have the power to assess, to re-assess, to influence and to self-direct
- You can enable others to achieve empowerment, to take charge of their lives and influence the arenas in which they are living

Underlying the concept of self-empowerment, is the belief that no matter what, there is always an alternative and we can choose.

(Source: adapted from Hopson and Scally, 1981, p. 57)

An empowering approach to health education may be the person who sits and listens to a dying relative, seeking to understand their feelings and needs, asking what they are worried about and what would help, respecting their wishes and allowing them to be in control of their life and their death. It may be the community worker who regularly attends to rough sleepers, empathically listening to their life stories and helping them to enter a relationship in which they learn to trust, to communicate, to share their concerns and identify what they need. It may be the telephone helpline where volunteers provide tailored support for each caller (Figure 7.10). If a need is met, the learner experiences the positive feedback that trust and communication can be beneficial, which encourages repetition. Their emotions are calmed, they feel valued, can think, clarify what they want, feel more in control, begin to believe choices are possible, articulate what additional knowledge or skills they need and then work towards putting their choices into action. They are better equipped to relate to people and to participate in groups. Groups can work together to lobby for change such as homeless shelters, accommodation and employment opportunities. Green and colleagues (2019) suggest that empowered individuals are more likely to

- choose to engage with services that support health
- be self-motivated to engage with disease-preventing and health-enhancing behaviours
- contribute to community action, which adds to their own individual empowerment

Community empowerment

Community empowerment is a continuum from personal action to small mutual group action, to the action of community organisations and then to action across a wider partnership which may bring about social and political action (Laverack, 2013). Social support itself is generally good for people's health and collectively people can drive forward their health-related agendas such as fighting for disability rights or

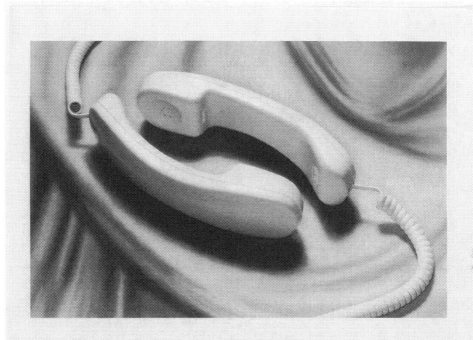

IF YOU'RE
JUST COMING OUT,
ASK A HELPLINE
ABOUT ABSOLUTELY
ANYTHING.
INCLUDING SEX.

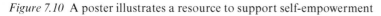

Figure 7.10 A poster illustrates a resource to support self-empowerment

Source: Health Education Authority, 1987–1995 Science Museum Group Collection made available under a CC BY 4.0 licence.

environmental sustainability. The additional skills needed to bring about environmental or social change include

- lobbying
- campaigning
- networking
- interpersonal skills and influence
- media skills
- advocacy
- policymaking

Health literacy is critical to empowerment. It means people have the cognitive and social skills to motivate and enable,

> "... individuals to gain access to, understand and use information in ways which promote and maintain good health ... it implies the achievement of a level of knowledge, personal skills and confidence to take action to improve personal and community health by changing lifestyles and living conditions ..."
>
> (WHO, 2012, pp. 61, 62)

Paulo Freire, an educator working in Brazil with the poor and illiterate in the 1960s, used community education to raise people's political consciousness. Learning to read and write was a first step to, as he saw it, regaining their full humanity and becoming aware of a social system which kept them oppressed. He argued education was inherently political because the more a person understands reality, the more they are able to change it. He prioritised reflection and action. For example, Freire set up literacy classes which he preferred to call culture circles. Led by facilitators, learners were presented with pictures or a sentence that would trigger a discussion and develop their problem-solving skills. The group may

- reflect on an aspect of their daily reality, such as limited food
- search for the root cause of the problem
- consider various solutions with their implications and consequences
- make an action plan

> (Green *et al.*, 2019)

In 1964, Friere lost his job, was interrogated, spent time in jail and was exiled from Brazil until 1980. Critical pedagogy, which his work championed, is the idea that education is never neutral and learning should build on people's own experiences, encourage critical reflection and then bring about the changes needed to reduce inequity and oppression.

Thinking point:

> Consider a group of people who meet to learn about healthier eating in an area of high deprivation.
>
> - What reflections might they share?
> - What might emerge as the main factors which influence their current eating?
> - What solutions might they suggest, and what might be the consequences?
> - What might their action plan say?
> - How might participating in this group change the participants?

Pros and cons of the empowerment model

The empowerment model aims for individuals and communities to achieve true autonomy, to reach their full potential. It emphasises active, participatory learning; building self-efficacy, that is belief in oneself to be successful, and a range of skills from life skills to community activism. This type of learning is potentially life-changing and life enhancing. It shows respect for people and their concept of health. It can encourage creative, innovative thinking and the emergence of the change-makers who are vital to an evolving democracy. Face-to-face communication, at least in formal settings, may make this type of learning time consuming and expensive though self-help and on-line resources, especially those that can be flexible and tailored to need, can help to keep costs down. In cultures that expect success to be measured in numbers, for example the number of early deaths or healthcare costs, personal accounts of feeling in control may have less value, though demonstrating the bringing about of social change is clearer to see. Educators wedded to the process of empowerment may find themselves in conflict with managers who want quick, tangible or different results based on 'absence of disease' and learners who simply want to be told what to do. Community activism can be highly motivating, but it can spawn leaders who may not accurately represent the views of all, and it can be politically contentious because it challenges those who believe in, or benefit from, the status quo.

Thinking point:

> Consider the core aims of a university or a hospital. Consider the challenges faced by a member of staff who wants to work in an empowering way with individuals.
>
> *The empowerment model is where people choose what to learn and ask an educator to facilitate their learning in the direction they choose. The aim is to develop personal insight, and the transferable knowledge and skills which can enhance their sense of personal power, their ability act and to take long-term control of their health and their lives.*

Social change model: health education becomes health promotion

The educational and empowerment models of health education gained popularity during the 1970s and 1980s alongside more holistic understandings of health. They influenced the health education practice of counsellors, health education officers, youth workers, teachers, lecturers, trades unions, consumer organisations, self-help groups, the police, drug and alcohol workers, charities, advocacy workers and some areas of health and social care. Instructing people was slowly replaced with more discussion and a respect for people's abilities to understand and make decisions for themselves. Self-help books and self-help groups multiplied. The preventive model remained strong within healthcare because it reflected the approach favoured by most of the medical profession. Most professions 'allied' to medicine broadly followed their lead. Political and social pressure to improve patients' rights (Mold, 2012) helped some healthcare professions, such as occupational therapists, hospital chaplains, palliative care nurses, midwives and health visitors to work with people in a relatively more educational and empowering way, but this could be difficult within the medical culture.

In the early 1980s, health educators, including the Health Education Council for England, Wales and Northern Ireland and the Scottish Health Education Group, became increasingly aware of the socio-economic causes of ill health. People may be informed, educated and even empowered, but many started to recognise that, against enormously powerful forces such as the tobacco industry and poverty, it was not a fair fight. Too many people were being enticed into life-long nicotine addiction and even more were destined to experience poorer health and a shorter life due to being born into poorer circumstances than others (Black *et al.*, 1982). These social determinants of health were significant drivers behind stark inequalities in health. They were socially unjust. This new knowledge undermined the notion that health-related behaviours were always a free choice. For example, people with limited income had no choice but to buy the cheap high-fat and sugar long-life foods which were offered in the local shops accessible by foot. As health educators focused 'upstream' to these deep underlying causes of poor health and disease, they called for governments, industries and businesses to introduce policies that would 'make healthy choices easier choices'. This model was called social change (Ewles and Simnett, 1985). Policies may be broad guidelines within which decisions and actions are taken; others may become finalised as

- workplace rules
- occupational health standards
- safeguarding procedures
- food hygiene standards
- the Equality Act 2010
- sugar tax
- banning types of advertising
- town planning
- banning sales of petrol and diesel cars by 2030 in the UK
- legal enforcement of COVID-19 coronavirus regulations

Pros and cons of the social change model

In a democracy, a new policy may come about through the 'bottom up' empowerment model. People get together, sign petitions, lobby for change in the workplace or vote for their government. At the point this is agreed, it becomes a 'top down' intervention. A policy is imposed on people and there may be sanctions for disobedience. Policies can 'make healthy choices easier choices', which can help to improve the health of the most disadvantaged and reduce health inequalities. However, we need to consider who the policymakers are and their agenda. They may have vested interests, they may not truly represent the majority and disregarding the views of the minority may have undesirable consequences. Policymakers may be authoritarian leaders who use coercion to enforce their vision of a healthy society. The 'healthy' choice may become the 'only' choice (Green *et al.*, 2019).

Health promotion

The action of planning and implementing a policy may change someone's experience of an environment, but is a policy an 'intentional activity designed to achieve health or illness related learning' to 'change a person's capability or disposition'? Was this health *education*? It was widely agreed that it was not. However, if we make the setting, that is the place and culture, conducive to making 'healthy choices easier choices', it becomes much easier for the people who live and work there to experience health, to learn about health and to make genuine, free, autonomous choices about their health. The setting and the learning are synergistic; one enhances the other. Keith Tones (Green *et al.*, 2019) summarised this in his formula:

$$\text{health promotion} = \text{health education} \times \text{healthy public policy}$$

In other words,

$$\text{health promotion} = \text{health education (preventive, educational and empowerment)} \times \text{social change}$$

Like the Victorians and Edwardians, we need both health education and a healthy social and physical environment to work together if we are to prevent disease and enhance people's health. We called this health promotion. We kept the three models, added social change, and called them four models of health promotion.

- Preventive model of health promotion
- Educational model of health promotion
- Empowerment model of health promotion
- Social change model of health promotion

Summary

This chapter has

- outlined the origins of educating the public about health using propaganda, coercion and instruction
- examined modern health education as three models: preventive, educational and empowerment
- defined learning processes such as persuasion, training, education, enablement and empowerment
- demonstrated how the process of learning determines whether the educator keeps or gives away power to the learner
- explained why health education became augmented into health promotion in the 1980s

Further reading

Green, J., Cross, R., Woodall, J. and Tones, K. (2019) *Health promotion. Planning and strategies.* 4th edn. London: Sage

Mittlemark, M.B., Sagy, S., Eriksson, M., Bauer, G.F., Pelikan, J.M., Lindström, B. and Espnes, G.A. (eds) (2015) *The handbook of salutogenesis.* New York: Springer

World Health Organization (2012) *Health education: theoretical concepts, effective strategies and core competencies.* Cairo: World Health Organization

Useful websites

European Commission *EPALE – Electronic Platform for Adult Learning in Europe: Life skills.* Available at: https://epale.ec.europa.eu/en/themes/life-skills
NHS *Health A to Z.* Available at: https://www.nhs.uk/conditions
World Health Organization *Health promotion.* Available at: https://www.who.int/health-topics/health-promotion

References

Aked, J., Marks, N., Cordon, C. and Thompson, S. (2008) *Five ways to wellbeing: a report presented to the foresight project on communicating the evidence base for improving people's well-being.* London: New Economics Foundation. Available at: https://neweconomics.org/2008/10/five-ways-to-wellbeing (Accessed 29th May 2022)
Antonovsky, A. (1987) *Unravelling the mysteries of health. How people manage stress and stay well.* San Francisco: Jossey-Bass
Black, D., Morris, J.N., Smith, C. and Townsend, P. (1982) 'The Black report', in Townsend, P., Davidson, N. and Whitehead, M. (eds) *Inequalities in health.* London: Penguin, pp. 29–213
Blythe, M. (1987) *A history of the central council for health education, 1927–1968.* Dissertation submitted for the Degree of doctor of philosophy. Faculty of Modern History University of Oxford Available at: https://ora.ox.ac.uk/objects/uuid:b6e412ea-c4de-4029-bf3f-5ec41cc9dc17 (Accessed 29th May 2022)
Cancer Research UK (2014) *Be clear on cancer evaluation update 2014.* Available at: https://www.cancerresearchuk.org/sites/default/files/evaluation_results_2014.pdf (Accessed 29th May 2022)
Cancer Research UK (2021) *Be clear on cancer.* Available at: https://www.cancerresearchuk.org/health-professional/awareness-and-prevention/be-clear-on-cancer (Accessed 29th May 2022)
Collins dictionary (2021) *Definition of 'disease'.* Available at: https://www.collinsdictionary.com/dictionary/english/disease (Accessed 29th May 2022)
Davin, A. (1978) 'Imperialism and motherhood', *History Workshop,* 5, pp. 9–65
Eriksson, M. (2017) 'The sense of coherence in the salutogenic model of health', in Mittlemark, M.B., Sagy, S., Eriksson, M., Bauer, G.F., Pelikan, J.M., Lindström, B. and Espnes, G.A. (eds) *The handbook of salutogenesis.* New York: Springer, pp. 91–96
Ewles, L. and Simnett, I. (1985) *Promoting health. A practical guide to health education.* Chichester: John Wiley
Faculty of Public Health and Mental Health Foundation (2016) *Better mental health for all. A public health approach to mental health improvement.* London: Faculty of Public Health and Mental Health Foundation
Family Links: The Centre for Emotional Health (2018) *Emotional health at work: why it matters and how you can support it.* London: Family Links: The Centre for Emotional Health and Institute for Public Policy Research
Fee, E. and Brown, T.M. (2005) 'The Public Health Act of 1848', *Bulletin of the World Health Organization,* 83(1), pp. 866–867
Green, J., Cross, R., Woodall, J. and Tones, K. (2019) *Health promotion. Planning and strategies.* 4th edn. London: Sage
Hamlin, C. and Sheard, S. (1998) 'Revolutions in public health: 1848, and 1998?', *BMJ,* 317(7158), pp. 587–591
Haynes, J.R. (2006) *Sanitary ladies and friendly visitors: women public health officers in London, 1890–1930.* Submitted for degree of PhD, University of London. Available at: www.semanticscholar.org/paper/sanitary-ladies-and-friendly-visitors-%3A-women-in-Haynes/2844c-faac3782d83e862b3e1850cb636d388697e (Accessed 29th May 2022)
Holdsworth, A. (1988) *Out of the doll's house.* London: BBC Books.
Hopson, B. and Scally, M. (1981) *Lifeskills teaching.* Maidenhead: McGraw-Hill
Illich., I. (1971) *Deschooling society.* New York: Harper and Row

Illich, I. (1976) *Limits to medicine. Medical nemesis: the expropriation of health.* London: Marion Boyars

Jensen, B.B., Dür, W. and Buijs, G. (2017) 'The application of salutogenesis in schools', in Mittlemark, M.B., Sagy, S., Eriksson, M., Bauer, G.F., Pelikan, J.M., Lindström, B. and Espnes, G.A. (eds) *The handbook of salutogenesis.* New York: Springer, pp. 225–235

Ladies Sanitary Association (1850) *The sick child's cry: and other household verses on health and happiness.* London: The Ladies' Sanitary Association

Laverack, G. (2013) *Health activism. Foundations and strategies.* London: Sage

Minkowski, W.L. (1992) 'Women healers of the middle ages: selected aspects of history', *American Journal of Public Health*, 82(2), pp. 288–295

Mold, A. (2012) 'Patients' rights and the National Health Service in Britain, 1960s–1980s', *American Journal of Public Health*, 102(11) doi:10.2105/AJPH.2012.300728

Naidoo, J. and Wills, J. (2009) *Foundations for health promotion.* London: Elsevier

National Archives (undated) *Catalogue description: Central Council for Health Education: Minutes and Papers.* Available at: https://discovery.nationalarchives.gov.uk/details/r/C10925 (Accessed 29th May 2022)

National Records of Scotland (2020) *Catalogue description: infectious diseases and public health files. 1843–1974.* Available at: https://www.nrscotland.gov.uk/research/catalogues-and-indexes (Accessed 29th May 2022)

Nelson-Jones, R. (1986) *Human relationship skills. Training and self-help.* London: Cassell

Oakley, A. (1980) *Women confined: towards a sociology of childbirth.* Oxford: Martin Robinson

PSHE Association (2014) *Ten principles of PSHE education.* Available at: https://www.ghll.org.uk/Ten%20Principles%20of%20PSHE%20Education.pdf (Accessed 29th May 2022)

Robinson, S. (2021) 'Social context of health and illness', in Robinson, S. (ed) *Priorities for health promotion and public health.* London: Routledge, pp. 3–33

Rogers, C.R. (1957) 'The necessary and sufficient conditions of therapeutic personality change', *Journal of Consulting Psychology*, 21(2), pp. 95–103

Rogers, C. (1983) *Freedom to learn for the 80s.* Columbus, Ohio: Merrill

Scriven, A. (2017) *Ewles and Simnett's promoting health. A practical guide.* London: Elsevier

Smith, B.J., Tang, C.T. and Nutbeam, D. (2006) 'WHO health promotion glossary: new terms', *Health Promotion International*, 21(4), pp. 340–345

Sutherland, I. (1987) 'History and background', in Sutherland, I. (ed) *Health education. Perspectives and choices.* London: NEC publications, pp. 1–19

Tones, K. and Tilford, S. (1994) *Health education: effectiveness, efficiency and equity.* London: Chapman Hall

Townsend, A. (1985) *Assertion training.* London: Family Planning Association Education Unit

Ussher, J. (1991) *Women's madness: misogyny or mental illness?* London: Harvester Wheatsheaf

Warne, S. (undated) *How to survive and illness – and begin to live.* Swansea: West Glamorgan Health Authority

Weare, K. (1992) 'The contribution of education to health promotion', in Bunton, R. and Macdonald, G. (eds) *Health promotion. Disciplines and diversity.* London: Routledge, pp. 66–85

Weare, K. (2019) 'Mindfulness and contemplative approaches in education', *Current Opinion in Psychology*, 28, pp. 321–326

Wolfe, R.M. and Sharp, L.K. (2002) 'Anti-vaccinationists past and present', *BJM*, 325(7361), pp. 430–432

World Health Organization (1978) *Declaration of Alma-Ata.* Available at: https://cdn.who.int/media/docs/default-source/documents/almaata-declaration-en.pdf?sfvrsn=7b3c2167_2 (Accessed 29th May 2022)

World Health Organization (1981) *Global strategy for health for all by the year 2000.* Geneva: World Health Organization

World Health Organization (2003) *Skills for health.* Geneva: World Health Organization

World Health Organization (2012) *Health education: theoretical concepts, effective strategies and core competencies.* Cairo: World Health Organization

8 Health promotion

Sally Robinson

Key points

- Introduction
- Health promotion models
- Ottawa Charter for Health Promotion
- Core characteristics of health promotion
- Planning health promotion for individuals, groups or communities
- Health promotion and public health
- Summary

Introduction

This chapter needs to be read alongside, preferably after, Chapter 7 because health promotion emerged from and augmented health education. In summary, health education is

- about fostering health-related learning, which may result from coercion, propaganda, indoctrination, instruction, training, education, facilitation, enablement, self-empowerment and community empowerment
- is concerned with disease prevention and salutogenesis across the whole health continuum (Figure 7.6, Table 7.1)
- about health-related awareness, knowledge, beliefs, self-awareness, attitudes, values, motivations, decisions, skills and behaviour
- is practised by many practitioners across a wide range of sectors and millions of individuals every day
- is at the heart of health promotion (Figure 8.1). Without it, we are left with policies designed for compliance. These neither enable nor empower people to make informed, free choices and actions

This chapter adds to these by explaining the four models of health promotion, the *Ottawa Charter for Health Promotion*, some additional characteristics of health promotion and how we approach planning health promotion for individuals, groups and communities.

DOI: 10.4324/9780367823696-10

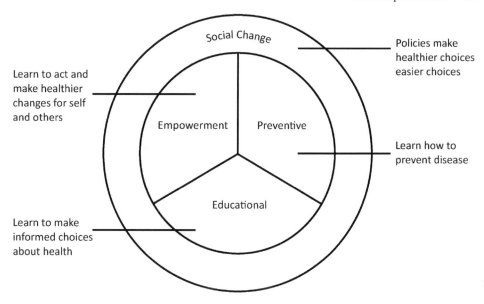

Figure 8.1 Health promotion comprises four models

Health promotion models

Much health promotion is about health education, a process of learning, to which we add policy because policy can help 'healthy choices to become easier choices' for people. If the policy enables people to live and work in a healthy environment, such as one that sells fruit and vegetables at a cheaper price than chocolate, then people are more easily able to put their healthy choices into action, should they wish to do so (Figure 8.1). Health promotion can be described as comprising four models, communication processes, where the first three are educational and the fourth, social change, is about making or changing policies.

- Preventive model, which includes the medical approach and the behaviour change approach
- Educational model
- Empowerment model
- Social change model

> Health promotion = health education (preventive, educational and empowerment)
> × social change

These health promotion models have slightly different names, according to different authors (Table 8.1). People have different views about which model they prefer. Often, these are influenced by their own vision of health, which means their values and their understanding of what health and a healthy society look like, as discussed in Chapter 1. Also, these are influenced by their own experiences as citizens, educators, policymakers, clients, students, patients or customers. We have described and discussed the pros and cons of each model in Chapter 7.

Table 8.1 Models of health promotion

	Preventive		Educational	Empowerment	Social change
	Medical	Behaviour change			
Naidoo and Wills (2016)	Medical	Behaviour change	Educational	Empowerment	Social change
Scriven (2017)	Medical	Behaviour change	Educational	Client-centred	Societal change
Beattie (1991)	Individual risk-reduction		Personal counselling	Community development	Social advocacy
Green *et al.* (2019)	Preventive		Empowerment		Healthy public policy
Direction of communication	Top down, one-way, expert leads		Side to side, two way, educator leads	Bottom up, two way, learner leads	Top-down, policymaker leads
Role of client	Compliance	Compliance	Active, questioning, decision-making	Active, questioning, personal reflection, decision-making, action	Compliance
Aim	Absence of disease due to compliance with screening or treatment	Adoption of healthy behaviour to prevent disease	Autonomy, people make informed choices about their health	Autonomy and empowerment, people have the knowledge and skills to take control of their health and reach their full potential	Make healthy choices easier choices through policy changes

Thinking point:

Consider which health promotion model best reflects the dominant way in which you would like to work with

- an individual who is at an increased risk of developing cardiovascular disease
- a couple stuck in a mutually abusive relationship
- a family living in poverty and hunger
- a large population during a pandemic

Try to identify the values and beliefs about health that underpin your choices.

Box 8.1 How health promotion models work together

Scenario A An expert tells Ricky that his cancer may return if he continues to drink large amounts of alcohol (preventive). Ricky looks at the Alcohol Education Trust website and discusses his thoughts and concerns with three friends. Ricky makes an informed choice to decrease his drinking (educational). Six months later, Ricky becomes aware of how easy it is to drink large amounts of cheap and accessible alcohol. Ricky and his friends start to lobby the supermarkets to increase their prices. This develops into a national movement (empowerment). The supermarkets agree to increase alcohol prices (social change). Alcohol sales fall and, after some time, so do the number of alcohol-related cancers.

Scenario B In 2020, during the COVID-19 coronavirus pandemic, the law stated that face coverings must be worn in indoor spaces to prevent the transmission of the virus across the UK (social change). In July 2021, the wearing of face coverings became a free choice (educational) in England, while in Scotland it remained mandatory (social change). Meanwhile, the scientists continued to warn that the virus spread most efficiently from person to person within the air of crowded indoor spaces. They strongly encouraged people to wear face coverings (preventive). There was much debate across the UK about whether face coverings should be mandatory (social change) or an informed choice (educational). Another debate was whether those who did not wear a face covering were making an uninformed choice or an informed choice.

Models of health promotion reflect the ways in which we promote people's health using communication, education and/or social change.

Ottawa Charter for Health Promotion

In 1986, the international community signed the *Ottawa Charter for Health Promotion*. Health promotion was described as a new type of public health, it set out how the world could work to meet the World Health Organization's *Global Strategy for Health for All by the Year 2000* (WHO, 1981). An accumulation of evidence showed

- people's experience of health and illness was influenced by much more than genetics, germs, malfunctions within the body and the healthcare system
- it was also shaped by people's health-related behaviours such as smoking
- these behaviours were shaped by the wider social, economic and cultural environment
- these social determinants of health affected people psychologically, socially and biologically and largely determined who kept healthy for most of their life, who developed disease and who died early, e.g. the poor
- inequalities in health, that is, 'the cards being stacked in favour or against' some people from before birth and throughout their life was unfair; it was a major social injustice
- reducing inequities (unfair inequalities) in health required government leadership and partnerships across all sectors, not merely the healthcare system, though this system needed reform to play its part

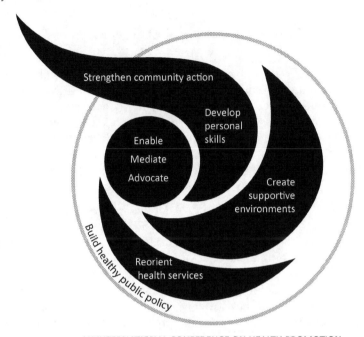

AN INTERNATIONAL CONFERENCE ON HEALTH PROMOTION
The move towards a new public health
November 17-21, 1986 Ottawa, Ontario, Canada

Figure 8.2 Ottawa Charter for Health Promotion

Source: WHO, 1986. Reproduced with permission from the World Health Organization

Jake Epp, a Canadian minister for health, was aware of the World Health Organization's *Global Strategy for Health for All by the Year 2000* (WHO, 1981) and produced his model for *Achieving Health for All: A Framework for Health Promotion* in early 1986 (Epp, 1986). He called it a 'new vision of health'. He recognised that both education and empowerment for individuals and communities were important, but if we were to reduce health inequities, more attention needed to be given to communities and to partnerships working alongside public policies that would create healthy settings/environments in which people could live and work. His work influenced the main points of the Ottawa Charter (Figure 8.2).

The Ottawa Charter states,

> "Health promotion is the process of enabling people to increase control over, and to improve, their health. To reach a state of complete physical, mental and social wellbeing, an individual or group must be able to identify and realize aspirations, to satisfy needs, and to change or cope with the environment. Health is, therefore, seen as a resource for everyday life, not the objective of living. Health is a positive concept emphasizing social and personal resources, as well as physical capacities. Therefore, health promotion is not just the responsibility of the health sector but goes beyond healthy lifestyles to wellbeing."
>
> (WHO, 1986, p. 1. Reproduced with permission from the
> World Health Organization Europe)

The Charter identifies the prerequisites for health as

- peace
- shelter
- food
- income
- education
- sustainable resources
- a stable ecosystem
- social justice and equity

It identifies three strategies for promoting health

- *Advocacy* – we must advocate for health because it is vital for personal, social and economic development. We need to make the biological, behavioural, social, cultural, political, economic and environmental factors favourable to health
- *Enablement* – people need to be able to take control over the factors that affect their health if they are to reach their fullest health potential. This includes ensuring people have equal opportunities and health equity
- *Mediation* – we need coordinated action for health by governments; the health, social and economic sectors; non-governmental and voluntary organisations; industry, local authorities and media. We need to involve professionals, social groups, individuals, families and communities. Health promotion needs to be flexible and adapted to local needs and systems

The Charter identifies five areas for action.

- Build healthy public policy, e.g. legal and tax measures that foster equity, policies to assure safe and healthier goods and services, and policies to support healthy environments which 'make the healthy choice the easier choice'
  This reflects the social change model of health promotion and the importance of reducing health inequities.
- Create supportive environments, e.g. we need to work together to conserve natural resources and make places where people live and work healthy, safe and enjoyable
  This reflects the social change model of health promotion, partnership working and sustainability.
- Strengthen community action, e.g. allowing communities ownership and control of their endeavours and destinies through community development and empowerment. This includes public participation, social support, learning opportunities and funding
  This reflects the empowerment model of health promotion, partnership working, health literacy and community empowerment.
- Develop personal skills, e.g. information, education and enhancing life skills, because these enable people to make informed choices about their health and to take control over their environment
  This reflects the educational and empowerment models of health promotion and health literacy.

Table 8.2 Global conferences on health promotion

Each conference includes a re-commitment to the 'Health for All' movement and to health promotion, as set out in the Ottawa Charter

			Main focus
1st	1986	Ottawa, Canada	Defined health promotion and its purpose in terms of strategies and five core areas of action to achieve 'health for all'
2nd	1988	Adelaide, Australia	Building healthy public policy as a means to achieving health and equity; health is a human right
3rd	1991	Sundsvall, Sweden	Supportive environments and sustainable development
4th	1997	Jakarta, Indonesia	Promote social responsibility for health; increase investment in health development; partnerships; community empowerment; settings for health as the core infrastructure for health promotion; formation of a global health promotion alliance
5th	2000	Mexico City	How to achieve health equity, strengthen the evidence-base of health promotion, strengthen political skills and actions for health promotion, a framework for countrywide plans for action on health promotion
6th	2005	Bangkok, Thailand	*The Bangkok Charter for Health Promotion in a Globalised World*, health promotion needs to be central to global development and foreign policy and is the responsibility of governments, communities, civil society and the private sector
7th	2009	Nairobi, Kenya	*Nairobi Call to Action*, urgency of health promotion becoming part of mainstream policy, financial crisis, global warming, non-communicable diseases. Community empowerment and the application of knowledge
8th	2013	Helsinki, Finland	*Health in All Policies*, intersectoral collaboration, health and equity as a political priority
9th	2016	Shanghai, China	*Shanghai Declaration on Promoting Health in the 2030 Agenda for Sustainable Development*
10th	2021	Virtual event and Geneva, Switzerland	*Geneva Charter for Well-being* calls for policies which: • support a positive vision of health which integrates physical, mental, spiritual and social wellbeing • are based on human rights, justice, solidarity, inter-generational and gender equity and peace • are committed to sustainability and respect humans and nature • measure success in ways that include human and planetary wellbeing, not merely gross domestic product • focus on empowerment, inclusivity, equity and meaningful participation

- Reorient the health services, e.g. move beyond healthcare, clinical and curative services, and include the pursuit of health. This means being more culturally sensitive, working with other sectors, supporting health- (in addition to disease-) related research and professional education, as well as working with the needs of an individual as a whole person

    This reflects the social change model of health promotion, the role of policy and partnership working.

The Charter says,

"Health is created and lived by people within settings of their everyday life: where they learn, work, play and love. Health is created by caring for oneself and others, by being able to take decisions and have control over one's life circumstances, and by ensuring that the society one lives in creates conditions that allow the attainment of health ... Caring, holism and ecology are essential issues in developing strategies for health promotion. Therefore ... in each phase of planning, implementation and evaluation of health promotion activities, women and men should become equal partners."

(WHO, 1986, p. 2. Reproduced with permission from the World Health Organization Europe)

This demonstrates the introduction of the 'settings approach' to health promotion and equity.

Health promotion is the way in which the World Health Organization believes we can achieve 'health for all' people across the world. The Ottawa Charter clarified the aims, scope and broad principles of health promotion. It created international cohesion and a clear direction. This has continued through further global health promotion conferences (Table 8.2).

The Ottawa Charter for Health Promotion explained the purpose and scope of health promotion as the recipe for how the world may achieve 'health for all'. It remains at the heart of the World Health Organization's mission and subsequent international agreements which guide national policies.

Core characteristics of health promotion

Health promotion is a concept, a discipline, a movement and a profession (Green *et al.*, 2019). It has several characteristics, which we discussed in Chapters 1 and 7:

- verbal, written, visual or non-verbal communication
- a view of health that is holistic, a human right, personal, a collective endeavour and symbiotically linked to global sustainable development, equity and social justice
- the whole health continuum
- individuals, families, communities and populations across their life course
- disease prevention (communicable and non-communicable)
- salutogenesis, the enhancement of health
- autonomy, enablement and empowerment
- a holistic process of learning to develop health-related understanding, self-awareness, social-awareness, motivation and skills

Table 8.3 Political ideologies

	Liberalism/liberal democracy	Socialism	Conservatism
People	People are unique and capable individuals who need to be free to grow and fulfil their potential. Individuals are equal. Individuals have the right to make free choices about how they want to live provided this doesn't limit someone else's liberty.	People are bound together by what they have in common and their common goals. As people are shaped by their social experiences, they are inseparable from society.	People are creatures of habit who will give up some freedom to gain familiarity and security. People are imperfect, so regulation, such as the law, needs to provide deterrents against anti-social behaviour.
Society	Society is tolerant; it accepts differences of ideas and views. Individuals need to pursue common goals for a good society.	The collective group is powerful and can overcome social and economic problems. Equality of opportunity is central.	Society comprises individuals. Pragmatic approach that rejects ideology or abstract notions, such as rights or social justice, that seek to shape society.
Government	There needs to be a limited government/ state, ideally devolved to local communities, to act as a referee between individuals to prevent exploitation.	Assets, such as property, may be 'nationalised'/ owned by the state to benefit society and the disadvantaged.	Practical, looking for what works in a particular situation, often learning from the past. Seeks to minimise change and or to make changes with minimum disruption – 'change to conserve'.
Economy	Supports capitalism/the market, but some regulation is required to promote social justice and equality.	Seeks alternatives to capitalism, aims to reduce divisions and inequalities in society.	Supports capitalism/the market. Neoconservatives believe the market will deliver all goods and services if left alone. Others believe some state intervention is needed to support the vulnerable.
Preferred approach to health promotion	Individual and community empowerment Autonomy	Legislation and policies to improve equality Advocacy Activism for the disadvantaged	Individual responsibility Informed choice Autonomy

In addition, it is concerned with

- politics of health promotion
- ethics of health promotion
- building healthy public policy
- working in partnerships
- strengthening community action

- settings: creating supportive environments
- reorienting the healthcare services

We will discuss each of these.

Politics of health promotion

Health promotion is political because it concerns power. For example, health outcomes are influenced by

- the distribution of resources, who can access or afford health, e.g. prices and the costs of transport, care, wages and welfare
- the giving or withholding of education including health-related learning
- economic and social inequalities, e.g. social inclusion/exclusion and discrimination
- local, national and international government policies
- big business and global capitalism
- the balance of state control/legislation versus personal control and individual choices
- the collective needs of the group/society versus the needs of the individual
- the social and economic value placed on different health-related professions, disciplines and types of knowledge compared to others

Thinking point:

> Recall the model(s) of health promotion you preferred, above. Now identify which political ideology (Table 8.3), best reflects your views. If you had the political power to influence a community of people, what guiding principles would be informing your policies?

Ethics of health promotion

If the aim is to bring about better health in ways that protect and enhance individuals' power and to reduce health inequities, those who work in health promotion need to be constantly mindful of working in an ethical manner (Box 8.2). The four core ethical principles are

- respect for autonomy – respecting people as autonomous beings with the capacity to make their own decisions and informed choices
- beneficence – acting in ways that balance the costs of the intervention against the benefits and acting in ways that benefit people
- non-maleficence – the intervention should avoid harm, and if it involves some harm it should be minimal and not disproportionate to the benefits
- justice – a fair distribution of the risks and costs; similar people being treated in a similar way

(Beauchamp and Childress, 2001)

Building healthy public policy

The term 'policy' includes clarifying values that guide decisions, actions or inaction. Policymaking is a process of bringing expertise to a problem or a goal, setting priorities, setting agendas, identifying necessary resources, making decisions, and then developing guidelines, codes, projects, rules or legislation. Policymaking brings order

Box 8.2 Ethical health promotion practice

"Ethical health promotion practice is based on a commitment to

- health as a human right, which is central to human development
- respect for the rights, dignity, confidentiality and worth of individuals and groups
- respect for all aspects of diversity including gender, sexual orientation, age, religion, disability, ethnicity, race and cultural beliefs
- addressing health inequities, social justice and prioritising the needs of those experiencing poverty and social marginalisation
- addressing the political, economic, social, cultural, environmental, behavioural and biological determinants of health and wellbeing
- ensuring that health promotion action is beneficial and causes no harm
- being honest about what health promotion is and what it can and cannot achieve
- seeking the best available information and evidence needed to implement effective policies and programmes that influence health
- collaboration and partnership as the basis for health promotion action
- the empowerment of individuals and groups to build autonomy and self-respect as the basis for health promotion action
- sustainable development and sustainable health promotion action
- being accountable for the quality of one's own practice and taking responsibility for maintaining and improving knowledge and skills."

(Source: IUHPE, 2016, p. 6. Reproduced with permission from IUHPE)

and direction over the medium or longer term. In the context of health promotion, policies are often associated with the social change model, they seek to address underlying social and environmental determinants of health and make the 'healthy choice the easier choice'. As these determinants are located with sectors such as housing, employment, education, transport and the private and the voluntary sectors, we are more likely to achieve healthy public policy where sectors collaborate. Who makes policies, how they are made, what they seek to do, and how they are received and acted upon are closely tied to power, politics and ethics.

Health in All Policies

Health in All Policies is an international approach that encourages all policymakers to

- think through the health implications of a proposed policy, whether it could be health enhancing or health harming
- encourage synergies, that is joint policies which can have a greater health promoting impact than separate ones
- consider how all public policies impact on the underlying social and environmental determinants of people's health

(WHO, 2014)

Health impact assessments and environmental impact assessments are structured ways of identifying, predicting and evaluating the impact of a policy, plan or project on the health of a population or on the natural environment (see Chapter 9).

Partnership working

Working in partnerships, or alliances, with others implies working in an equal, non-hierarchical way. Partnerships may

- provide a more holistic and comprehensive understanding of the core issue
- utilise a broad range of expertise
- contribute to participants' learning and empowerment
- pool resources such as skills, knowledge, equipment and networks
- encourage a more efficient and effective use of resources
- break down barriers between sectors, professionals, agencies and people who live in the local community
- speed up communications and reduce bureaucracy between partners
- enable more ambitious projects, such addressing the underlying causes of poor health rather than individual symptoms and behaviours
- share the risks and rewards of a new, innovative endeavour
- reduce conflicting and confusing information as the partnership unites behind a consistent narrative to present to others

Partnerships may be based around types of expertise, resources, a geographical area or a network. They may be

- intersectoral, e.g. voluntary sector, private sector and public sector; or the housing sector, environment sector and care sector
- interagency/multi-agency, e.g. organisations and/or services such as the police, social services, district nursing, a charity and a local business
- interdisciplinary/multi-disciplinary, e.g. science, humanities and social science; or combinations of expertise in interdisciplinary applied subjects such as education, health and criminology
- interprofessional/multi-professional, e.g. an occupational therapist, geriatric nurse, geriatrician, social worker and a hospital chaplain
- a team, e.g. individuals with different expertise who may work in the same organisation, community or globally

'Partnership' is a word that takes away the labels 'professional', 'discipline' and 'agency'. It is generally preferred because health promotion, with its empowering ethos, is keen to include citizens, local people, clients, patients, service users and consumers. Those who live, work or experience the health issue are encouraged to participate, to be heard and to help create solutions.

Partnerships may

- be informal or formal
- be called forums, groups, federations etc.

- concern a single issue or a multi-layered project
- concern two people or a whole community
- focus on a place, neighbourhood, town, nation or international area
- have no timetable/be open-ended or have a fixed timetable with a clear end point
- be about bonding, learning, liaison, peer support, cooperation, commissioning or delivering services, lobbying, influencing, managing, planning, coordinating policies, finance etc.
- be strategic, e.g. coordinating policies, overseeing other partnerships as they all move towards a broad goal such as sustainability or regeneration

(Naidoo and Wills, 2011)

Setting up and working in partnership is challenging. Individuals bring their own culture, interests, assets and morals, perhaps shaped by the profession in which they work, the local area in which they live or the social group with whom they identify. They speak with their own language/jargon, assume certain understandings and may find it difficult to agree on goals. They may be long-standing rivals or, quite simply, may not be prepared to listen, learn or compromise in a spirit of equality. The partnership may be no more than a bureaucratic process, an illusion, set up to please others or to 'tick a box'. It may contain significant power imbalances, such as one agency who dominates and drives its own agenda. Between them, the partners may not have the life skills, including communication, conflict resolution and shared decision-making, to build mutual trust and enable the partnership to function well.

Partnerships are more likely to work well if they

- have a clear, shared vision
- have clear leadership
- are well managed, e.g. good planning and administrative tasks being completed in a timely manner
- set out clear roles and responsibilities for each member
- enjoy formal recognition, thus the work has worth to others
- have realistic aims and time frames
- share the risk, or stake, in the process
- have sufficient time and other resources for the task
- feel connected and trusting of one another in a non-hierarchical relationship
- build on the experience and assets that each partner brings
- have the life skills to enable harmonious and constructive communication
- encourage compromise and the give and take of knowledge, skills and resources
- enable flexibility, e.g. elements of both formal and informal working
- are perceived as fair in terms of processes and outcomes
- tap into each partner's enthusiasm and commitment

(Green *et al.*, 2019)

Strengthening community action

Community action is central to health promotion, and partnerships are at the heart of community action. A virtual or real community implies people are connected by a common interest. Most people will identify with more than one community, for example

- a community outside or around an organisation, e.g. outside a hospital or nightclub
- a community within a geographical area, e.g. a neighbourhood, an area of deprivation, a village or a university campus
- a community culture, heritage or religion, e.g. Hindu, Jewish, Christian, Chinese, Black or Asian
- a social group that has common concerns or interests, e.g. being gay, elderly, a mental health service user or trans gender; having learning disabilities or being interested in environmental protection or a type of music

Needs and assets

Community action, like all health promotion, comprises both disease prevention, focussing on deficits to be addressed, and salutogenesis, focussing on strengths and the enhancement of health (see Chapter 7). When working with a community or an individual, the starting point is an assessment of their needs and assets. The word 'need' puts the onus on providing support; as opposed to 'problem', which implies a deficit. An assessment of needs may begin with Maslow's hierarchy of needs (see Chapter 1) to inform priorities. For a larger population, a formalised public health needs assessment may be carried out (see Chapter 9). For individuals, groups and communities, Bradshaw's taxonomy of needs is often used as a loose framework for informal or more formal inquiries, such as interviews, questionnaires and focus groups. Community needs assessments often include activities which aim to encourage people to express their concerns. These include taking and sharing photographs, audio or video recordings; making art works or models; asking people to rank priorities in a list, to participate in a story dialogue or to contribute to discussions. It may be carried out by an outsider or by the community themselves. There are four types of need, which can overlap (Bradshaw, 1972).

- 'Normative need' means that which is defined by an expert or a professional against a desirable standard such as being within a 'normal' range of body mass index (BMI), a 'normal' body temperature or a standard of behaviour outlined by law. These may be presented as neutral or based on objective scientific evidence, but they are not. They are influenced by values, such as those of a profession, 'experts' or scientists who may be perceived as having more influence and power than others
- 'Felt need' is what people feel they need. It is influenced by real and perceived circumstances and expectations. If people believe something is easily accessible and available to others, this felt need is likely to be inflated. It becomes what they want rather than what they really need
- 'Expressed need' means the felt need is turned into a communication, what people say or demand they need, or into an action, what they show they need
- 'Comparative need' means that some individuals are in receipt of an intervention, such as a resource, service or education, and others are not. If we are aiming for equality, the latter has a comparative need

The assessment of assets reflects the salutogenic arm of health promotion. It includes a community's knowledge, skills and resources, as well as understanding their values,

---

Box 8.3 Singing to improve community cohesion in Italy during the COVID-19 pandemic, Spring 2020

The COVID-19 coronavirus pandemic forces Italy into its first national lockdown in Spring 2020. For many people, this means having no contact with family, friends or neighbours as they stay at home to keep safe. Their joint community activities and sources of interpersonal support, their social capital, have gone. The streets fall silent. Quite spontaneously, the Italians to start singing from their windows. In some cities, they sing contemporary songs full of meaning and emotion; in other cities, they sing the old, traditional songs associated with Italian culture. At times, it is the national anthem. At the windows are animated people of all ages, enjoying this moment of emotional exchange and community cohesion. Social media sends out videos to be shared among other communities. It is as if the individuals use what they have, their identity expressed as a song, to cope with their loss of freedom and feelings of loneliness. Community singing enhances their mood and helps them to cope during these times of uncertainty.

(Source: Corvo and De Caro, 2020)

---

attitudes, motivations, capabilities and social capital. Social capital refers to the social fabric of a community. There are three types/forms/functions/dimensions of social capital, which are often used interchangeably (Claridge, 2018).

- Bonding is about connections within a community, e.g. people who have similar backgrounds, characteristics and attitudes, 'people like us', perhaps people who live within the same village
- Bridging is about connections between communities, e.g. people with different cultural or socio-economic backgrounds, people with a shared interest though they may have different social identities, perhaps people with an interest in dementia who live in different villages

---

Box 8.4 Threats to community cohesion in the UK during the COVID-19 pandemic, January 2021

The COVID-19 coronavirus pandemic, first discovered in China, is fuelling hate crimes against Chinese and other people of South Asian origin in the UK. This is due to conspiracy theories, hateful online abuse and a tendency for news outlets to use images of Asian people to illustrate stories.

A blog on Stonewall's website, the charity that campaigns for the equality of lesbian, gay, bi and trans (LGBT) people, says domestic abuse, family rejection leading to homelessness and the loss of safe spaces/venues for LGBT people are increasing during the pandemic.

There are concerns that COVID-19 guidance is not being communicated properly across communities. These include people whose first language is not English and younger people who are less engaged with mainstream media.

(Source: NPC, 2021)

- Linking is a sub-theme of bridging and is about relations with those in authority, e.g. people of different social status. Linking may be a means of accessing power, wealth or advancement

Social capital is a measure of social cohesion, which means people can focus on the shared values that join them together (Boxes 8.3 and 8.4). They feel a sense of belonging, and have a mutual understanding and tolerance of differences. It is a strong basis on which to foster community engagement with initiatives and actions which may be health promoting.

Types of community action

There are many types and definitions of community-related activity, and one important distinction is how much power and control is given over to the community (Figure 8.3). Feeling a sense of control over one's life is vital to good health. Research shows how a low sense of control is associated with greater anxiety and stress which encourage chronic low grade inflammation, the progression of cardiovascular disease and damaging health-related behaviours (Kivimäki and Steptoe, 2018; McEwen, 2008). In turn, community control, social cohesion, a sense of belonging, trust, feeling heard and being capable of contributing to change is important to community health (Marmot *et al.*, 2020). Types of community action are named and defined in ways that can overlap with one another.

Community-based (Box 8.5)

- means the community is the medium, setting or venue for intervention
- means the problem, objectives or action is defined by a person, agency or 'other'
- suggests the concept of the community seems straightforward
- focusses on a group of individuals defined by a person/expert or agency
- includes activities that are, for the most part, directly health-related

(Naidoo and Wills, 2016)

Community consultation is,

> "An exchange that enables communities to input their views. Typically, this involves sharing information with people and seeking a response which is captured and listened to."

(Public Health Wales, 2019, p. 13)

Community development

- means a community is the target of an intervention to enhance capacity, capabilities and empowerment
- is where the problem, objectives and action are defined by the community
- recognises that the concept of community is complex and ever-changing with power imbalances and conflict
- focusses on community services, policies or structures that impact on the health of the community
- includes a broad range of activities which address indirect, underlying influences on health and outcomes such as enhancing social capital or empowerment

(Naidoo and Wills, 2016, p. 169)

Box 8.5 A community-based initiative using educational and empowerment models of health promotion

Action for Community Development, in London, runs a Community Health Project to support the local ethnic minority populations. It includes culturally sensitive workshops about healthy lifestyles and provides accessible information about disease prevention and local services.

Workshops include

- Healthy heart
- Healthy eating
- Diabetes awareness
- Glaucoma awareness
- HIV/AIDS prevention
- Mental health and wellbeing

They have a drop-in centre that provides a range of services provided in partnership with local organisations. One person wrote,

> "Thankyou for listening to me, your advice was helpful. I called … the CID (criminal investigation department) police and she listened and gave me advice, she is going to contact who she can and contact the ASB (anti-social behaviour) team. I didn't know help like this was available, thanks to victim support who led me to you."

They also help local people to access services such as

- GPs
- opticians
- dentists
- mental health and emotional support services
- disability and special needs services
- sexual health, family planning, HIV/AIDS services
- child health and women's services

and they include workshops and symposiums about Black organ donations.

(Source: Action for Community Development, 2021)

Community empowerment (Box 8.6) means,

> "A community takes action – that is, participates in action to influence policy or practice at local or national level – feels that it has actually achieved something, even if the outcome is not dramatic."

(Green *et al.*, 2019, pp. 54, 55)

Michael Marmot (2010) wrote about empowering communities creating,

> "… conditions for individuals to take control of their own lives. For some communities this will mean removing structural barriers to participation, for others facilitating and developing capacity and capability through personal and community development."

(p. 34)

Box 8.6 Healthy living centres

UK healthy living centres are designed to enable communities to bring together the services and activities which best support their own local community's needs. Centres vary, but they often combine leisure opportunities; education such as English language classes, adult reading classes and basic computing; support for sexual health or drug-related concerns; primary healthcare; social care; social support; complementary therapies and a wide range of community groups such as cookery, arts and crafts and groups for older people or for those who have recently immigrated to the UK. Local people are in charge, leading and participating in what the centre offers. Healthy living centres are based on the empowerment model of health promotion.

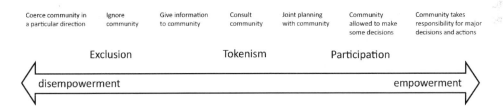

Figure 8.3 From community disempowerment to empowerment

Community empowerment fits within the empowerment model of health promotion (see Chapter 7 and Box 8.7). It rests on the premise that the more we support and enable communities, the greater their capacity to bring about the changes which improve their own health on their terms. Popay and colleagues (2020), writing about communities living in areas of deprivation, describe community empowerment as comprising an 'inward gaze' and an 'outward gaze'. An

- 'inward gaze' means the community focusses on living and working conditions in the local neighbourhood, the community's psychosocial capacities and health-related behaviours
- 'outward gaze' means the community focusses on the social and political context in which the community sits. This includes the wider social determinants of health such as employment, education and affordable food; and other forms of 'power over' such as the rules within which the community can work, the way resources are distributed and notions of what is acceptable to those with power

DIY welfare versus empowerment

Jennie Popay (2021) describes how, for many years, UK community development focussed on the deficit approach which identified community needs and sought to rectify them through a relatively disempowering process. Since 2010, the salutogenic,

---

Box 8.7 Examples of community action using an empowerment model of health promotion

Scotland passed the Community Empowerment Act in 2015. It aims to empower communities by strengthening their voices in decisions that they care about. The Scottish Development Centre is a charity that supports communities. Their work spans joint working with communities to enable communities to take full responsibility for their decisions and actions. Here are six examples of its work.

- *Scottish Co-production Network* enables those who use public services to share ideas and skills with those who run public services
- *Community Health Exchange* enables a network of community-led organisations and their public sector partners to work together to reduce health inequalities in communities across Scotland
- *Health Issues in the Community (HIIC)* provides training to enhance a community's participation, capacity and skills in relation to health, poverty, power and social justice
- *Supporting Communities* focusses on communities which face disadvantages such as poverty, being in a rural area or discrimination. It aims to build the community's confidence to develop ideas and skills to address the issues that are important to them
- *Visioning Outcomes in Community Engagement (VOiCE)* is a planning and recording computer software programme that supports communities with their reflection, planning, implementing and evaluating
- *Knowledge Is Power* supports communities to undertake research and develop their own evidence, which will be pooled to inform national policy

(Source: SCDC, 2021)

---

asset-based approaches accelerated and the phrase 'community empowerment' began to be used to reflect the greater participation and responsibility given to communities. By 2020, Popay suggests the process had gone too far and many low-income communities were being 'asset-assessed to death', a statement that was supported by an average fall in life expectancy in some lower-socio-economic groups. She argues that, since the global financial crash in 2007/08, and what was called the 'era of austerity' that followed, local groups and communities, under the political rhetoric of being empowered, were, in reality, being encouraged to fill the gaps left by depleted public services. This is summed up as 'do it yourself welfare'. Communities are sometimes encouraged to focus on the 'inward gaze' not the 'outward gaze', and this discourages the community from examining the wider social, political and economic environment in which it sits. Popay's recommendation is to promote more collective action. To achieve true community empowerment, she advocates

- 'power-within' – communities need to work to enhance their own sense of personal and psychological power; a belief in themselves and their abilities to take control
- 'power-over' – communities should take power from others, so they gain power over themselves
- 'power-with' – communities should work collectively to gain power and work towards goals. Communities with power deliberately use it to increase the power of other communities

Together, these provide the 'power to' take collective decisions and action for themselves (see Chapter 7, Box 7.1 p.158).

Settings: creating supportive environments

The Healthy Settings movement began with the Ottawa Charter. It adopts a social-ecological model of health, which means people and their setting are an ecosystem, and each element of the ecosystem plays a role in keeping the people and the setting healthy (Robinson, 2021). The setting may be social or physical, and the settings approach emphasises partnerships, community participation, equity and empowerment. In Chapter 1 (Box 1.5) we included one example of a social setting, the working culture of social workers. The World Health Organization (2022) supports the following settings:

- Healthy cities
- Healthy villages
- Healthy municipalities and communities
- Health promoting schools
- Healthy workplaces
- Healthy markets
- Healthy homes
- Healthy islands
- Health promoting hospitals and health services
- Health promoting prisons
- Health promoting universities

Healthy Cities

Healthy Cities was the first settings project, starting in 1986. It aimed to put health on the agenda of cities. It spread rapidly across Europe and then the rest of the world. Healthy cities,

> "... foster health and well-being through governance, empowerment and participation, creating urban places for equity and community prosperity, and investing in people for a peaceful planet. Healthy cities lead by example, tackling inequalities and promoting governance and leadership for health and well-being through innovation, knowledge sharing and city health diplomacy. Healthy cities act as leaders and partners in tackling our common public health challenges ..."
> (WHO, 2018, p. 3. Reproduced with permission from the World Health Organization Europe)

The World Health Organization (2022) reports more people live in urban areas than in rural areas. Cities may offer access to education, health and social protection, but they can sprawl into overcrowded slums with poor access to clean water, poor sanitation, high rates of infectious disease, violence and poor mental health. Only 12% of cities have reached targets for reduced air pollution. By 2050, 70% of the world's population will live in cities. The ninth global conference on health promotion in Shanghai in 2016 explicitly linked the Healthy Cities movement to the United Nations *2030 Agenda for Sustainable Development*. Sustainable Development Goal 11 is to make cities and human settlements inclusive, safe, resilient and sustainable.

Box 8.8 Belfast Healthy City

Belfast became a healthy city in 1988. It was among the first 15 to be designated as a WHO healthy city. Today there are over a hundred. Belfast Healthy Cities puts addressing health inequalities at the core of its work. It encourages government departments, local public health bodies and organisations in the public sector to consider the health impact of all their policies and actions. It pioneered a range of new concepts which have now become mainstream in the city such as healthy ageing, healthy urban planning, health impact assessments, health literacy, active living and healthy places. In 2018, Belfast hosted 600 international delegates for the WHO International Healthy Cities Conference *Changing cities to change the world*. It was a double celebration to mark 30 years of the European Healthy Cities Network and 30 years of Belfast being a member.

(Source: Belfast Healthy Cities, 2022)

The World Health Organization European Healthy Cities Network is a partnership of cities committed to health and sustainable development across Europe. Every five years, a city (a loose term that can include towns, regions and counties) can join the European Healthy Cities Network and benefit from its support if they meet certain criteria. These normally include having political support and adequate resources to meet the goals set out by the World Health Organization's Regional Office for Europe for the next five years. In 2019, UK healthy cities included Belfast (Box 8.8), Carlisle, Derry City, Liverpool, Newcastle, Sunderland and Swansea. The *Copenhagen Consensus of Mayors* (WHO, 2018) presents the priorities for 2019 to 2024 (Figure 8.4).

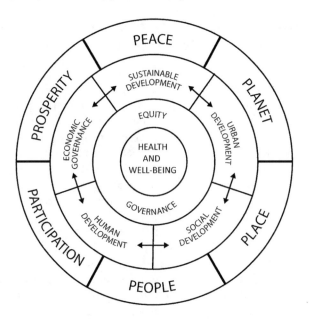

Figure 8.4 Priorities for the European Healthy Cities Network 2019 to 2024

Source: WHO, 2018, p. 2. Reproduced with permission from the World Health Organization Europe

It states healthy cities will foster health and wellbeing for all and reduce health inequities; lead by example, nationally, regionally and locally; and support the implementation of the World Health Organization's strategic priorities, which are

- investing in the *people* who make up our cities
- designing urban *places* that improve health and wellbeing
- greater *participation* and partnerships for health and wellbeing
- improved community *prosperity* and access to common goods and services
- promoting *peace* and security through inclusive societies
- protecting the *planet* from degradation including through sustainable consumption and production

National Healthy Cities Networks are national networks made up of each city's representatives. They collectively hold their nation's accumulated knowledge, experience and resources. These national networks support their cities and towns with political, strategic and technical support. They provide a single forum for their own governments to work with, and they give their nation's Healthy Cities movement a voice on the international stage. In 2019, the UK national network comprised Chelmsford, Glasgow, Lancashire, Manchester, Norwich, Tamworth, Wakefield and Warrington. The Network of European National Healthy Cities Networks comprises the representatives from *countries,* and they work directly with the World Health Organization (WHO, 2015).

Place-based approaches

Place-based partnerships across the UK are not part of the World Health Organization Healthy Settings movement, but they have emerged due to its influence and the global priorities for health promotion. The aim is to foster a collaborative approach to preventing, or providing early intervention for, a physical, social or psychological health concern in a geographical area using local, tailored approaches. They emphasise

- building on people's strengths/assets
- reciprocal relationships between local people and professionals
- building support networks
- facilitation and encouraging local people to be active participants

(Baczyk *et al.*, 2016)

For example, representatives from the local healthcare service, local government, the voluntary sector and others may work together to tackle obesity in a town, reduce health inequalities, regenerate a small local area, reduce alcohol and drug dependency, support mental health or create a new Healthy New Town (Box 8.9). For instance, healthcare practitioners may contribute to a partnership to reduce obesity by drawing attention to the social and economic causes of weight gain in the area, supporting initiatives for healthy eating and active travel, offering weight management services in local venues and using social prescribing to enable people to attend cookery classes, walking groups and so forth.

Box 8.9 A Healthy New Town: Bicester, Oxfordshire

Bicester's vision is to,

"To create a healthy community by making it easy, attractive and affordable for people of all ages to live healthy, sustainable lifestyles and to replicate the learning elsewhere. The aim is that Bicester becomes a place where healthy behaviour is easy, fun and affordable – where being active, eating healthy food and being a good neighbour are just part of normal daily life … The programme … [is]… working closely with a wide range of partners including schools, businesses, health and care providers, the voluntary sector, housing developers and academic partners, with Cherwell District Council acting at the lead organisation."

(Source: NHS England, 2022. Reproduced under the terms of the Open Government Licence v.3.0)

Reorienting healthcare services

Healthcare services are powerful settings because they enjoy a long established, and largely respected, reputation for being at the forefront of health matters. Healthcare services need to become promoters of health as opposed to providers of care and become fully integrated into the wider health system. This is discussed in more detail in Chapter 15. In summary, a health promoting healthcare service

- recognises that it is one part of the health system, not the whole health system
- puts health at the heart of what it does, alongside care
- is a healthy setting where the whole service, its physical and social environment, are health promoting for staff, visitors and patients/service users
- is integrated into a health system which comprises all those organisations, people and activities which share the primary aim of promoting, maintaining and restoring health
- works in partnership with other agencies within the care sector, e.g. integrated care systems
- works in partnership with a range of different sectors and agencies across society, e.g. local government departments, private businesses, charities and education
- recognises the value of primary healthcare being at the interface of the whole healthcare service and all other agencies and sectors
- is person-centred, where individuals have a right to participate in the design of the service and are at the heart of decisions about their personal healthcare
- supports the population's health from pre-conception to death and bereavement
- draws attention to the social and environmental determinants of health and supports social and environmental changes for better population health

Health promotion is a concept, discipline, movement and profession underpinned by internationally agreed aims, values, principles and characteristics.

Planning health promotion for individuals, groups or communities

Planning health promotion is about clarifying the purpose and outcome and then thinking through all the practical steps in a logical manner.

Stage 1 Identify who is the focus, their needs and assets

Who is the focus for the health promotion?
    a person, group or community
    those with a disease, disorder, distress, a health-related behaviour
    those who live or work in a place, a setting, an environment, a culture

What definition of health are we working with?

Whose definition of health are we working with?

Who identifies there is a need?
    the person, group, community, leader, professional, practitioner

What type of need?
    normative need
    felt need
    expressed need
    comparative need

    Maslow's hierarchy of needs

    Do needs relate to knowledge, beliefs, attitudes, motivations, skills/behaviours, resources, the social or physical environment?

What methods will identify needs?
    e.g. interviews, focus groups, photographs, health needs assessment

Who identifies assets?
    the person, group, community, leader, professional, practitioner

What types of assets?
    personal assets, e.g. cognitive, physical, emotional, spiritual, behavioural
    material assets, e.g. resources, wealth, location
    social assets, e.g. friends, colleagues, networks, social capital

Stage 2 Clarify the approach, aims and objectives

Which health promotion model most clearly frames the general approach and the desired outcome?
    preventive (medical approach/behaviour change approach)
    educational
    empowerment
    social change

Keep ethical principles in mind
    respect for autonomy
    beneficence
    non-maleficence
    justice

Who sets the aims and objectives?
    the person, group, community, leader, professional, practitioner

How are the aims and objectives set?
    coercion, instruction, information, education, consultation, partnership/joint
        working, enablement, empowerment

Clarify aims
    A health promotion project may have one aim, or it may have a few. An aim is a
        broad goal of what we are trying to achieve, e.g. to reduce cocaine consump-
        tion, to improve social and emotional health, to create a communal garden

Set out objectives
    Objectives (targets or outcomes) set out how the aim is to be met. Start with
        the aim and break it into small steps. Objectives often focus on the health-
        related education or policy outcomes of the work, but objectives may also
        relate to the process of the work.

Objectives are
    specific, e.g. to walk to the bus stop and back, twice a day for two weeks
    measurable, e.g. number of times the walk was successfully completed as
        planned
    achievable/realistic, e.g. has managed to complete this walk once already
    challenging, e.g. this will slowly build up walking ability and confidence

Educational objectives (preventive, educational and empowerment models)
    to become aware of …
    to know …
    to understand …
    to feel …
    to clarify …
    to motivate …
    to share …
    to collaborate …
    to decide …
    to create …
    to be able to …
    to maintain …

Non-educational objectives (social change model)
    to increase price
    to improve accessibility
    to advertise
    to 'place a product'
    to implement a policy
    to change the physical, social or cultural environment

Stage 3 Methods to achieve objectives

Who decides the methods?
    the person, group, community, leader, professional, practitioner

The methods need to
> meet the objectives/produce the specific outcome
> fit within the preferred health promotion model
> be ethical
> be acceptable
> be realistic in terms of time and other resources

Methods may include
> leaflets, lectures, media, counselling/therapy, one-to-one discussion, group work, life skills, role play, community development/empowerment, lobbying, advocacy, policymaking and law enforcement. Educational methods are also discussed in Chapter 7.

Stage 4 Identify resources

Resources include
> the person, group, community, population, clients, patients
> practitioners, professionals, influencers, leaders
> research, evidence, existing policies, publications, online resources
> people's time, finance, meeting places, expertise, services, equipment

Stage 5 Plan the evaluation

Evaluation is a type of research. We gather evidence. Thinking about evaluation early in the process is helpful because it may reveal that the objectives need adjusting. Measurable objectives are those that can be evaluated.

Consider
> Who is to conduct the evaluation? Someone 'inside' the work or 'outside' the work? It may be individual self-evaluation.
> Where will the evaluation focus attention? The plans, the action, post-action?
> What is to be evaluated? These should relate to the outcomes/objectives; it is the way we know whether, or to what degree, they have been met.
> Why evaluate? For reasons of accountability to someone or for learning purposes?
> When will the evaluator report? At points during the work, formative, or at the end of the work, summative?
> Who is the evaluation for? Self, participants, sponsor, clients, managers or members of the community?
> What will be the style of the evaluator? Participative/joint/democratic, autocratic or bureaucratic?
> What form will the evaluation take? Will it be a description or a judgement of the work?
> How will the evaluation be carried out? Collecting quantitative or qualitative information; studying a sample or cases, will it be retrospective or predictive?
>
> (Ebbut, 1987)

These questions may inform an informal interview, a simple questionnaire or something larger such as a structured health impact assessment or an environmental impact assessment.

Stage 6 Set out the action plan

Having clarified what is to be done, how it is to be done and what resources are available, the action plan is a very detailed breakdown of all the practical tasks, who is responsible for these and a clear timeline. Action plans may be compiled in the form of list(s), grid(s) or Gantt charts. They include preparatory tasks, including those relating to the evaluation, the tasks associated with the health promotion activity, the tasks following the activity and sometimes long-term communication or follow-up. A large health promotion initiative can be complex, and there may be several action plans that are timed to run simultaneously or in a sequence.

Stage 7 Action: implement the plan

Deliver the action plan. Health promotion is always a learning activity for everyone involved. Reflecting, listening, evaluating and sometimes modifying elements are all part of the process. The learning informs the next health promotion plan.

Planning a health promotion intervention requires careful thinking about priorities and how both the process of promoting health and its outcomes can affect people and settings.

Health promotion and public health

Health promotion and public health have different roots and core values, but during the 1980s and 1990s they came closer together when both traditions recognised the importance of the social determinants of health and tackling inequalities in health. The World Health Organization provides the following definitions of health promotion and public health.

> "Health promotion is the process of enabling people to increase control over, and to improve their health … Health promotion represents a comprehensive social and political process. It not only embraces actions directed at strengthening the skills and capabilities of individuals, but also action directed towards changing social, environmental and economic determinants of health so as to optimise their positive impact on public and personal health. Health promotion is the process of enabling people, individually and collectively, to increase control over the determinants of health and thereby improve their health … The Ottawa charter identifies three basic strategies for health promotion … advocacy… enabling … mediating … [and] … five priority action areas: to build healthy public policy; create supportive environments; strengthen community action; develop personal skills; and re-orient health services."
>
> (WHO, 2021, p. 4. Reproduced with permission
> from the World Health Organization)

Public health is,

> "… an organized activity of society to promote, protect, improve, and - when necessary - restore the health of individuals, specified groups, or the entire population. It is a combination of sciences, skills and values that function through collective societal activities and involve programmes, services and institutions aimed at protecting and improving the health of all people … Public health is a social

and political concept aimed at improving health, prolonging life and improving the quality of life among whole populations through health promotion, disease prevention and other forms of health intervention. The Ottawa Charter advocates significantly different approaches to the description and analysis of the determinants of health, and the methods of solving public health problems. These methods include the strategies and action areas in the Ottawa Charter."

(WHO, 2021, pp. 27–28. Reproduced with permission from the World Health Organization)

In some countries, health promotion is the 'overarching umbrella term' within which sits public health, often characterised as health protection, disease prevention, epidemiology, environmental health and centralised services. For other countries, public health has become the 'overarching umbrella term' within which sits health promotion with its emphasis on education, empowerment and community development. The choice is often influenced by those with the greatest power to influence governments, for example the education or medical professions; the health authorities or the local authorities. For example across the four nations of the UK, over the last 20 years, we have seen the emergence of 'public health' being used as the 'overarching umbrella term' in which sits the domains: health protection, healthcare public health and health improvement (see Chapters 2 and 9). In 2005, 'health improvement' explicitly included health education and health promotion (Griffiths *et al.*, 2005), yet these two terms are no longer used in national policy documents. In March 2021, the Government announced a new Office for Health Promotion to be set up for England, but by October it was launched as the Office for Health Improvement and Disparities (Gov.UK, 2021a; 2021b).

Thinking point:

Consider the comparison of health promotion with public health shown in Table 8.4. Does this reflect your understanding and experience? What might explain decisions to use the terms health promotion, health improvement or public health in your nation's policies?

Table 8.4 Comparing health promotion with public health

Health promotion	*Public health*
Emerged from, and augmented, personal and social health education	Emerged from environmental health/structural engineering/sanitary reform and then epidemiology/public health medicine
A comprehensive social and political process	A social and political concept
Process of enabling people	Organised activity of society
Aims to enable people, individually and collectively, to increase control over the determinants of health	Aims to improve health, prolong life and improve the quality of life among populations through health promotion, disease prevention and other forms of health intervention
Advocacy, enabling and mediating	Collective societal activities which include programmes, services and institutions

(Continued)

Table 8.4 Comparing health promotion with public health *(Continued)*

Health promotion	Public health
Uses preventive, educational, empowerment and social change models	Emphasises 'top down' preventive and social change models
Emphasises individuals, groups and populations	Emphasises population health
Values empowerment and autonomy as integral to preventing disease and promoting health. These help to create, and are supported by, healthy settings	Prime focus is on disease prevention, risky health-related behaviour, health protection and improving health and social care services
Emphasises processes; 'how' we promote health is a key influence on outcomes	Emphasises surveillance and measurable population outcomes
Often person- and community-centred, pathogenic and salutogenic	Often disease centred, pathogenic
Outcomes are usually measured using a holistic model of health, e.g. morbidity, mortality, health-related behaviours, evidence of learning knowledge and skills, empowerment/taking control and social change. Health as a positive concept	Outcomes are usually measured using a medical model of health, e.g. morbidity, mortality and risky health-related behaviours. Health as absence of disease
Politically more contentious because the attainment of health is bound to human rights, justice, peace and equity	Politically less contentious

Both aim to reduce early death, preventable diseases and reduce inequalities in health through partnership working across disciplines and sectors

Summary

This chapter has

- described and applied four models of health promotion
- discussed the Ottawa Charter for Health Promotion and its significance
- considered the scope and characteristics of health promotion
- examined health promotion in relation to politics, policy, partnerships, community action, the settings approach and reorientation of health services
- outlined the key stages of planning a health promotion activity
- considered the relationship between health promotion and public health

Further reading

Laverack, G. (2014) *The pocket guide to health promotion.* Maidenhead: Open University Press
Scriven, A. (2017) *Promoting health. A practical guide.* 7th edn. London: Elsevier
Scriven, A. and Hodgins (2012) *Health promotion settings. Principles and practice.* London: Sage

Useful websites

EuroHealthNet. Available at: https://eurohealthnet.eu (Accessed 29th May 2022)
Institute of Health Promotion and Education (IHPE). Available at: https://ihpe.org.uk (Accessed 29th May 2022)
Integrity Action. Available at: http://www.integrityaction.org (Accessed 29th May 2022)

References

Action for Community Development (2021) *Community health project*. Available at: https://www.actionforcd.org/community-health-project (Accessed 29th May 2022)

Baczyk, M., Schenk, K., McLaughlin, D., McGuire, A. and Gadsden, S. (2016) *Place-based approaches to joint planning, resourcing and delivery. An overview of current practice in Scotland*. Improvement Service, Livingston. Available at: https://www.improvementservice.org.uk/__data/assets/pdf_file/0016/10744/place-based-approaches-report.pdf (Accessed 29th May 2022)

Beattie, A. (1991) 'Knowledge and control in health promotion: a test case for social policy and social theory', in Calnan, M., Gabe, J. and Bury, M. (eds) *The sociology of the health service*. London: Routledge, pp. 162–202

Beauchamp, T.L. and Childress, J.F. (2001) *Principles of biomedical ethics*. 5th edn. Oxford: Oxford University Press

Belfast Healthy Cities (2022) *Belfast healthy cities*. Available at: https://www.belfasthealthycities.com (Accessed 29th May 2022)

Bradshaw, J. (1972) 'Taxonomy of social need', in McLachlan, G. (ed) *Problems and progress in medical care: essays on current research* (7th series). London: Oxford Press, pp. 71–82

Claridge, T. (2018) 'Functions of social capital – bonding, bridging, linking', *Social Capital Research, Dunedin, New Zealand*, 20th January. Available at: https://www.socialcapitalresearch.com/wp-content/uploads/2018/11/Functions-of-Social-Capital.pdf?x92028 (Accessed 31st May 2022)

Corvo, E. and De Caro, W. (2020) 'COVID-19 and spontaneous singing to decrease loneliness, improve cohesion and mental well-being: an Italian experience', *Psychological Trauma: Theory, Research, Practice and Policy*, 12(S1), pp. S247–S248

Ebbut, C. (1987) 'Signposts on the road to the bottomless pool', in Campbell, G. (ed) *Health education and community: a review of research and developments*. London: The Falmer Press

Epp, J. (1986) *Achieving health for all: a framework for health promotion*. Ottawa Health and Welfare Canada. Available at: https://www.canada.ca/en/health-canada/services/health-care-system/reports-publications/health-care-system/achieving-health-framework-health-promotion.html#conc (Accessed 29th May 2022)

Gov.UK (2021a) *New office for health promotion to drive improvement of nation's health*. Available at: https://www.gov.uk/government/news/new-office-for-health-promotion-to-drive-improvement-of-nations-health (Accessed 24th May 2022)

Gov.UK (2021b) *New body to tackle health disparities will launch 1 October, co-headed by new deputy chief medical officer*. Available at: https://www.gov.uk/government/news/new-body-to-tackle-health-disparities-will-launch-1-october-co-headed-by-new-dcmo-2 (Accessed 24th May 2022)

Green, J., Cross, R., Woodall, J. and Tones, K. (2019) *Health promotion. Planning and strategies*. London: Sage

Griffiths, S., Jewell, T. and Donnelly, P. (2005) 'Public health in practice: the three domains of public health', *Public Health*, 119(10), pp. 907–913

International Union for Health Promotion and Education (2016) *Core competencies and professional standards for health promotion*. Available at: https://www.iuhpe.org/images/JC-Accreditation/Core_Competencies_Standards_linkE.pdf (Accessed 29th May 2022)

Kivimäki, M. and Steptoe, A. (2018) 'Effects of stress on the development and progression of cardiovascular disease', *Nature Reviews Cardiology*, 15(4), pp. 215–229

Marmot, M. (2010) *Fair society, healthy lives. The Marmot review.* London: H.M. Government

Marmot, M., Allen, J., Boyce, J., Boyce, T., Goldblatt, P. and Morrison, J. (2020) *Health equity in England. The Marmot review 10 years on.* London: Institute of Health Equity

McEwen, B.S. (2008) 'Central effects of stress hormones in health and disease: understanding the protective and damaging effects of stress and stress mediators', *European Journal of Pharmacology*, 583(2–3), pp. 174–185

Naidoo, J. and Wills, J. (2011) *Developing practice for public health and health promotion.* London: Elsevier

Naidoo, J. and Wills, J. (2016) *Foundations for health promotion.* 4th edn. London: Elsevier

New Philanthropy Capital (2021) *How philanthropists should respond to coronavirus. Consequences, crises and opportunities for charities.* Available at: https://www.thinknpc.org/resource-hub/coronavirus-guide (Accessed 29th May 2022)

NHS England (2022) *Bicester, Oxfordshire.* Available at: https://www.england.nhs.uk/ourwork/innovation/healthy-new-towns/demonstrator-sites/eco-bicester (Accessed 29th May 2022)

Popay, J. (2021) *Power, politics and community assets.* Local Government Association Available at: https://www.local.gov.uk/power-politics-and-community-assets (Accessed 29th May 2022)

Popay, J., Whitehead, M., Ponsford, R., Egan, M. and Mead, R. (2020) 'Power control communities and health inequalities 1: theories, concepts and analytical frameworks', *Health Promotion International*, 36(5), pp. 1253–1263

Public Health Wales (2019) *Principles of community engagement for empowerment.* Cardiff: Public Health Wales

Robinson, S. (2021) 'Social context of health and illness', in Robinson, S. (ed) *Priorities for health promotion and public health.* London: Routledge, pp. 3–33

Scottish Community Development Centre (2021) *What we do.* Available at: https://www.scdc.org.uk/what (Accessed 29th May 2022)

Scriven, A. (2017) *Promoting health. A practical guide.* 7th edn. London: Elsevier

World Health Organization (1981) *Global strategy for health for all by the year 2000.* Geneva: World Health Organization

World Health Organization (1986) *Ottawa charter for health promotion, 1986.* Available at: https://www.euro.who.int/en/publications/policy-documents/ottawa-charter-for-health-promotion,-1986 (Accessed 29th May 2022)

World Health Organization (2014) *The Helsinki statement on health in all policies.* Available at: https://www.who.int/publications/i/item/9789241506908 (Accessed 29th May 2022)

World Health Organization (2015) *National healthy cities networks in the WHO European region.* Copenhagen: World Health Organization (Europe)

World Health Organization (2018) *Copenhagen consensus of mayors. Healthier and happier cities for all.* Available at: https://www.euro.who.int/__data/assets/pdf_file/0003/361434/consensus-eng.pdf (Accessed 29th May 2022)

World Health Organization (2021) *Health promotion glossary of terms 2021.* Geneva: World Health Organization

World Health Organization (2022) *Health promotion. Healthy settings.* Available at: https://www.who.int/teams/health-promotion/enhanced-wellbeing/healthy-settings (Accessed 29th May 2022)

9 Public health

*Rajeeb Kumar Sah, Devendra Raj Singh,
Lalita Kumari Sah and Sally Robinson*

Key points

- Introduction
- History of public health
- Defining public health
- Public health reports
- Annual public health reports
- National public health profiles
- Health needs assessment
- Health impact assessment
- Summary

Introduction

This chapter explains the historical origins and contemporary practice of public health in the UK. Public health is concerned with protecting and improving the health of populations. The chapter will define public health and its three domains of practice: health protection, health improvement and healthcare public health. It discusses the background to public health reporting and describes annual public health reports and public health profiles. The chapter explains the purpose of health needs assessments and health impact assessments and how they are undertaken.

History of public health

Although the concept of public health originates from early civilisation, for example the sanitation systems of the Romans, modern public health emerged in the 19th century. In the UK, the industrial revolution encouraged people to move from rural to urban areas where there were opportunities to work in industry and commerce. This rapid movement led to urban areas becoming densely populated with poor access to clean water, adequate drainage systems, suitable housing and good quality food. Communicable diseases, also called infectious diseases, such as cholera, typhoid, tuberculosis and smallpox spread quickly through the overcrowded and insanitary conditions and became epidemics. The cholera epidemic of 1831 to 1832 killed over 32,000 people in Britain (UK Parliament, 2022) and was a key reason for the emergence of the sanitary movement across the UK. In 1842, Edwin Chadwick (1800–1890) (Figure 9.1), secretary to the Poor Law Commission, published the *Report on the sanitary condition of the labouring population of Great Britain*. It described the appalling

DOI: 10.4324/9780367823696-11

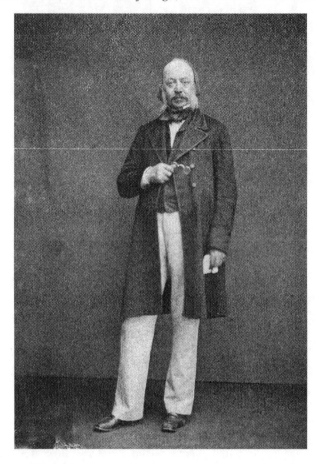

Figure 9.1 Sir Edwin Chadwick

Source: Wellcome collection made available under a CC BY 4.0 licence

conditions in which many people lived. Chadwick paid for the costs of publication himself, as the Poor Law Commission did not want to be associated with it. The report strongly argued that the diseases could be eliminated if the environmental conditions were improved. The report gained widespread publicity and initiated a debate about the link between the physical environment and disease while the rates of communicable diseases continued to rise. Following a second cholera epidemic, the first Public Health Act was passed by Parliament in 1848. It marked the beginning of the modern public health movement.

The 1848 Public Health Act provided legislation to improve the sanitary conditions in England and Wales. It established the General Board of Health, a central authority, and local health boards. The health boards were to advise on public health matters such as ensuring the adequate supply of clean water, sewerage, drainage and the regulations of slaughterhouses and other practices which could be harmful to health. Key players were the sanitary inspectors, inspectors of nuisances and medical officers for health. In 1854, John Snow (1813–1858) traced an outbreak of cholera to the contaminated water coming from the pump on Broad Street in central London.

His work represented a turning point in understanding the cause of the disease, and it is regarded as the event that founded the science of epidemiology (see Chapter 3). In 1857, Louis Pasteur (1849–1895) demonstrated that toxins caused certain diseases and developed what became known as 'germ theory'. Robert Koch (1843–1910) identified the bacteria that causes tuberculosis and cholera in 1882 and 1884, which provided further evidence that germs cause disease. Together, Snow, Pasteur and Koch helped to provide the scientific evidence for public health action.

From the 1860s, public health reforms were favoured by most politicians and the press. The 1875 Public Health Act consolidated all the previous public health measures and established named local authorities as the sanitary authorities with responsibility to provide clean water, dispose of all sewage and refuse, and ensure the sale of safe food. These sanitary authorities, now led by medical officers of health, had the power to provide medicines and to use measures to prevent and control epidemics of infectious diseases. By the later years of the 19th century, the sanitation movement was replaced by a greater emphasis on health education and disease prevention, and medical professionals began to have a greater influence over public health matters (see Chapter 7).

During the Boer War (1899–1902), in South Africa, more than a quarter of the volunteers who came forward to join the British army were rejected on health grounds. This drew attention to the health of school children and the need to improve health during pregnancy, infancy and early childhood. The infant and child mortality rates had not improved over the previous century (Phin, 2009). The Ministry of Health Act 1919 gave the Ministry of Health responsibility for all aspects of health, including the provision of public health services. The Local Government Act 1929 transferred the administration of the Poor Law to local authorities. This also included responsibility for vaccinations, hospitals and health-related institutions. In 1948, the National Health Service (NHS) brought healthcare services under the control of central government, starting with hospitals, followed by family practitioner services such as general practitioners and pharmacists, and community-based services including district nursing and some public health services such as health visiting. Other public health services, such as environmental health, stayed within local authorities. There have been several reorganisations of the NHS since. Meanwhile, health education was led by the Central Council for Health Education and the Department of Health for Scotland, and later the Health Education Council for England, Wales and Northern Ireland and the Scottish Health Education Group (see Chapter 7).

By the mid-20th century, mass mortality from communicable diseases had been falling for some time. The transition from communicable to non-communicable diseases, known as the epidemiological transition, seemed complete (see Chapter 3). As the focus shifted towards the causes of these non-communicable diseases, attention was drawn to health-related behaviours such as smoking, use of alcohol, poor diet and sedentary behaviour. By the 1980s, research into the underlying causes of such behaviours led to a greater awareness of the social, cultural, economic, political and environmental determinants of health and disease, and subsequent health inequalities (Marmot, 2010; Townsend *et al.*, 1992). Although health education, and the work of health education officers, continued, health in the UK meant 'healthcare' to most. The first public health White Paper for more than a century was published in 1992 as *The Health of the Nation* (DH, 1992) and successive UK, and later national, governments have produced public health White Papers thereafter. In 2013, in England,

Table 9.1 A summary of the five waves of public health

Five waves	Key ideas and developments
The First Wave (1830–1900)	Structural approach, e.g. changing the environment. Chadwick reported the relationship between unsanitary living conditions and patterns of disease. Great public health works, e.g. creation of reservoirs for clean water for urban populations and building sewers. Growth of municipal/local powers leading to improvements in housing, living and working conditions. Addressed the concerns of civil and social disorder, e.g. alcohol consumption, crime and illegitimacy. Development of municipal/local authorities, embryonic emergency services and an emergent voluntary/charity sector.
The Second Wave (1890–1950)	Biomedical/medical approach. Rationalist philosophies of the enlightenment period. Scientific discoveries, e.g. a shift from miasmic to germ-based theories of disease, disease prevention and treatment. Health became associated with the perception of body as a machine. Genesis of modern emergency services.
The Third Wave (1940–1980)	Clinical approach. Materialist philosophies, e.g. believing material changes drive history and that society's institutions and other modes of operation are shaped by the structure of class relations. Health was the result of the conditions of everyday life. Emergence of the welfare state, e.g. large-scale social housing and other welfare benefits. Universal education. Establishment of the National Health Service.
The Fourth Wave (1960–2000 and continuing)	Social approach, e.g. recognising the social determinants of health. Emergence of modern society. Health/epidemiological transition from infectious diseases to chronic diseases. Health risks associated with consumer choices and risky health-related behaviours associated with poor diet, inactivity, tobacco, alcohol and drugs. Effective healthcare interventions to prolong life. Emergence of social inequalities in health.
The Fifth Wave (2000 onwards)	Culture of health, e.g. encouraging a culture where healthy behaviours are the norm and the social and physical environment supports this while discouraging unhealthy behaviours. Shared responsibility for health, e.g. health as a common good, achieved by working together with shared norms, values, beliefs and behaviours. Intersectoral working; taking a positive, holistic and collaborative approach involving a range of stakeholders such as employers or private businesses. Effective health communication. Integrated public health services. Addressing persistent health inequalities and the burden of chronic/non-communicable diseases.

Sources: Davies *et al.*, 2014; Hanlon *et al.*, 2011; Hanlon *et al.*, 2012; Scottish Government, 2016.

Public Health England was established as an executive agency of the Department of Health and the public health functions which had been previously located within the NHS moved back to local authorities.

Today, Public Health Wales is part of NHS Wales, the Northern Ireland Public Health Agency reports to the Health and Social Care Board and Public Health Scotland is located within NHS Scotland. Public Health England was responsible for coordinating UK-wide responses to emergencies, including the COVID-19 coronavirus pandemic which began in late 2019. The pandemic shifted the focus back to the threat of communicable diseases and led to a reorganisation whereby Public Health England's health protection functions were transferred to the new UK Health Security Agency (UKHSA) (see Chapter 10). Its health improvement and healthcare public health functions were transferred to the new Office for Health Improvement and Disparities (England); and to NHS England, NHS Improvement and NHS Digital (DHSC, 2021).

Hanlon and colleagues (2011) describe the UK as having experienced at least four waves of improvements to public health since the industrial revolution. Each wave has comprised a range of developments. The current fifth wave is debated. These waves are loosely described, interlinked and have had a cumulative effect. They indicate the major shifts in thinking about the health of the population alongside changes in society (Table 9.1).

> *Modern public health in the UK is a multi-disciplinary and multi-sectoral endeavour that has its roots in environmental, epidemiological, educational and social research, reform and actions undertaken by a wide range of practitioners over the last 200 years.*

Defining public health

There are many factors which shape, or determine, a population's health. These include social, cultural, economic, political, genetic and environmental factors. Public health is about understanding, and then engaging with, the determinants of health to protect and improve the population's health to enable people to live longer lives free from disease and disability.

> "The distinguishing feature of public health is its focus on populations rather than individuals."
>
> (Baum, 2016, p. 14)

There have been several attempts to define public health, but there is no agreed definition. One that is still quoted was proposed by Charles-Edward A. Winslow in 1920, and it reflects contemporary thinking at that time. He defined public health as,

> "… the science and art of preventing disease, prolonging life, and promoting physical health and efficiency through organized community efforts for the sanitation of the environment, the control of community infections, the education of the individual in principles of personal hygiene, the organization of medical and nursing service for the early diagnosis and preventive treatment of disease, and the development of the social machinery which will ensure to every individual in the community a standard of living adequate for the maintenance of health."
>
> (Winslow, 1920, p. 23)

In 1988, the Acheson Report provided a more contemporary definition of public health as,

> "The science and art of preventing disease, prolonging life and promoting health through the organised efforts of society."
>
> (Acheson, 1988, p. 1)

In the UK, public health is

- focussed on the health of the community or population
- seeks to prevent or reduce harm
- requires collective efforts to make changes to bring about public health improvements

(Dawson, 2011)

There are three domains of work (Figure 9.2).

- Health improvement, also called 'health and wellbeing', is concerned with improving the health and wellbeing of people by encouraging health-related behaviours and tackling the wider determinants of health such as housing, employment and the environment. It includes health education and health promotion, which are discussed in Chapters 7 and 8

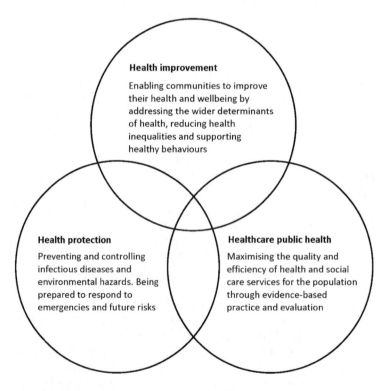

Figure 9.2 Three domains of public health practice

Sources: Griffiths *et al.* (2005); PHS (2021a)

- Health protection concerns the prevention and control of infectious diseases and protecting people from chemical, radiological and environmental health hazards. It includes enforcing regulations for clean air and water, and safe food. It also includes preparedness for disasters and emergency responses to prevent people from disease or injury. This is discussed in Chapter 10
- Healthcare public health, also called 'health services', 'health and social care services' or 'health service delivery and quality' concerns prioritising available resources, planning for efficient and good quality care services and improving health-related outcomes for the population. It also supports clinical governance, the systems for improving the quality of care; evidence-based clinical practice; research and evaluation

(FPH, 2020; Griffiths *et al.*, 2005; PHS, 2021a)

UK public health practice is organised in three domains: health improvement, health protection and healthcare public health.

Public health reports

Directors of public health, and their teams of public health specialists and practitioners, produce a wide range of reports including various types of health profiles, annual public health reports, health needs assessments and health impact assessments. All are supported by evidence obtained from epidemiological and other research studies. Collecting large-scale health-related population data began with the Census, introduced in 1801. It provided the first comprehensive record of births, deaths, employment, and the inhabited and empty houses in each parish. From this, the State became increasingly interested in recording more about its citizens, including their health and welfare (Crook, 2007). Factories and prisons were inspected from 1833 and 1836 respectively, followed by the mines in 1842. Inspectors of nuisances and sanitary inspectors, the equivalent of today's environmental health officers, both inspected and reported. The new police force reported crime. The clergy had kept records for each parish since 1538. These are examples of the wide range of collected data that informed Chadwick's *Report on the sanitary condition of the labouring population of Great Britain* in 1842, which recommended local authorities appoint medical officers for health. These posts became mandatory in 1872. Medical officers undertook the work to collect local data and produce annual reports on the physical environment, the 'sanitary state', of their district. They reported on living conditions but also the causes and ages of deaths. These reports marked the beginning of the transition towards the medicalisation of public health, away from the environment, and provided early examples of the epidemiological reporting, meaning rates of death and disease, which came to characterise these reports in later decades (Gorsky, 2007). Meanwhile, in 1893 Charles Booth, a sociologist, presented his first report of his systematic analysis of census data showing the relationship between housing and poverty, street by street in London, accompanied by his 'poverty maps' (Booth, 1893).

By the 1970s, medical officers were community physicians, described as epidemiologists and administrators of medical/healthcare services, led by the Faculty of Community Medicine, later the Faculty of Public Health Medicine (Warren, 1997). 'Community profiles', that is the collection of information about very small local areas, were undertaken by community nurses and community physicians to support

NHS primary healthcare. The concept of a holistic 'health needs' assessment, based on a modern, positive and holistic understanding of health, was well understood by health education practitioners and then by the specialist health promotion workforce working in local health promotion units, but its implementation was limited by the context in which they worked and the pervasive shadow of medical influence (Duncan, 2013; Ewles and Simnett, 1985). In the late 1980s, the outbreak of bovine spongiform encephalopathy (BSE) among cattle and its link to variant Creutzfeldt-Jakob disease (vCJD) in humans was the first major warning that public health had been neglected for too long. Donald Acheson (1988), the chief medical officer, argued the collection of comprehensive, regional and national epidemiological data was woeful, and his work led to the establishment of several public health observatories across the country to collect data and to publish annual public health reports. The 'Lalonde Report' (Lalonde, 1974), the World Health Organization's *Health for All by the Year 2000* (WHO, 1981) and the *Ottawa Charter for Health Promotion* (WHO, 1986) described as 'the new public health', were influential in changing 'public health medicine' with its focus on epidemiology, back towards the origins of 'public health' (and the name change to the current Faculty of Public Health which sets standards for today's multi-professional public health specialists) (Duncan, 2013). It took until the late 1990s for the new public health departments, into which some health promotion specialists were gradually subsumed, to start to produce public health reports that included health-related behaviours, reference to the social determinants of health and health inequalities, as well as the usual local death and disease statistics.

Annual public health reports

Directors of public health are responsible for the public's health in a geographical area, usually a local authority. This includes setting local public health objectives, presenting annual reports on the health of the population and identifying the key determinants of their health. Each year, some choose to provide an overview but many choose to focus their report on a few priorities within their area, such as local inequalities in health, vulnerable people or a topic such as obesity or deprivation. Over the last three decades, these reports have changed from tables of epidemiological data to varied, online, colourfully presented, accessible reports or slides with summaries and pictures, which mean they can be widely accessed and understood. As the director of public health in Peterborough wrote,

> "The Annual Public Health Report (APHR) is designed to convey information about health in Peterborough in a form which is clear and understandable for the public."
>
> (Peterborough.gov.uk, 2019)

The annual public health report provides key information to the wider public health workforce, those who may be able to act and improve the public's health (see Chapter 2). These include those who work in environmental health departments; local transport; education; healthcare, social care and emergency services; local businesses; charities and so forth.

National public health profiles

National public health profiles emerged from *Securing good health for the whole population* (Wanless, 2004) which argued the UK National Health Service would not be able to cope with the demand for treatment and care if we did not reduce the demand by investing in prevention and public health, and to do this we needed to improve the monitoring of the population's health. National health profiling began a few years later. It is led by the Scottish Public Health Observatory, England's Office for Health Improvement and Disparities, the Public Health Wales Observatory and

Table 9.2 Examples of health indicators for England

Domain	Examples of health indicators
Overarching indicators	Life expectancy at birth Healthy life expectancy at birth Disability-free life expectancy at birth Inequality in healthy life expectancy at birth Inequality in life expectancy at 65
Wider determinants of health	Children in relatively low-income families (under 16) Adults with a learning disability who live in stable and appropriate accommodation Percentage of people in employment Domestic abuse-related incidents and crimes Homelessness – households in temporary accommodation Social isolation – percentage of adult carers who have as much social contact as they would like Killed and seriously injured casualties on England's roads
Health improvement	Obesity in early pregnancy Smoking status at time of delivery Hospital admissions caused by unintentional and deliberate injuries in young people (15 to 24 years) Percentage of physically inactive adults Successful completion of drug treatment – opiate users Estimated diabetes diagnosis rate Cancer screening coverage Sickle cell and thalassaemia screening – coverage Self-reported wellbeing – people with a high anxiety score
Health protection	Population vaccination coverage, e.g. flu (aged 65+) TB incidence HIV late diagnosis NHS organisations with a board approved sustainable development management plan Adjusted antibiotic prescribing in primary care by NHS
Healthcare and premature mortality	Infant mortality rate Under 75 mortality rate from cancer Under 75 mortality rate from all cardiovascular disease Premature mortality in adults with severe mental illness Preventable sight loss, e.g. glaucoma Hip fractures in people aged 65 and over Excess winter deaths index

Source: OHID (2022).

the Public Health Agency of Northern Ireland. Profiles provide population data for a geographical area, such as a local authority or region, and show whether that population's health is worse than, similar to or better than the average for the nation. Over the years, trends can be spotted and priorities for action identified.

National public health profiles comprise a range of health indicators. These can be measured using data that can be easily collected from a wide range of surveys and records. Health indicators include health-related behaviours, prevalence of disease, life expectancy and the use of services. Indicators of the determinants of health include deprivation, housing and the environment, education and crime. The choice of indicators is influenced by government policy. For example, in England there are over 160 indicators, determined by the *Public Health Outcomes Framework*, which are regularly updated (Gov.UK, 2022). Indicators are grouped into domains: overarching indicators, wider determinants of health, health improvement, health protection, and healthcare and premature mortality (Table 9.2). The collated data helps to identify to what degree England is meeting its current national public health policy goals: to increase healthy life expectancy and to reduce inequalities in health.

> *Directors of public health are required to publish local health-related data. These data are used for local and national profiles and for their own annual public health reports.*

Health needs assessment

Identifying health needs is about identifying what people need to remain, or to become, healthy. Bradshaw (1972) presented a 'taxonomy of social need' which set out four types of need: normative, felt, expressed and comparative.

- *Normative need* is that which is defined by 'experts', perhaps professionals or policymakers. A desirable standard is set based on their experience, evidence and consultation. For example, nutritional standards and criteria for screening. Where a population's health falls short of these standards identifies a health need. Normative needs are not absolute in that they may vary according to changes in evidence, changes in society and its values, as well as judgements about the available resources to tackle a health need. For example, guidelines to protect the UK population from the spread of COVID-19 coronavirus changed many times from 2020 to 2022
- *Felt need* concerns the subjective perceptions of people, and they equate with their wants, wishes and desires. People's felt needs are mostly based on their beliefs, knowledge and experiences, and relate to perceptions of what others have and what is available. Felt needs can be inflated and unrealistic. For example, a community living in an inner city may feel a need for an Olympic village
- *Expressed need* is a felt need that is translated into a demand for action. The need is communicated to others. Policymakers may interpret 'no demand' as 'no need', but there may be various reasons why a felt need is not expressed such as having no resources or expertise, or it may be deemed culturally inappropriate
- *Comparative need* means when we compare two populations of similar characteristics, one is receiving an intervention or a service that supports their health and the other is not. The latter has a comparative need. The population of town X may have access to health-related adult education courses and town Y does not. Town Y may be identified as having a comparative need for such education

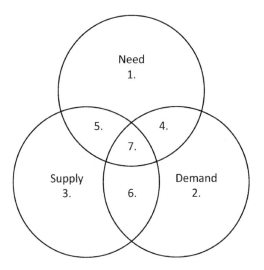

Figure 9.3 Healthcare need, supply and demand

Sources: Adapted from Wright *et al.* (1998, p. 1311); Stevens *et al.* (2004, p. 4).

Health needs can be considered from different perspectives. For example, in the context of healthcare public health, we may undertake a 'healthcare' needs assessment, and an economist may weigh up the costs and benefits of providing extra healthcare services. Limited resources mean the demand for healthcare, that is the expressed need of the public, often outstrips the supply of healthcare services. Need, supply and demand are interrelated and they intersect to form seven distinct outcomes (Figure 9.3). There is a

1 need, but neither demand nor supply
2 demand, but neither need nor supply
3 supply, but neither need nor demand
4 need and demand, but no supply
5 need and supply, but no demand
6 supply and demand, but no need
7 need, demand and supply

Health needs assessment process

For assessing the public health needs of a population, a health needs assessment (HNA) can be a powerful tool for decision making, setting priorities, allocating resources, evaluating health-related interventions and accomplishing goals. The World Health Organization defines HNA as,

> "The process of systematically collecting information to enable the practitioner, team and policy makers to identify, analyse, prioritise and meet the health needs of an individual, family or population."

> (WHO, 2001, p. 43)

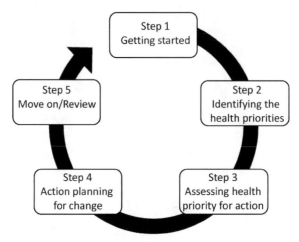

Figure 9.4 Five steps of a health needs assessment

It is a systematic process of gathering evidence to identify a population's health needs and the availability of resources to meet those needs (Reed and Fleming, 2014). The HNA is used for planning interventions to support the public's health. Today's public health needs assessments comprise a process of five steps, shown in Figure 9.4.

Step 1: Getting started

Getting started with a HNA is a task to be undertaken by a multi-disciplinary team. The involvement of stakeholders, meaning those people or institutions with a particular interest in the work, is crucial and they should be included in identifying who will carry out which elements of the HNA. The team identifies the population of interest, the aim of the HNA, the objectives of the HNA, the methods to be used, the resources needed and a plan for how the results will be used. The population needs to be clearly identified, for example it might be a sample of adults aged 20 to 30 years residing in Caernarfon. The HNA may wish to focus on a specific health indicator such as sexual behaviour, high blood pressure, injuries or breastfeeding. The HNA might focus on a population whose overall health status is poorer than populations in other regions. The aim of a HNA could be to inform and shape local or national public health priorities, but in UK public health it is often carried out to provide information to monitor and support existing local or national broad priorities, such as reducing health inequalities or improving the health status of a targeted population. Key considerations for Step 1 are

- the aims and objectives of the assessment
- identifying the target population
- identifying the sites for the assessment
- identifying who needs to be involved
- resources
- relevant information that is already available
- potential risks
- deciding how the assessment results are to be used

Step 2: Identifying the health priorities

Many health issues will be present within a population and the HNA needs to prioritise. Research is carried out to collect data about health concerns and the determinants of health which might be affecting the population. Research methods may include literature reviews, surveys and qualitative methods. The data is analysed to produce a profile of the population's health and to identify potentially important determinants of their health. For example, the profile might show rates of respiratory disease and potential determinants might include information about air quality and local occupations. The fieldwork can produce a huge amount of data. Commonly used criteria for prioritising health needs are

- the relevance of the health need
- the impact, the magnitude and severity of the health need
- changeability, the community's capacity and willingness to act on the health need
- the ability to have a measurable impact on the health need
- the availability of health resources
- any existing interventions and policies
- trending health concerns in the community
- the need among vulnerable populations

Some useful techniques for prioritising needs are shown in Box 9.1.

Box 9.1 Techniques for prioritising needs

Multi-voting technique

- Round one – participants vote for as many priorities as they wish
- All votes are tallied, the areas receiving three or more votes are re-presented
- Round two – all participants can vote up to three times on the remaining priorities
- All votes are tallied and the three priorities receiving three or more votes are re-presented
- Round three – all participants can vote twice
- Repeat until a desirable number of priorities is selected

Nominal group technique

- The group is given the topic and individuals are asked to silently jot their preferred priorities on paper
- A moderator asks for one priority from each participant and lists them on a flip chart
- Repeat until all preferred priorities are listed
- A moderator encourages discussion with the aim of clarifying, simplifying and grouping the list
- A moderator facilitates discussion about how each of the priorities meets other agreed criteria such as feasibility, cost and so forth
- All participants rank each of the priorities from one to 10
- Repeat until a desirable number of priorities are selected

The Hanlon method

- Rate, from 0 to 10, each priority against agreed criteria, e.g. the size of the health need, seriousness of the health need and the effectiveness of potential interventions
- Apply the 'PEARL' test:

Propriety – is the intervention for addressing the health need suitable?
Economics – does it make economic sense to address this need and what are the economic consequences of not doing so?
Acceptability – is the intervention acceptable to the community?
Resources – are the resources, including finances, available for the intervention?
Legality – are there any legal impediments to the intervention?

- Calculate scores for each priority using the ratings in step one and the formula

$[A + (2 \times B)] \times C = D$ where

A is the rating for size of the health need
B is the rating for the seriousness of the health need
C is the rating for the effectiveness of potential interventions
D is the score for that priority

- Based on the priority scores, rank the priorities

(Source: NACCHO, 2013)

Key considerations for Step 2 are

- methods for health profiling, how to gather the information
- the availability of the population's health-related data
- methods for gathering information about the population's needs
- methods for gathering information about the perceptions of potential health providers, e.g. perceptions of service providers or business leaders
- strategies for overcoming the challenges of data collection
- identifying health priorities with a rationale for the decisions made

Step 3: Assessing a health priority for action

Not all health priorities can be acted upon simultaneously. Deciding which to act upon first requires a more detailed assessment, being clear about whether there is a shared understanding of the health issue in the population, what interventions are possible and potentially effective, what changes would be required and, basically, what would work. The choice of the selected priority needs to be justified, and the implications of taking action need to be identified. This process needs to consider acceptability, which includes identifying the anticipated changes required by people or organisations if tackling this priority is to have a positive impact on health. It also needs to consider what resources are available and would be needed. This Step includes the same considerations as Steps 1 and 2, and also includes identifying

- who is to be assessed, by whom and why
- what health conditions and determinants of health have the most significant impact on this health priority

- which interventions would be the most effective and acceptable to the population
- how feasible are the proposed interventions to address the priority
- whether tackling this priority contributes to national goals such as reducing inequalities in health
- the resources needed to address the priority and how accessible they are

Step 4: Action planning for change

At this point, the project team is brought together to agree a plan of action to improve the health of the population. It has clear aim(s); objectives; indicators to monitor progress; targets such as time targets to implement the changes/interventions and sustainable actions. The overall timeline for the project is agreed and tasks are assigned, often to smaller working groups. Indicators to monitor progress could include planning to collect quantitative data to measure inputs, processes, outputs and impacts. Qualitative research may also be incorporated, perhaps to evaluate people's perceptions. In planning the evaluation of an intervention, the team might consider

- relevance – the extent to which the intervention will meet the need. How well will the objectives of the intervention, and its design, respond to the health needs identified? Will it continue to do so if there is a change in circumstances?
- coherence – how well does the intervention fit with other interventions in the local setting
- effectiveness – the extent to which the intervention will achieve its objectives
- efficiency – to what extent will the intervention deliver results in an economic and timely way
- impact – the extent to which the intervention will make a difference and generate positive, negative, intended or unintended outcomes; and whether it will have an effect at a broader or higher level
- sustainability – the length of time that the benefits of the intervention are likely to last

(OECD, 2022)

The final action plan will be detailed and logical. Key considerations for Step 4 are

- clear aims, objectives, indicators and targets
- leadership and delegation, giving people clear roles and responsibilities
- clear timelines with the required resources
- built-in monitoring and evaluation of the intervention
- decisions to justify the relevance of the intervention to meeting the aims
- using the indicators to measure progress
- risk assessments to identify potential challenges to the intervention
- work out an alternative plan in case of failure

Step 5: Move on/review

The final stage is about reflection and evaluation after the intervention has taken place. The team revisits its evaluation criteria and discusses what it has learnt from the experience, reflects on what went well, what did not go well and why. This includes understanding the effectiveness of the intervention, the enabling factors and the challenges. Decisions are made about whether the intervention is complete, is to continue or is to be discontinued. The HNA process is ready for the next cycle, starting with Step 1. Key considerations for Step 5 are

- evaluating how well the action plan was implemented
- whether the project met its original aims, objectives, indicators and targets
- whether it contributed to improving the population's health or reducing health inequalities
- learning from the project's success and challenges
- identifying the key messages to take forward
- deciding what happens next

Joint strategic needs assessments

Across the four nations of the UK, legislation has supported better integration of health and care. This comprises public health, healthcare and social care. In England, the Health and Social Care Act 2012 introduced local joint strategic needs assessments to support the work of local health and wellbeing boards. Local authorities were to work with their corresponding clinical commissioning groups (the local NHS services) to assess the health needs of the local population and to use this evidence to commission services to improve its health and wellbeing. The Public Bodies (Joint Working) Scotland Act 2014 and the Social Services and Well-being (Wales) Act 2014 also made 'local strategic needs assessments' or 'population needs assessments' a legal requirement for the same purpose of bringing together health boards and local authorities. In Northern Ireland, the integration of health and social care has been in place for longer. The Health and Social Care Board and Public Health Agency produce annual reports, and health needs assessments focus on specific topics such as homelessness (HSC and PHA, 2017).

In England, the Department of Health directs joint strategic needs assessments (JSNAs) to focus on the,

> "... needs that could be met by the local authority, CCGs, or the NHS ... JSNAs are produced by health and wellbeing boards ... Local areas are free to undertake JSNAs in the best way suited to their local circumstances – there is no template or format that must be used and no mandatory data ...[they] can be ... informed by ... looking at specific groups ... or on wider issues that affect health such as employment, crime, community safety, transport, planning or housing ..."
>
> (DH, 2013, p. 6)

For example, Devon County Council explains that a JSNA is,

> "... concerned with social factors ... such as housing, poverty and employment ... looks at the health of the population with a focus on behaviours which affect health ... provides a common view of health and care needs ... identifies health inequalities ... provides evidence for ... health and care interventions."
>
> (DCC, 2022)

In Scotland, the Act says that a local strategic needs assessment should inform local joint working, with no further guidance about what it should contain. In East Dunbartonshire,

> "The JSNA provides an overview of the current and projected population demographic across East Dunbartonshire. It also provides information relating to life circumstances, health behaviours, and health and social care status."
>
> (EDHSCP, 2021, p. 3)

In Wales, the Act,

> "... requires that local authorities and local health boards must jointly carry out an assessment of the needs for care and support, and the support needs of carers in the local authority areas."
>
> (GGHSCWP, 2016, p. 6)

Thinking point:

> Consider these quotes and compare the approaches to population-based health needs assessments across the UK.

These needs assessments all use the same principles of a health needs assessment, as described, to guide their local planning. Recent challenges have included the need to prioritise emergencies such as the COVID-19 pandemic and economic constraints such as the limited resources across healthcare and local authorities. Public health, especially its health improvement functions, can find itself being squeezed between the demands of urgent healthcare and urgent social care.

Health impact assessment

The *Ottawa Charter for Health Promotion* (WHO, 1986) made building healthy public policy one of its five key areas for action, meaning policies must support and not undermine healthy environments, equity and the safety of goods and services. They should encourage the 'healthy choice to be the easier choice' (see Chapter 8). Environmental impact assessments became a legal requirement in the UK in 1988. When a local planning authority is deciding whether to grant permission for a building or other environmental project, it must demonstrate its potential impacts on the environment and include opportunities for the public to participate in the process (Gov.UK, 2014). Social impact assessments, which were established in the United States of America, were introduced to the UK to analyse the positive or negative social, cultural and economic impacts of planning policies and other development projects on communities, and these were followed by legal requirements for community safety impact assessments and equality impact assessments in the Crime and Disorder Act 1998, Policy and Justice Act 2006 and Equality Act 2010 (Lipietz *et al.*, 2017). The requirement for health impact assessments emerged during the 1990s when they were included within several national and local public health policy documents across the UK and the European Union's *Maastricht Treaty* and *Amsterdam Treaties* both required that policy proposals were checked to ensure their impacts that would not undermine population health (Lock, 2000). Today, impact assessments are legally required as part of policy development across all the UK's healthcare, public health and social care systems. These include health inequalities impact assessments. England's *Health and Care Bill*, published in January 2022, included 36 impact assessments ranging from water fluoridation, food information, collaborative commissioning, adult social care, professional regulation, joint committees and joint appointments, and the merger of NHS England and NHS Improvement (DHSC, 2022).

A health impact assessment is a,

> "... practical systematic approach to judge the potential and unintended health effects of a policy, programme or project on a population, particularly on vulnerable or disadvantaged groups."
>
> (WHO, 2022)

It is,

> "A combination of procedures, methods and tools by which a policy, programme or project may be judged as to its potential effects on the health of a population, and the distribution of those effects within the population."
>
> (ECHP, 1999, p. 4)

Health impact assessments have many strengths. They can

- inform the design and development of policies, plans and strategies
- provide a framework for monitoring and evaluating changes in population health
- generate evidence which can be used to mitigate health risks
- generate evidence which can be used to maximise health potential
- contribute to the evidence that supports improving health in ethical and sustainable ways
- be used to hold policymakers to account for decisions that impact a population's health or the determinants of health
- provide an opportunity to engage stakeholders, service-users and others in planning processes
- illuminate alternative or better choices of action
- be used to argue for resources, including in funding applications, and to enable community participation

(Davenport *et al.*, 2006; Herriott and Williams, 2010; Marmot *et al.*, 2020; Thomson *et al.*, 2018; WHO, 2014; 2022; Winkler *et al.*, 2021)

In the UK, there is much guidance about how to conduct health impact assessments. These include guidance from the lead Wales, Scotland, England and Northern Ireland public health departments and agencies (Green *et al.*, 2020; 2021; IPH, 2020; PHE, 2020; PHS, 2021b). Examples include *Health Impact Assessment of Government Policy* (Herriott and Williams, 2010), *Rapid Health Assessment Tool* (NHSLHUDU, 2017), *Health Impact Assessment (HIA) and Local Development Plans (LDPs): A Toolkit for Practice* (Green *et al.*, 2021). The quality assurance of the HIA can be ensured by using the *Quality Assurance Review Framework for Health Impact Assessment* (Green *et al.*, 2020).

Health impact assessments will be tailored according to the focus, scale and scope of the project and the available resources such as time. There are three types of health impact assessments (HIAs)

- *Desk-based HIAs* are those that mostly rely on existing knowledge and evidence, a literature review, and can be completed within days. They comprise a brief written report which may recommend a more comprehensive HIA. Desk-based HIAs are used for policy reviews, assessment of service plans, outlines of planning applications or proposals for new interventions where there are a limited number of potential health outcomes and a fuller HIA is not possible
- *Rapid or intermediate HIAs* include a literature review and evidence collected from local stakeholders, often brought together by a steering group. These are normally completed within weeks and comprises a full report containing recommendations. These are used for service reviews and modifications, and for new interventions including those initially recommended for a comprehensive HIA but this was not conducted due to limited resources
- *Comprehensive or detailed HIAs* include literature reviews, public and stakeholder engagement, and substantial quantitative and qualitative evidence from a range of research studies. This type of HIA is the most resource intensive and produces an in-depth report with recommendations. These are normally undertaken for major projects such as a housing development or regeneration proposals where there can be significant health impacts and/or there is considerable uncertainty about the impacts of a proposed policy

Health impact assessment process

A HIA follows a systematic process using different tools and techniques including literature reviews, public engagement opportunities, stakeholder workshops, quantitative surveys, interviews with key people, focus groups with those who might be affected by the intervention and so forth. It is usually described as a series of four, five or six stages which are flexible, stand-alone or integrated (PHE, 2020; Pyper *et al.*, 2021). Here we describe five stages (Figure 9.5). We use the word 'intervention' to mean a policy, a programme or a project.

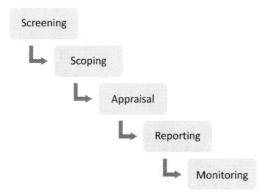

Figure 9.5 Five stages of a health impact assessment

Stage 1: Screening

Screening means deciding whether to undertake a HIA and whether it would be viable. It involves identifying the intervention and then providing a rationale for a HIA. Screening includes considering the context, such as the place, population and existing health data, and what is known about the intervention's potential effects on people's health and the determinants of health. It may include asking key questions within the local population and stakeholders, and using formal screening tools/checklists to assess the viability of the HIA for the selected intervention.

Stage 2: Scoping

Scoping is setting out a plan for conducting the HIA. It includes deciding what type of HIA will be conducted, depending on need and resources, and setting up a team, a 'steering group', with defined roles and responsibilities. The plan will include the timeframe, the geographical boundaries and the skills of those who will participate. Towards the end of this stage, a list of potential impacts will be identified. These will include the potential risks and benefits of the intervention on the health of the population and on the determinants of their health.

Stage 3: Appraisal

Appraisal concerns the collection of data and a detailed analysis of potential health impacts. This includes gaining an in-depth understanding of the intervention and carrying out quantitative and qualitative research such as surveys, focus groups and field observations. Potential outcomes relating to how many people would be affected, the environment, health hazards and the impact on health inequalities are often included. The appraisal articulates the nature, likelihood and extent of potential health impacts if the intervention is to go ahead.

Stage 4: Reporting

The findings from the previous stages are reported to the steering group which compiles a report comprising a description of the scope and the collected evidence. It identifies the evidence-based priorities and recommendations for how potential health problems might be avoided or minimised. The identification of priorities and recommendations are usually the result of much discussion around practicalities, resources, feasibility, intersectoral working and so forth, as they apply to the design and operational aspects of the proposed intervention.

Stage 5: Monitoring

The monitoring section of a HIA explains how the health impacts of the intervention will need to be monitored if it progresses. Once the intervention begins, such as the enacting of a policy or the start of a project, it is important to collect ongoing evaluation data using a range of research methods to compare its real health impacts against the predictions in the HIA. This data contributes to measuring the intervention's effectiveness and the learning can be used to inform future HIAs.

Thinking point:

> A new airport is to be built in a rural area and a steering group has been set up to carry out a health impact assessment. What type of documents and data would they need to consult, who might they consult and what do they need to find out?

Health needs assessments assess the needs of a population and determine the priorities for interventions to improve the population's health. Health impact assessments predict how a proposed intervention may affect the population's health.

Summary

This chapter has

- described the historical context of public health
- defined public health in the UK and identified its three domains
- described examples of public health reporting requirements in the UK
- explained the purpose of health needs assessments and health impact assessments, and how they are undertaken

Further reading

Baum, F. (2016) *The new public health.* 4th edn. Oxford: Oxford University Press
Deveaux, T. (2020) *Bassett's environmental health procedures.* 9th edn. London: Routledge
Donaldson, L.J. and Rutter, P.D. (2018) *Donaldsons' essential public health.* 4th edn. London: CRC Press
Krentel, A. and McKee, M. (eds) (2022) *Issues in public health. Challenges for the 21st century.* 3rd edn. London: Open University Press/McGraw Hill

Useful websites

Chartered Institute of Environmental Health. Available at: https://www.cieh.org
Faculty of Public Health. Available at: www.fph.org.uk
UK Public Health Association. Available at: https://ukpha.org.uk
UK Public Health Network. Available at: https://ukpublichealthnetwork.org.uk

References

Acheson, D. (1988) *Public health in England: the report of the committee of inquiry into the future development of the public health function.* London: Her Majesty's Stationery Office
Baum, F. (2016) *The new public health.* 4th edn. Oxford: Oxford University Press
Booth, C. (1893) 'Life and labour of the people in London: first inquiry based on the 1891 census', *Journal of the Royal Statistical Society*, 56(4), pp. 557–593
Bradshaw, J. (1972) 'Taxonomy of social need', in McLachlan, G. (ed.) *Problems and progress in medical care: essays on current research.* 7th series. London: Oxford University Press, pp. 71–82
Crook, T. (2007) 'Sanitary inspection and the public sphere in late Victorian and Edwardian Britain: a case study in liberal governance', *Social History*, 32(4), pp. 369–393
Davenport, C., Mathers, J. and Parry, J. (2006) 'Use of health impact assessment in incorporating health considerations in decision making', *Journal of Epidemiology and Community Health*, 60(3), pp. 196–201

Davies, S.C., Winpenny, E., Ball, S., Fowler, T., Rubin, J. and Nolte, E. (2014) 'For debate: a new wave in public health improvement', *The Lancet*, 384(9957), pp. 1889–1895

Dawson, A. (2011) 'Resetting the parameters: public health as the foundation for public health ethics', in Dawson, A. (ed) *Public health ethics: key concepts and issues in policy and practice.* Cambridge: Cambridge University Press, pp. 1–19

Department of Health (1992) *The health of the nation.* London: Her Majesty's Stationery Office

Department of Health (2013) *Statutory guidance on joint strategic needs assessments and joint health and wellbeing strategies.* Available at: https://assets.publishing.service.gov.uk/government/uploads/system/uploads/attachment_data/file/223842/Statutory-Guidance-on-Joint-Strategic-Needs-Assessments-and-Joint-Health-and-Wellbeing-Strategies-March-2013.pdf (Accessed 6th May 2022)

Department of Health and Social Care (2021) *Public health system reforms: location of Public Health England functions from 1 October.* Available at: https://www.gov.uk/government/publications/location-of-public-health-england-phe-functions-from-1-october-2021/public-health-system-reforms-location-of-public-health-england-functions-from-1-october (Accessed 9th May 2022)

Department of Health and Social Care (2022) *Health and care bill.* Available at: https://assets.publishing.service.gov.uk/government/uploads/system/uploads/attachment_data/file/1045623/combined-summary-document-impact-assessement-health-and-care-bill-v2.pdf (Accessed 7th May 2022)

Devon County Council (2022) *What is the joint strategic needs assessment (JSNA)?* Available at: https://www.devonhealthandwellbeing.org.uk/jsna/about (Accessed 9th May 2022)

Duncan, P. (2013) 'Failing to professionalise, struggling to specialise: the rise and fall of health promotion as a putative specialism in England, 1980–2000', *Medical History*, 57(3), pp. 377–396

East Dunbartonshire Health and Social Care Partnership (2021) *Joint strategic needs assessment.* Available at: https://www.eastdunbarton.gov.uk/health-and-social-care/health-and-social-care-services/east-dunbartonshire-health-and-social-care (Accessed 6th May 2022)

European Centre for Health Policy (1999) *Health impact assessment.* Available at: http://www.healthedpartners.org/ceu/hia/hia01/01_02_gothenburg_paper_on_hia_1999.pdf (Accessed 9th May 2022)

Ewles, L. and Simnett, I. (1985) *Promoting health. A practical guide to health education.* Chichester: John Wiley

Faculty of Public Health (2020) *Functions and standards of a public health system.* Available at: https://www.fph.org.uk/media/3031/fph_systems_and_function-final-v2.pdf (Accessed 4th May 2022)

Green, L., Parry-Williams, L. and Edmonds, N. (2020) *Quality assurance review framework for health impact assessment (HIA).* Wales Heath Impact Assessment Support Unit. Available at: https://phwwhocc.co.uk/whiasu/wp-content/uploads/sites/3/2021/05/QA_Interactive_PDF_version_eng.pdf (Accessed 9th May 2022)

Green, L., Parry-Williams, L. and Huckle E. (2021) *Health impact assessment (HIA) and local development plans (LDPs): a toolkit for practice.* Wales Health Impact Assessment Support Unit. Available at: https://phw.nhs.wales/publications/publications1/health-impact-assessment-hia-and-local-development-plans-ldps-a-toolkit-for-practice (Accessed 7th May 2022)

Griffiths, S., Jewell, T. and Donnelly, P. (2005) 'Public health in practice: the three domains of public health', *Public Health*, 119(10), pp. 907–913

Gorsky, M. (2007) 'Local leadership in public health: the role of the medical officer of health in Britain, 1872–1974', *Journal of Epidemiology and Community Health*, 61(6), pp. 468–472

Gov.UK (2014) *Environmental impact assessment.* Available at: https://www.gov.uk/guidance/environmental-impact-assessment#the-purpose-of-environmental-impact-assessment (Accessed 7th May 2022)

Gov.UK (2022) *Public health outcomes framework: indicator updates.* Available at: https://www.gov.uk/government/publications/public-health-outcomes-framework-indicator-updates (Accessed 7th May 2022)

Greater Gwent Health, Social Care and Well-being Partnership (2016) *Population needs assessment Gwent region report.* Available at: http://www.gwentrpb.wales/SharedFiles/Download.aspx?pageid=30&mid=174&fileid=82 (Accessed 6th May 2022)

Hanlon, P., Carlisle, S., Hannah, M., Lyon, A. and Reilly, D. (2012) 'A perspective on the future public health: an integrative and ecological framework', *Perspectives in Public Health*, 132(6), pp. 313–319

Hanlon, P., Carlisle, S., Hannah, M., Reilly, D. and Lyon, A. (2011) 'Making the case for a "fifth wave" in public health', *Public Health*, 125(1), pp. 30–36

Health and Social Care and Public Health Agency (2017) *A picture of health.* Available at: https://www.publichealth.hscni.net/sites/default/files/A%20Picture%20of%20Health%20Dec%202017_0.pdf (Accessed 6th May 2022)

Herriott, N. and Williams, C. (2010) *Health impact assessment of government policy.* London: Department of Health.

Institute of Public Health (2020) *Health impact assessment (HIA).* Available at: https://publichealth.ie/hia-guidance (Accessed 7th May 2022)

Lalonde, M. (1974) *A new perspective on the health of Canadians. A working document.* Ottawa: Government of Canada

Lipietz, B., Wickson, T., Diaconescu, I. and Lee, R. (eds) (2017) *Social impact assessment in London planning.* Available at: https://www.ucl.ac.uk/bartlett/development/sites/bartlett/files/social_impact_assessment_in_london_planning.pdf (Accessed 7th May 2022)

Lock, K. (2000) 'Health impact assessment', *BMJ*, 320(7246), pp. 1395–1398

Marmot, M. (2010) *Fair society, healthy lives. The Marmot review.* H.M. Government: London

Marmot, M., Allen, J., Boyce, T., Golblatt, P. and Morrison, J. (2020) *Health equity in England: the Marmot review 10 years on.* Available at: https://www.health.org.uk/publications/reports/the-marmot-review-10-years-on (Accessed 9th May 2022)

National Association of County and City Health Officials (2013) *Guide to prioritization techniques.* Available at: https://www.naccho.org/uploads/downloadable-resources/Gudie-to-Prioritization-Techniques.pdf (Accessed 7th May 2022)

NHS London Healthy Urban Development Unit (2017) *Rapid health impact assessment tool.* 3rd edn. Available at: https://www.healthyurbandevelopment.nhs.uk/wp-content/uploads/2017/05/HUDU-Rapid-HIA-Tool-3rd-edition-April-2017.pdf (Accessed 14th May 2022)

Office for Health Improvement and Disparities (2022) *Local authority health profiles.* Available at: https://fingertips.phe.org.uk/profile/health-profiles (Accessed 7th May 2022)

Organization for Economic Co-operation and Development (2022) *Evaluation criteria.* Available at: https://www.oecd.org/dac/evaluation/daccriteriaforevaluatingdevelopmentassistance.htm (Accessed 6th May 2022)

Peterborough.gov.uk (2019) *Annual public health report.* Available at: https://www.peterborough.gov.uk/healthcare/public-health/annual-public-health-report (Accessed 7th May 2022)

Phin, N.F. (2009) 'The historical development of public health', in Wilson, F. and Mabhala, A. (eds) *Key concepts in public health.* London: Sage Publications, pp. 5–10

Public Health England (2020) *Health impact assessment in spatial planning: a guide for local authority public health and planning teams.* Available at: https://www.gov.uk/government/publications/health-impact-assessment-in-spatial-planning (Accessed 9th May 2022)

Public Health Scotland (2021a) *Our context – public health in Scotland.* Available at: http://www.healthscotland.scot/our-organisation/our-context-public-health-in-scotland/public-health-overview (Accessed 4th May 2022)

Public Health Scotland (2021b) *Health inequalities impact assessment (HIIA).* Available at: http://www.healthscotland.scot/tools-and-resources/health-inequalities-impact-assessment-hiia/what-is-an-hiia (Accessed 7th May 2022)

Pyper, R., Cave, B., Purdy, J. and McAvoy, H. (2021) *Health impact assessment guidance: the case for HIA*. Dublin and Belfast: The Institute of Public Health in Ireland

Reed, J.F. and Fleming, E. (2014) 'Using community health needs assessments to improve population health', *North Carolina Medical Journal*, 75(6), pp. 403–406

Scottish Government (2016) *2015 review of public health in Scotland: strengthening the function and re-focussing action for a healthier Scotland*. Available at: https://www.gov.scot/publications/2015-review-public-health-scotland-strengthening-function-re-focusing-action-healthier-scotland/documents (Accessed 9th May 2022)

Stevens, A., Raftery, J. and Mant, J. (2004), 'An introduction to health care needs assessment', in Stevens, A., Raftery, J., Mant, J. and Simpson, S. (eds) *Health care needs assessment. The epidemiologically based needs assessment reviews*, Florida: CRC Press, *First series, volume 1*. 2nd edn. pp. 1–17

Thomson, K., Hillier-Brown, F., Todd, A., McNamara, C., Huijts, T. and Bambra, C. (2018) 'The effects of public health policies on health inequalities in high-income countries: an umbrella review', *BMC Public Health*, 18(859) doi:10.1186/s12889-018-5677-1

Townsend, P., Davidson, N., Black, D. and Whitehead, M. (eds) (1992) *Inequalities in health*. London: Penguin

UK Parliament (2022) *Cholera in Sunderland*. Available at: https://www.parliament.uk/about/living-heritage/transformingsociety/towncountry/towns/tyne-and-wear-case-study/introduction/cholera-in-sunderland/#:~:text=In%20Britain%2C%2032%2C000%20people%20died,done%20to%20prevent%20its%20recurrence (Accessed 28th April 2022)

Wanless, D. (2004) *Securing good health for the whole population*. Available at: https://www.southampton.gov.uk/moderngov/documents/s19272/prevention-appx%201%20wanless%20summary.pdf (Accessed 7th May 2022)

Warren, M.D. (1997) 'The creation of the faculty of community medicine (now the faculty of public health medicine) of the royal colleges of physicians of the United Kingdom', *Journal of Public Health Medicine*, 19(1), pp. 93–105

Winkler, M.S., Viliani, F., Knoblauch, A.M., Cave, B., Divall, M., Ramesh, G., Harris-Roxas, B. and Furu, P. (2021) *Health impact assessment. International best practice principles*. International Association for Impact Association. Available at: https://www.researchgate.net/publication/352573139_Health_impact_assessment_international_best_practice_principles_International_Association_for_Impact_Assessment (Accessed 9th May 2022)

Winslow, C.E. (1920) 'The untilled fields of public health', *Science*, 51(1306), pp. 23–33

Wright, J., Williams, R. and Wilkinson, J.R. (1998) 'Development and importance of health needs assessment', *BMJ*, 316(7140), pp. 1310–1313

World Health Organization (1981) *Global strategy for health for all by the year 2000*. Geneva: World Health Organization

World Health Organization (1986) *Ottawa charter for health promotion, 1986*. Available at: https://www.euro.who.int/__data/assets/pdf_file/0004/129532/Ottawa_Charter.pdf (Accessed 5th May 2022)

World Health Organization (2001) *Community health needs assessment*. Available at: https://www.euro.who.int/__data/assets/pdf_file/0018/102249/E73494.pdf (Accessed 9th May 2022)

World Health Organization (2014) *Health in all policies: Helsinki statement. Framework for country action*. Available at: https://www.who.int/publications/i/item/9789241506908 (Accessed 9th May 2022)

World Health Organization (2022) *Health impact assessment*. Available at: https://www.who.int/health-topics/health-impact-assessment#tab=tab_1 (Accessed 6th May 2022)

10 Health protection

Meradin Peachey

Key points

- Introduction
- Communicable diseases
- Vaccination
- Food safety and micro-biological hazards
- Chemical, biological, radiological and nuclear hazards
- Risk assessment in the workplace
- Screening
- Summary

Introduction

This chapter will demonstrate how health protection makes an important contribution to public health. Health protection protects the health of individuals, groups and populations by taking action to prevent, control and manage communicable diseases and microbiological hazards. It also includes emergency response and planning for chemical, biological, radiological and nuclear hazards, advising on risk assessments in the workplace, and preventing disease through vaccination and screening programmes. The chapter will cover the key concepts, definitions, terminologies and tools that are used to manage and reduce risks of disease, and it will explain how health protection is organised in the UK.

Communicable diseases

'Communicable diseases' is the generic term for all infectious or transmissible diseases that spread from one person or animal to another causing illness, death and disability. The terms 'communicable' and 'infectious' are often used interchangeably. They are caused by pathogens which can be viruses, bacteria, fungi or protists. The development of a communicable disease can be illustrated as 'the disease triangle' (Figure 10.1). For an infection to occur, the pathogen needs to identify a vulnerable host in the right environmental, including socio-economic, conditions. The host provides nourishment and shelter for the pathogen. For example, in malaria the host is a human who is susceptible to a mosquito bite. The pathogen is a parasite that infects the mosquito and the environment is where the mosquito lives and breeds, often in hot and damp conditions in places like sub-Saharan Africa (Figure 10.2). Some diseases emanate from animals

DOI: 10.4324/9780367823696-12

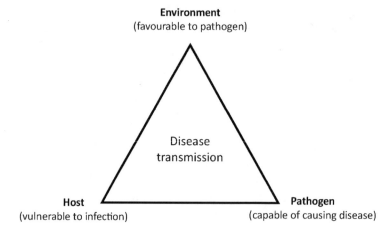

Figure 10.1 The disease triangle

and can be transferred to humans. Then, if the pathogen mutates, it can cause human-to-human transmission. Good standards of animal health and safety, and human hygiene, can help to prevent the transmission of disease from animals to humans.

We can catch a communicable disease by

- direct contact with a person carrying the pathogen, e.g. measles or mumps
- contact with contaminated fluids, e.g. human immunodeficiency virus (HIV) in human blood, mucous or saliva
- inhaling contaminated droplets from another person's cough or sneeze, e.g. cold, influenza or pneumonia

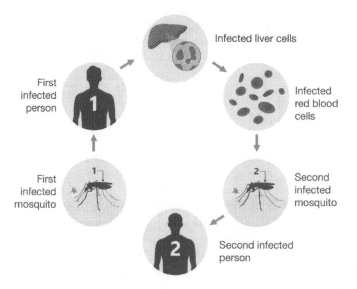

Figure 10.2 Transmission cycle of malaria

Source: solar22/Shutterstock.com

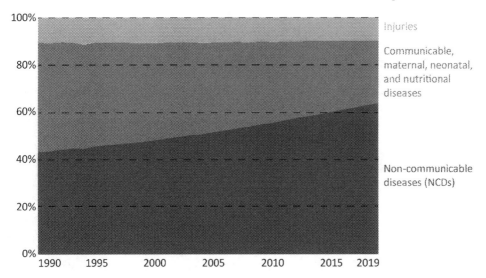

Figure 10.3 Global disease burden by cause, 1990 to 2019, measured as disability-adjusted-life years per year

Source: Institute for Health Metrics and Evaluation (IHME) in Roser and Ritchie, 2021. Reproduced under a Creative Commons BY license

- receiving a bite from an animal or insect carrying the pathogen, e.g. malaria or Zika
- consuming contaminated water or foods, e.g. legionnaires disease or salmonella poisoning

Thinking point:

With reference to a local and familiar communicable disease, identify its pathogen, the environment in which it thrives and the host.

Building the knowledge, understanding and skills to track communicable disease patterns is an important component of public health because they cause significant illness (morbidity) and death (mortality) across the world (Roser and Ritchie, 2021). In 1990, over 1.1 billion people were living with a communicable disease; by 2016 this had fallen to below 670,000, a reduction of about 40%. Among the under-fives, between 2000 and 2019, there was a 63.3% reduction in mortality from communicable diseases (Perin *et al.*, 2022). These reductions are mainly due to public health measures such as sanitation and immunisation. Even though cases of communicable diseases are reducing, they are still a significant burden on the world (Figure 10.3).

Surveillance and management of communicable diseases

Global travel, population mobility, global commodities and global trade are part of modern life. Communicable diseases in one country affect another, so understanding global patterns of disease is an important part of how we detect and control them. There are two components to managing communicable diseases: surveillance and managing an outbreak.

Surveillance

Surveillance is how we routinely monitor levels of communicable disease, maintain an overview, identify new and emerging diseases, identify higher levels of disease than might be expected and identify new outbreaks. One of the priorities of the World Health Organization (WHO), with its membership of 194 countries, is to reduce communicable diseases across the world through surveillance, planning and regular guidance. It has been successful in eradicating smallpox, reducing HIV and tuberculosis, as well as reducing childhood diseases through vaccination programmes. The WHO works in partnership with each country's communicable disease agency providing support with surveillance and management. Communicable disease agencies include the Chinese Center for Disease Control and Prevention (CCDC); the Centers for Disease Control and Prevention (CDC) in the United States of America, the Public Health Agency of Canada, the European Centre for Disease Prevention and Control (ECDC), Singapore's National Centre for Infectious Diseases, Taiwan Centers for Disease Control, the Communicable Diseases Network Australia (CDNA) and the UK Health Security Agency (UKHSA). It is through these worldwide systems that new and emerging diseases can be detected, such as the Zika virus in South America, Ebola in African countries and the COVID-19 coronavirus in China.

The UK Health Security Agency (UKHSA) was established in 2021 to replace the health protection work of Public Health England. It is supported by Public Health Wales (PHW), the Communicable Diseases Scotland Unit (CDSU) and the HSC Public Health Agency Northern Ireland. The UK system for reporting communicable diseases is through the statutory 'notification of infectious diseases' under the Public Health (Control of Disease) Act 1984. Data is collected by the UKHSA, and reports are published weekly by the UK Government (Gov.UK, 2021a).

Outbreak management

An outbreak of a communicable disease is commonly defined as an incident in which two or more people experiencing a similar illness are linked in time and place. More specifically, this includes

- a greater than expected incidence of infection compared to the usual background rate for that particular location
- a single case for certain rare diseases
- a suspected, anticipated or actual event involving microbial or chemical contamination of food or water

(PHE, 2014)

For example, an outbreak may be the hundreds of cases of flu expected during the winter in the UK, or it may be two cases of legionnaires disease linked to the same source of infection.

In the UK, an outbreak is identified and confirmed by public health professionals. It is common for environmental health officers and communicable disease consultants to manage and control outbreaks, such as food poisoning or measles, every day. Depending on the nature of the outbreak, an incident team comprising multiple agencies may manage the outbreak or undertake an extended research programme. The process of managing an outbreak is to

- identify the disease (cases), the diagnostic characteristics, the incubation period, the mode of transmission and the infectivity
- confirm the outbreak is present
- trace the contacts of people with the disease
- isolate cases and contacts to restrict the spread of the disease
(Donaldson and Rutter, 2018; PHE, 2014; Rubin *et al.*, 2020a).

Next, the appropriate policies and procedures are followed to control, minimise or eradicate the outbreak. The aim is to interrupt the 'disease triangle' between the host, the pathogen and the environment which is allowing the disease to spread. For example, measles is a highly contagious virus, the host is the nose or throat of a human and it is spread from person to person through respiratory droplets. The measles vaccination is the most effective way to break the cycle.

Point source outbreak

A point source outbreak means everyone is exposed to the same pathogen. This is common in food poisoning, where we see a rapidly rising number of cases followed by a sudden drop in cases. For example, this occurred during the outbreak of campylobacter food poisoning from pâté served in a Scottish restaurant in 2006 (Figure 10.4).

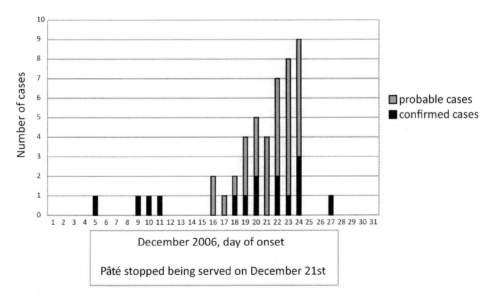

Figure 10.4 Campylobacter gastroenteritis poisoning from restaurant pâté, Scotland 2006 (*n* = 47 diners)

Source: Adapted from O'Leary *et al.*, 2009, p. 385

Steps of managing an outbreak

1. Prepare for field work
2. Confirm existence of a communicable disease
3. Verify the diagnosis
4. Identify and count the number of cases. Create a case definition
5. Record the data in terms of time, place and person
6. Introduce immediate control measures if indicated
7. Formulate a hypothesis (e.g. the cause)
8. Test the hypothesis
9. Plan additional systematic studies
10. Implement and evaluate control (and preventative) measures
11. Initiate surveillance
12. Communicate findings e.g. write a report and disseminate

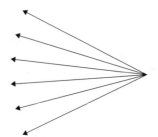

Controls can be introduced
at any step

Figure 10.5 Control measures may be introduced at any step of managing an outbreak

Source: Adapted from Goodman *et al.*, 1990, p. 10

Control measures

To manage the outbreak, the multi-agency incident team will implement control meas-ures. These can range from removing the source of contaminated food, like the pâté in Scotland, closing a business that is serving food, changing hygiene measures, and providing health education, treatment and/or vaccinations. Control measures can be introduced at any step of managing an outbreak of communicable disease to protect the public, as shown in Figure 10.5.

Managing pandemics

The term 'epidemic' is used when the number of new cases of a specific communi-cable disease exceeds expected numbers. A 'pandemic' extends this definition to include a multi-national, or even global, distribution of a new communicable disease (Donaldson and Rutter, 2018). The Black Death, the bubonic plague of 1347, was responsible for 200 million deaths, which is the highest death toll from a pandemic to date. Other pandemics have included 56 million deaths from smallpox in 1520 and 40 to 50 million deaths from Spanish flu in 1918. Recent pandemics include Severe Acute Respiratory Syndrome (SARS) in 2002, Swine Flu in 2009 and Middle Eastern Respiratory Syndrome (MERS) in 2012 (Table 10.1). Swine Flu is an influenza virus,

Table 10.1 Worldwide distribution, infections and deaths in recent pandemics

Virus	Dates	Number of infections/cases	Number of deaths	Number of countries
SARS	2002–2004	8,000	774	29
Swine flu	2009–2010	34,000,000	151,000–575,000	58
MERS	2012–2020	2,519	866	27
COVID-19	January 22nd 2020 to February 4th 2022	391,040,000	5,730,000	223

Sources: Abdelrahman *et al.*, 2020; Our World in Data, 2022; Worldometer, 2022.

whereas MERS and SARS are from the coronavirus family where the virus is transmitted from animal to human, then human to human (Abdelrahman *et al.*, 2020).

The Chinese Government notified the WHO on December 31st 2019 of an atypical virus in Wuhan, in Hubei Province, causing pneumonia. The WHO named the virus COVID-19 (Corona Virus Disease 2019) on February 11th 2020, and confirmed it was transmitting human-to-human, though it emanated from animals. They declared it to be a pandemic on March 11th 2020. In the UK, the first two cases of COVID-19 were confirmed on January 31st 2020 by the Chief Medical Officer for England. By February 4th 2022, there were over 391 million cases and 5.7 million deaths attributed to COVID-19 across 223 countries. The UK had experienced 157,865 deaths, one of the highest death rates in the world for any country with a population of over 12 million (Our World in Data, 2022).

Outbreak management in a pandemic

Pandemics require a different approach to the usual management of an outbreak and measures of control. The processes of surveillance will identify whether the level of disease and mortality is more than expected; the level of transmissibility, and whether treatment or vaccination is available. These help to determine whether a pandemic requires local or worldwide action. Managing the pandemic needs to take account of the global nature of society, worldwide trade, tourism, migration and air travel. It requires:

- *testing*, which includes testing for those with symptoms (symptomatic) and those without (asymptomatic); mass testing for whole populations and testing at international or national borders
- *contact tracing*, which includes tracing the close contacts of people with the disease. This could be carried out using phone calls, apps, e-mails or texts
- *isolating cases and contacts*, which includes isolating at home and hotels. This needs to be enforced, perhaps by law, alongside further testing and, ideally, with financial support
- *quarantine* to prevent further spread of infection. This includes quarantining one country from another through border controls and quarantine at home or in hotels. Quarantine requires enforcement and further testing
- *non-pharmaceutical/societal interventions* include restrictions on socialising and the work of business. These are challenging because they put pressure on individuals and their income. Unless there is financial support, they might not comply with testing, tracing or isolation
- *communication* is important when governments are restricting people's lives and choices. People need to understand the science behind the pandemic and the behaviours they need to adopt to avoid contracting and spreading the infection. One challenge can be an infodemic of too much information, both accurate and inaccurate, which can make it difficult for people to know the correct course of action (PAHO/WHO, 2020) (see Chapter 6, Box 6.3)

Health protection includes the surveillance and management of communicable diseases.

Vaccination

Vulnerable hosts, such as humans, can protect themselves from pathogens and disease through good nutrition, which supports their immune response, and by

- using mosquito nets to protect against malaria carrying mosquitos
- avoiding contact with sexually transmitted infection by using condoms
- good hygiene practices such as hand washing and using personal protective equipment
- vaccination

The terms 'vaccination' and 'immunisation' are often used interchangeably.

- Vaccination is the process of giving a vaccine, which increases a person's immunity
- Immunisation is the process of developing immunity in populations and individuals

Immunity

We can gain active or passive immunity.

- *Active immunity* is when the body develops its own immune system, either by itself or through vaccination. This is long lasting
- *Passive immunity* is when the body is protected by antibodies that come from immune individuals. These can be transferred during the transfusion of blood or blood products such as immunoglobulin, and, more often, they are transferred across the placenta during pregnancy. The protection provided by the mother to her baby is more effective for some infections, such as tetanus and measles, than for others, such as polio or whooping cough. This type of protection only lasts for a few weeks or months

The World Health Organization (2022) explains how a pathogen is made up of several parts which are usually unique to that pathogen and the disease it causes. Each pathogen contains an antigen. The human body's immune system includes thousands of antibodies, and each antibody is trained to recognise one specific antigen. When the human body is exposed to an antigen for the first time, it takes time for the immune system to respond and produce the antibodies that are specific to that antigen (Figure 10.6). In the meantime, the person is susceptible to becoming ill. Once the antigen-specific antibodies are produced, they work with the rest of the immune system to destroy the pathogen and stop the disease. The body also creates antibody-producing memory cells, which remain alive even after the pathogen has been defeated by the antibodies. If the body is exposed to the same pathogen again, the antibody response is quicker and more effective because the memory cells are in situ, ready to pump out the correct antibodies. In this way, the immune system protects a person from disease.

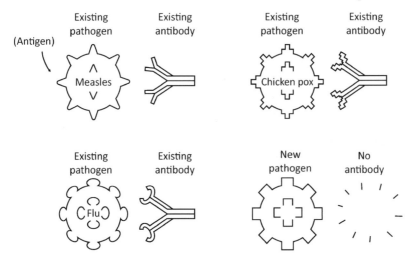

Figure 10.6 The body produces a specific antibody for every new antigen

Source: WHO, 2022. Reproduced with permission from the World Health Organization

How vaccination works

A vaccination protects the host who is exposed to a pathogen from a specific disease. It breaks the 'disease triangle' and enables the body to develop immunity. Vaccines contain either a weakened form of the pathogen, which is sometimes called 'live attenuated'; an inactive form of the pathogen; or a blueprint which tells the body how to produce the antigen. The vaccination will not cause disease in the individual, but it will prompt the body's immune system to respond in the same way as it would to any new pathogen/antigen and produce the specific antibody (WHO, 2022). For example, the measles, mumps and rubella (MMR) vaccine contains a weakened, live attenuated pathogen which encourages the body to develop its own antibodies. Two doses of the vaccine will provide long lasting immunity. The vaccines for whooping cough, diphtheria, tetanus and polio, given in childhood, contain an inactive form of the pathogen. They produce an initial response to the antigen, but this 'primary course of the vaccination' will need to be boosted with further doses later. No vaccine is 100% effective, and we do not yet have vaccines for all communicable diseases, for example human immunodeficiency virus (HIV).

Herd immunity

Herd immunity means the pathogen is unable to find a host because so many people are vaccinated. Herd immunity protects all individuals in a community, including those who are unvaccinated, perhaps for clinical reasons. For example, polio was a devastating disease in the early 1900s. By 1950, polio-related death and disability had dramatically reduced across the world due to high vaccination rates and herd immunity. Recently, Africa was able to declare itself to be polio-free after an international commitment to widespread vaccination programmes in all communities across the continent. Smallpox was eradicated across the world in 1980 and Dowdle and Cochi (2011) believe this was due to four conditions which need to be part of any public health action aimed at eradicating future communicable diseases. These are

- biological feasibility, e.g. intervention measures such as drugs, vaccines and clean environments, need to be safe and effective
- sustained political and societal will, e.g. support from the national government and from the local community
- satisfactory infrastructure for the public health work, e.g. sound management and sufficient capacity
- enough funding for the work

Public health challenges

Vaccination rates need to be high in all countries if we are to achieve widespread herd immunity and reduce outbreaks of communicable diseases. In the UK, there are several reasons why vaccination rates are not sufficiently high. For example, Public Health England has estimated that the measles vaccine, introduced in 1968, has prevented 20 million cases of measles and 4,500 deaths, but measles has not been eradicated (OVG, 2020). In 1988, the vaccination for measles was included in the combined measles, mumps and rubella (MMR) vaccine. The UK is reaching the World Health Organization's target of 95% of five-year-olds for the first vaccination but only achieves 87.4% for the second, and this has enabled the virus to circulate (UKHSA, 2019). Secondly, not all countries have high vaccination rates so global travel puts UK residents at risk from outbreaks in other countries. In addition, Professor Wakefield published his poorly conducted, inaccurate research in 1998 which suggested the MMR vaccination was causing autism. This created global scepticism and reduced the uptake of the vaccine (WHO 2001).

In 2013, the UK had a significant outbreak of measles centred around Swansea (Figure 10.7). Out of the 447 cases confirmed in Mid and West Wales, 64 were admitted

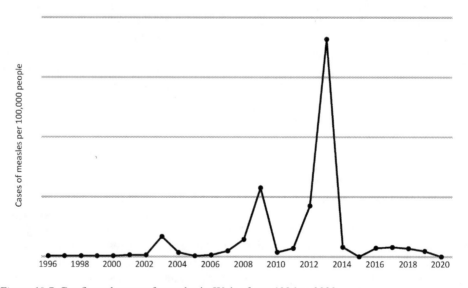

Figure 10.7 Confirmed cases of measles in Wales from 1996 to 2020

Source: Adapted from Public Health Wales, 2021

to hospital and there was one death. A 'catch up' programme of first and second vaccinations for secondary school pupils was introduced, which substantially reduced the number of cases. A similar, but smaller, outbreak was seen in London at the same time. In 2020, there were 79 cases of measles compared to 2,002 in 2012 (Gov.UK, 2021b).

> *Vaccination provides immunity against pathogens. If enough people are vaccinated, herd immunity will protect all people in that community, even the unvaccinated.*

Food safety and micro-biological hazards

Most food in the UK can potentially become contaminated and cause mild to severe gastrointestinal illness, commonly known as food poisoning. The most common pathogens are bacteria, but food poisoning can be caused by viruses and parasites. The public are responsible for their own food standards in the home, but outside the home the standards are set by the Food Standards Agency for England, Wales and Northern Ireland, and Food Standards Scotland. These agencies are responsible for food safety and food hygiene. In addition to providing advice and training, they work with local authorities to enforce food safety regulations. For example, local authorities employ environmental health officers (EHOs) who visit business premises, provide licences to operate, give advice, carry out regular inspections and, if necessary, use their powers to close a business if it does not meet minimum standards (CIEH, 2018). The agencies also employ meat inspectors in meat plants, something that was introduced after the outbreak of bovine spongiform encephalopathy (BSE), 'mad cow disease', in the late 1980s and 1990s.

Common diseases from food

In the UK, campylobacter and salmonella cause the highest number of food-related cases of disease each year, while listeria monocytogenes and *E. coli* 0157 cause more severe disease which can lead to hospitalisation and death. Other common pathogens include norovirus, sometimes called the 'vomiting bug', hepatitis A, cryptosporidium and clostridium (Gov.UK, 2021c). A less common source of infection is the parasite Cylospora, which is more common in contaminated food in developing countries. It can infect travellers who are vulnerable hosts, causing mild gastrointestinal symptoms which can be treated with antibiotics (NHS, 2018).

Campylobacter and salmonella

Campylobacter bacteria are normally found in raw and uncooked meat and poultry. It is estimated there were over 600,000 cases in the UK in 2019 (Gov.UK, 2021c). Salmonella bacteria are found in raw and uncooked meats, eggs, poultry and dairy products. There were about 45,703 cases in the UK in 2019 (Gov.UK, 2021c). Both bacteria cause gastrointestinal symptoms such as nausea, vomiting, abdominal pain, diarrhoea and sometimes a fever. Drinking plenty of fluids is advised, and only rarely is hospitalisation required (NHS, 2021a). Therefore, it is important to avoid storing raw meat above other foods in the fridge and to avoid using the same work surfaces for the preparation of raw meat as well as other foods.

E. coli 0157

E. coli 0157 bacteria have been causing disease since 1980 across the world and since 1983 in the UK (Pennington, 2014). It is relatively rare but becoming increasingly common. It can cause organ failure and death and is associated with food contaminated with animal faeces or from petting animals. In 2016, there was an outbreak of 161 cases in England (154), Wales (6) and Scotland (1) linked to eating mixed salad leaves. The advice to the public included to wash all loose soil from salad and raw vegetables unless it was labelled 'ready to eat' (Gov.UK, 2016). The largest outbreak in the world was recorded at Godstone, Surrey in 1991, where there were 91 cases. This led to significant changes including minimising contact with animal faeces, limiting the number of animals available for petting, instructions for washing hands before and after petting animals and the introduction of procedures to ensure faster intervention by public health professionals (Pennington, 2014).

Cross contamination

Cross contamination is where harmful bacteria is transferred to food. This will not be visible to the naked eye, nor does it affect the taste, smell or texture of the food. Foods which need to be handled with care include raw meat and poultry, fish, eggs and those vegetables and fruit which are not labelled as being 'ready to eat' (Table 10.2).

Table 10.2 Preventing food poisoning from fruit and vegetables

Fruit and vegetables		
	'Ready to eat'	*Not 'ready to eat'*
Examples	Pre-packed vegetables, salad and fruit which are labelled 'ready to eat'. Vegetables, salad and fruit which have been washed and prepared on the premises.	Visibly dirty vegetables, e.g. carrots, potatoes, leeks and lettuce. Vegetables, salad and fruit which is *not* labelled as 'ready to eat', e.g. tomatoes, lettuce, apples, white cabbage and spinach.
Risk	Pre-packed vegetables, salad and fruit which are labelled 'ready to eat' have been through procedures which mean they are safe to eat. Vegetables, salad and fruit which have been prepared on the premises need to be protected from contamination, particularly if they are to be eaten raw.	Visibly dirty vegetables are likely to present a risk of *E. coli* 0157 contamination. Vegetables and fruit which are *not* labelled as 'ready to eat' might have been contaminated with *E. coli* 0157 depending on how they were grown and harvested.
Washing	These foods require no washing before consuming.	These foods must be washed in running water, and peeled, if necessary, before consumption or the next step of processing/cooking.
Storage	Store as 'ready to eat'.	Store separately from the 'ready to eat' fruit, salad and vegetables.

Source: Adapted from Food Standards Agency Scotland, 2012, p. 69).

Businesses that handle food have a duty to protect the public. Guidance for businesses includes:

Stage 1: Think about the raw food that comes into your business.

Who handles the food?
Where is the food received?
Where do you store the food?
Where is the food prepared?
Is the raw food kept separate from 'ready to eat' food?
What utensils or equipment come into contact with the raw food?

Stage 2: Introduce a permanent physical separation between raw food and other food

Limit the handling of raw food to specific members of staff
Create a permanent raw food area where only raw food is handled
Always keep the raw food separate from any 'ready to eat' food
Make the equipment and utensils used for raw food clearly identifiable, e.g. colour coding

Stage 3: Train all your staff in handling food safely
(Source: Food Standards Agency Scotland, 2012)

Vulnerable hosts

Some people are more at risk of illness from contaminated food than others. These are grouped into four risk groups.

- Those who are unable to perform adequate personal hygiene, e.g. due to a lack of ability or capacity, or those who lack access to hygiene facilities
- Children aged five or under who attend a school, nursery or similar childcare groups
- Those whose work involves preparing and serving unwrapped, 'ready to eat' food and drink
- Those who work in clinical, social care or nursery settings with young children, older people or vulnerable people, and whose work includes the potential to transfer infection via faecal-oral transmission
(Source: PHE and CIEH, 2020)

Antimicrobial resistance

Antimicrobial resistance (AMR) is where pathogens change over time and antimicrobial medicines become ineffective. The emergence and spread of drug-resistant pathogens mean common infections can no longer be treated. The World Health Organization (2021) has declared AMR as one of the top ten threats to humanity, with very few new effective antimicrobials, such as antibiotics, being developed. We reduce AMR by immunisation; using antibiotics only when needed for bacterial infection; always completing the course of antibiotics; and by carrying out safe food preparation and handwashing.

Thinking point:

> Consider some of the challenges to getting full population compliance with the measures needed to reduce antimicrobial resistance.

Chemical, biological, radiological and nuclear hazards

The public need to be protected from hazardous chemical, biological, radiological and nuclear (CBRN) events and accidents.

- Chemical hazards include harmful chemical substances, e.g. those used in warfare and industry, or household chemicals (Boxes 10.1 and 10.3)
- Biological hazards include the deliberate release of dangerous viruses, bacteria or biological toxins, e.g. ricin, found in castor oil beans, which was sent to American President Trump in 2020
- Radiological hazards include being exposed to harmful radioactive materials, e.g. polonium-210 which poisoned Alexander Litvinenko in London, 2006
- Nuclear hazards include exposure to harmful radiation and the thermal or blast effects from a nuclear detonation (Box 10.2)

(CPNI, 2021)

Emergency planning and response

The UK Civil Contingencies Act 2004 outlines the multi-agency responsibilities for emergency planning, risk assessment and emergency response. Agencies from across the UK, such as representatives from local authorities, emergency services, the National Health Service and the Environment Agency, come together to form local resilience

---

Box 10.1 Bhopal: the world's worst industrial disaster, 1984

The American-owned Union Carbide Corporation's factory in Bhopal, India, made pesticides for agriculture. At 11 pm on December 2nd 1984 an employee noticed that a storage tank was leaking methyl isocyanate gas, and that a safety device had been turned off. At 1 am, a loud rumbling was heard as 40 tons of toxic fumes escaped into the air forming a large grey cloud. Almost immediately, 3,800 people died along with thousands of animals. Gradually local hospitals were overwhelmed with the poisoned. Disease and disability continued for decades. Twenty years later, reports estimated the gas leak had caused between 15,000 and 20,000 premature deaths. The Corporation immediately tried to distance itself from legal responsibility, though it was eventually forced to pay some compensation to the Indian Government. The Corporation has not revealed exactly what was in the toxic cloud, but it is suspected that the methyl isocyanate was heated to a sufficiently high temperature to degrade to form hydrogen cyanide. The victims showed classic signs of cyanide poisoning. Although Union Carbide shut down its Bhopal factory, it did not clean up the site and it continues to leak toxic chemicals, some of which have been found in the water system.

(Source: Broughton, 2005)

Box 10.2 Chernobyl: the world's worst nuclear disaster, 1986

The Chernobyl nuclear power plant is situated in the north of Ukraine. In 1986, Ukraine was part of the Soviet Union (USSR). The operators decided to carry out an experiment to check the safety of the nuclear reactors if the electricity supply were to fail. On April 26th, at 1.23 am in number 4 reactor, the experiment started. Within seconds, an explosion of steam blew the lid off the reactor releasing radioactivity into the environment. The reactor burnt, and the radioactivity continued to escape across large areas of Europe for ten days. Between April 27th and May 6th 116,000 people were evacuated from an area 2,500 km^2. This rose to 350,000 evacuees from areas around Ukraine, Belarus and Russia. Many of these areas remain abandoned due to the continuing dangerous levels of radioactivity.

In addition to the adverse social, psychological and economic impact of the accident, the radioactive iodine contaminated food and milk. By 2015, there were more than 20,000 cases of thyroid cancer among those who were children at the time. Among those who were adults, rates of leukaemia and other types of cancer continue to rise, as do radiation-induced cataracts. The accident was attributed to poor reactor design, poor emergency planning procedures and a low level of skill among the reactor operators.

(Source: Beresford *et al.*, 2016; WHO, 2016; WNA, 2021)

forums (LRFs). These may be supported by other organisations such as National Highways, public utility companies, the military and the voluntary sector. Emergency plans will contain a risk assessment of the hazard. The initial response is to

- identify the agent
- identify the source
- identify the perimeter of the impact, such as a plume
- identify any affected individuals
- communicate with the public

Box 10.3 Emergency response to Novichok poisoning in Salisbury, 2018

Nerve agents disrupt nerve signals to the muscles causing problems with breathing, convulsions, sweating, wheezing and vomiting. As the nerves to the heart and lungs involuntarily contract, it leads to death. Novichok, which means 'newcomer', is a slow-acting chemical weapon/poison created by the Soviet Union, designed to be absorbed through the skin. In March 2018, two Russian citizens living in Salisbury, Wiltshire, were deliberately poisoned with Novichok which was later found on their front door. Months later, Dawn Sturgess, who touched the discarded perfume bottle in which the agent had been transported, died.

The emergency planning procedures were implemented immediately, as this was identified as a potential terrorist event. The Wiltshire and Swindon Local Resilience Forum comprised 26 partner agencies including Public Health Wiltshire,

Wiltshire Police, Wiltshire Council, Ministry of Defence, Defence Science and Technology Laboratory at Porton Down, Salisbury District Hospital Trust, South Western Ambulance Service, NHS England and Government Agencies: the Department for Environment, Food and Rural Affairs (DEFRA), Public Health England and the Environment Agency. Its aim was to preserve public safety and reassure the public alongside assisting the ongoing murder investigation led by the Counter Terrorism Network. Deputy Chief Constable Mills said, "Over six months, the [forum] developed an approach to public health risks which had never been encountered anywhere in the world." Tracy Daszkiewicz, director of public health, worked with the police and intelligence agencies to trace the movements of the two poisoned Russian citizens to prevent the spread of the nerve agent around the city.

James Rubin and colleagues carried out a study with 500 residents to record the public impact of the Novichok poisoning in Salisbury. He found 40.6% reported anxiety, 29.8% reported anger and 30.6% reported uncertainty. For the majority, the emotional impact was mild. However, a notable number of people avoided Salisbury. The researchers concluded that public trust and confidence could have been improved by explaining this was a targeted incident with specified contamination.

(Source: Rubin *et al.*, 2020b; Wiltshire Police Federation, 2019)

Common exposures in the UK

The UK Health Security Agency (UKHSA) is responsible for protecting the public from communicable diseases caused by chemical, biological, radiological and nuclear hazards. The Health and Safety Executive for Great Britain, and the equivalent for Northern Ireland, are independent regulators of health and safety in the workplace. They enforce the Control of Substances Hazardous to Health (COSHH) regulations which outline chemical controls, limits and standards. An employer is required to carry out their own risk assessments, monitor compliance and ensure their staff are appropriately trained. Accidents at work due to toxic chemicals or fumes can impact a person's health immediately or cause disease in later years, such as asbestosis. Further examples are discussed in Chapter 14. Harmful substances and activities include:

- dust or fumes in the air which can cause lung diseases
- fluids used in metal work, because they can grow fungi and bacteria, which cause dermatitis and asthma
- wet working, such as cleaning, because it can cause dermatitis
- prolonged contact with wet cement can cause dermatitis and chemical burns
- benzene, found in crude oil, can cause leukaemia
- a wide variety of other substances used at work including paint, glue, ink, lubricant, beauty products and detergent

(HSE, 2012)

In the early hours of Sunday morning December 5th 2005, there was an explosion and fire in the Buncefield oil storage depot in Hemel Hempstead, England. This was investigated by the Health and Safety Executive and the Environment Agency, working as the 'competent authority', that is the legally designated authority, for the regulation of major accident hazards. It identified several failings and learning points. Large quantities of petrol had overflowed causing a gas plume which then ignited into an explosion. The main recommendations related to the safety procedures and practices at sites which have major hazards. The report stated,

- "There should be a clear understanding of major accident risks, and the safety-critical equipment and systems designed to control them
- There should be systems and a culture in place to detect signals of failure in safety-critical equipment and to respond to them quickly and effectively
- Time and resources for process safety should be made available

Once all the above are in place:

- There should be effective auditing systems in place which test the quality of management systems and ensure that these systems are actually being used on the ground and [that they] are effective
- At the core of managing a major hazard business, [there] should be [a] clear and positive process [of] safety leadership, with board-level involvement and competence to ensure that major hazard risks are being properly managed"

(CASMG, 2011, p. 5. Reproduced under the terms
of the Open Government licence v3.0)

Health protection includes measures to protect the population's heath against food-related, chemical, biological, radiological and nuclear hazards.

Risk assessment in the workplace

Carrying out risk assessments is common practice in all industries. They include assessing the health and safety risks to the organisation and to the individual and then mitigating them with the appropriate action. The Health and Safety Executive (2015) works with four primary goals; these act as standards for health and safety in the workplace:

- the need for strong leadership
- involving the workforce
- building competence
- creating healthier, safer workplaces

Once a potential hazard has been identified, we assess the level of risk to an individual member of the workforce by asking,

- "Who might be harmed and how
- What you're already doing to control the risks
- What further action you need to take in order to control the risks
- Who needs to carry out the action
- When the action is needed by"

(HSE, 2022)

Recording workplace injuries

In the UK, it is a legal requirement that the Health and Safety Executive is notified about work-related accidents and incidents. In accordance with the Reporting of Injuries, Diseases and Dangerous Occurrences Regulations (RIDDOR), employers, and others who are in control of work premises, must keep records and report,

- "Work-related accidents which cause death
- work-related accidents which cause certain serious injuries (reportable injuries)
- diagnosed cases of certain industrial diseases

and

- certain 'dangerous occurrences' (incidents with the potential to cause harm)"

(HSE, 2013, p. 1)

Reporting incidents provides useful information on which to develop risk assessments in the workplace. Reports often relate to injuries (Figures 10.8 and 10.9).

Hazard analysis for food safety

In the UK, anyone who runs a food business, or premises where food is served, needs to have a Hazard Analysis and Critical Control Point (HACCP) plan to keep the

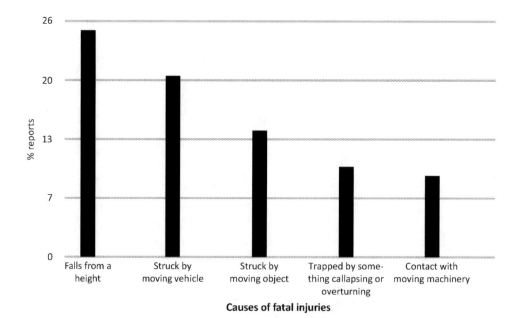

Figure 10.8 Fatal injuries to employees and the self-employed by the most common kinds of accidents, 2016/17 to 2020/21

Source: Adapted from HSE, 2021, p. 4

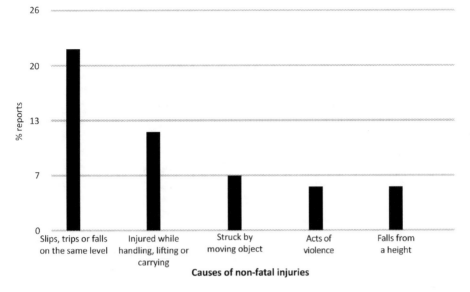

Figure 10.9 Non-fatal injuries to employees by the most common kinds of accidents, 2020 to 2021

Source: Adapted from HSE 2021, p. 4

food safe from biological, chemical and other physical hazards. To make the plan, a business must

- identify any hazards that must be avoided, reduced or removed
- identify the critical control points (CCPs). These are the points when a potential hazard needs to be prevented, removed or reduced, e.g. by cooking, cooling, heating to a minimum temperature or adding an ingredient
- set limits for the CCPs, e.g. something that can be measured such as a temperature or a length of time
- monitor the CCPs, e.g. observations and measurements which check that the CCPs are being met, such as checking and recording the fridge temperature every hour
- rectify any problems with CCPs, e.g. if the fridge temperature is found to be too high, identify to whom this should be immediately reported
- put checks in place to ensure the plan is working, e.g. annual meetings with an external consultant to discuss the plan and associated records
- keep records, e.g. records of temperature checks, staff training and checklists

(Gov.UK, 2022)

Health protection policies in workplaces help to protect the whole population.

Screening

Health protection includes offering screening to healthy populations, with no symptoms, to identify disease. A screening programme needs to be safe, cause no harm, be easily accessible and have a high degree of accuracy. The UK National Screening Committee (UKNSC) advises government ministers and the National Health Service for each of the four UK nations on all aspects of screening programmes, from research to implementation. Each nation sets its own screening policies and there are some differences across the UK. Wilson and Jungner (1968) set out the four types of screening:

- 'mass screening' refers to large-scale screening across the whole population, such as breast screening
- 'selective screening' is used for high-risk groups of the population. It may, or may not, involve mass screening. Chlamydia screening is an example of selective screening for the young, sexually active population
- 'case-finding' is where the purpose of the screening is to find cases of a disease where there are no symptoms, such as breast cancer
- 'screening tests' may be used in epidemiological surveys, which are purposefully looking for cases of disease that need to be treated

UK National Screening Committee criteria

The UKNSC has five criteria against which it judges a potential screening programme. All five need to be met for them to recommend it proceeds. In summary, these are:

- the condition is an important health problem in terms of its severity or frequency in the population
- the screening test is simple, safe, accurate and validated. There is agreement about the parameters of who the screening is suitable for, what constitutes a positive test and the policy concerning the further diagnostic investigations offered to those who are positive
- there should be an effective intervention, for example a treatment, for those who have a positive screening test; and this intervention should produce better outcomes compared to the usual care given to individuals who have no screening
- the evidence that the screening programme will reduce mortality and morbidity needs to be based on high-quality research. Where the purpose of screening is to enable someone to make an informed choice, the evidence must accurately measure risk. There needs to be evidence that the screening programme is ethically, clinically and socially acceptable to the public and to health professionals
- there must be sufficient resources available to implement the screening programme including resources for testing, diagnosis and treatment; information to allow participants to make informed choices; and a plan for monitoring and quality assurance standards

(UKNSC, 2015)

Prostate cancer

There are over 52,000 cases of prostate cancer each year, but there is no screening programme in place. The UKNSC evaluated the prostate-specific antigen (PSA) blood test against their screening criteria and concluded:

- the test measures the amount of prostate specific antigen in the blood, but it is not sufficiently accurate to detect who needs treatment. It can miss men who *do* have cancer; and falsely identify men who *do not* have cancer who then undergo unnecessary, and sometimes unpleasant, tests and treatment. (The accuracy of tests is discussed in Chapter 3.)

- where early-stage prostate cancer is identified, its treatment needs to be weighed up against its side effects. It is known that some men have prostate cancer which causes them no problems during their lifetime
- it is unclear how PSA screening would impact the death rates due to prostate cancer
- on balance, the UKNSC concluded a PSA-based screening programme does not meet their criteria

(UKNSC, 2022)

UK mass screening programmes

There are 11 mass screening programmes in the UK (Table 10.3). The challenges for screening programmes include maintaining a high uptake of screening, building confidence with the public and enabling them to make informed choices, and maintaining high-quality standards across all screening programmes. For example, errors in the cervical screening programme at the Kent and Canterbury hospitals laboratory, which became public from 1996 to 1998, led to

- eight deaths from cervical cancer
- a decrease in the accuracy of local women's knowledge about screening; for example confusion about the recommended frequency of tests, and muddling cervical screening with investigations such as a colposcopy or laser treatment
- reduced confidence about the reliability of the test among local women, which was thought to be related to the press coverage

(Houston *et al.*, 2001)

Quality assurance systems, to monitor the quality of each type of screening service, operate across the UK and reports are available online. Details about routine screening for trans and non-binary people are available online (PHE, 2021). We will describe breast screening and cervical screening.

Table 10.3 UK mass screening programmes offered through the National Health Service

Type of mass screening	Condition
Screening in pregnancy	Infectious diseases (hepatitis B, HIV and syphilis)
	Sickle cell disease and thalassaemia
	Physical development/foetal anomaly (20-week scan)
Screening for newborn babies	Physical examination
	Hearing test
	Blood spot test
Diabetic eye screening	Early signs of diabetic retinopathy
Cervical screening	Human papillomavirus (HPV) which can lead to cancer
Breast screening	Early signs of breast cancer
Bowel cancer screening	Early signs of bowel cancer
Abdominal aortic aneurysm (AAA) screening	Dangerous swelling of the aorta, a major artery

Source: NHS, 2021b.

Breast screening

Breast cancer is the commonest cancer in the UK, accounting for 15% of all cancer cases (Cancer Research UK, 2022). Breast screening is routinely offered to women, trans women, trans men who have breast tissue and non-binary people between 50 and 70 years old, every three years across the UK. Additional selective and case finding screening is available for those deemed at greater risk. The screening comprises a mammogram, that is an X-ray of the breasts, which aims to detect cancers that are too small to see or feel. The mammogram is approved, validated and safe, though uncomfortable. An individual will receive the results of the mammogram about two weeks later. If a *potential* abnormality is seen, follow-up tests to *confirm* a diagnosis of the presence of cancer cells are offered. England's mass screening programme, offered from 2018 to 2019, was evaluated and it found

- the screening test was effective
- 2.23 million people over the age of 45 were screened, which means there was a 71% response rate
- cancers were diagnosed in 19,558 women, which was 8.8 per 1000 of the women screened

(NHS Digital, 2020)

There has been a significant reduction in morbidity and mortality from breast cancer. One study found that breast screening attendance in England led to a reduction in death rates by 39% (Massat *et al.*, 2016).

Cervical screening

There are about 3,200 cases of cervical cancer diagnosed in the UK every year (Cancer Research UK, 2022). Although cases of cervical cancer decreased by 25% during the 1990s, the rates have remained stable since 2006. There are about 850 deaths per year, which is more than two per day. Cervical screening was introduced in 1998, and it is routinely offered to all women, trans men and non-binary people who were assigned female at birth and who are registered with a General Practitioner as female, between the ages of 25 and 64 every three to five years. The cervical smear test comprises a small sample of cells being wiped from the cervix using a soft brush. The sample is checked for the human papillomavirus (HPV). The test is approved, validated and safe, though uncomfortable. The individual will receive the results about two weeks later. A positive test shows (i) HPV is present but there are no abnormal cells, or (ii) HPV is present and there are abnormal cells. The individual might be invited for follow-up tests to investigate further.

There has been a decline in the uptake of adult cervical screening across the UK over the last decade. For example, in Scotland the government target is for 80% of the eligible population to take up the screening opportunity, but only 69.3% did so during the year ending 31st March 2021 with particularly low uptake in the younger age groups (PHS, 2021) (Figure 10.10). Health promotion campaigns involve working with communities, health professionals and selected health-related services.

Since 2008, vaccination for the HPV virus has been routinely offered to 12 to 13 year olds. Falcaro and colleagues. (2021) studied a sample of those vaccinated when 12 or 13 years old and those who were vaccinated at 14 to 18 years old during a special 'catch-up' programme. They found the vaccine reduced cervical cancer by between

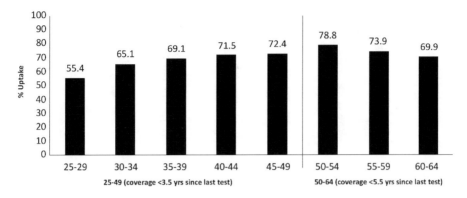

Figure 10.10 Percentage uptake of cervical screening among women (25 to 64 years), Scotland 2020 to 2021

Source: PHS, 2021. Reproduced under the terms of the Open Government Licence v.3.0

34% and 87% among those in their twenties depending when they were vaccinated. The combination of cervical screening and the HPV vaccination programme has the potential to almost eradicate cervical cancer.

A screening programme needs to be evidence-based, safe, easily accessible and accurate.

Summary

This chapter has

- described a range of health protection threats and how to prevent and manage them
- showed how communicable diseases are spread and outbreaks managed
- discussed the threat to society from pandemics and how outbreaks are managed
- described how vaccination works
- detailed common food safety hazards and how to prevent food poisoning
- outlined how the public are protected from major chemical, biological, radiological and nuclear hazards
- explained the principles of risk assessments and incident recording in the workplace
- presented an overview of UK screening programmes with examples of success

Further reading

Bonita, R., Beaglehole, R. and Kjellström, T. and World Health Organization (2006) *Basic epidemiology.* 2nd edn. Geneva: World Health Organization (Chapter 7)

Ghebrehewet, S., Stewart, A.G., Baxter, D., Shears, P., Conrad, D. and Kliner, M. (eds) (2016) *Health protection: principles and practice.* Oxford: Oxford University Press

Useful websites

Health and Safety Executive (GB). Available at: https://www.hse.gov.uk
The Global Health Observatory. Available at: https://www.who.int/data/gho

UK Health Security Agency. Available at: https://www.gov.uk/government/organisations/uk-health-security-agency

UK National Screening Committee. Available at: https://www.gov.uk/government/organisations/uk-national-screening-committee

References

Abdelrahman, A., Li, M. and Wang, X. (2020) 'Comparative reviews of SARS-CoV-2, SARS-CoV, MERS-CoV, and influenza a respiratory viruses', *Frontiers in Immunology*, 11 doi:10.3389/fimmu.2020.552909

Beresford, N.A., Fesenko, S., Konoplev, A., Skuterud, L., Smith, J.T. and Voigt, G. (2016) 'Thirty years after the Chernobyl accident: what lessons have we learnt?', *Journal of Environmental Radioactivity*, 157(2016), pp. 77–89

Broughton, E. (2005) 'The Bhopal disaster and its aftermath: a review', *Environmental Health*, 4(6) doi:10.1186/1476-069X-4-6

Cancer Research UK (2022) *Cancer statistics for the UK*. Available at: https://www.cancer-researchuk.org/health-professional/cancer-statistics-for-the-uk (Accessed 21st June 2022)

Centre for the Protection of National Infrastructure (2021) *Chemical, biological, radiological and nuclear (CBRN) threats*. Available at: https://www.cpni.gov.uk/chemical-biological-radiological-and-nuclear-cbrn-threats (Accessed 21st June 2022)

Chartered Institute of Environmental Health (2018) *Food safety*. Available at: https://www.cieh.org/training-and-courses/work-based-training/food-safety (Accessed 21st June 2022)

Competent Authority Strategic Management Group (2011) *Buncefield: why did it happen?* Health and Safety Executive. Available at: https://www.hse.gov.uk/comah/buncefield/buncefield-report.pdf (Accessed 7th June 2022)

Donaldson, L.J. and Rutter, P.D. (2018) *Donaldsons' essential public health*. 4th edn. Florida: CRC Press

Dowdle, W.R. and Cochi, S.L. (2011) 'The principles and feasibility of disease eradication', *Vaccine*, 29, Suppl 4, D70–D73 doi:10.1016/j.vaccine.2011.04.006

Falcaro, M., Castañon, A., Ndlela, B., Checchi, M., Soldan, K., Lopez-Bernal, J., Elliss-Brookes, L. and Sasieni, P. (2021) 'The effects of the national HPV vaccination programme in England, UK, on cervical cancer and grade 3 cervical intraepithelial neoplasia incidence: a register-based observational study', *The Lancet*, 398(10316) doi:10.1016/S0140-6736(21)02178-4

Food Standards Agency Scotland (2012) *CookSafe. Food safety assurance system*, Issue 1.2 May. Available at: https://www.foodstandards.gov.scot/downloads/CookSafe_Manual_Complete_September_2021.pdf (Accessed 21st June 2022)

Goodman, R.A., Buehler, J.W. and Koplan, J.P. (1990) 'The epidemiological field investigation: science and judgment in public health practice', *American Journal of Epidemiology*, 132(1), pp. 9–16

Gov.UK (2016) *News story. E. coli 0157 national outbreak update*. Available at: https://www.gov.uk/government/news/update-as-e-coli-o157-investigation-continues (Accessed 21st June 2022)

Gov.UK (2021a) *Notifications of infectious diseases (NOIDs)*. Available at: https://www.gov.uk/government/collections/notifications-of-infectious-diseases-noids (Accessed 4th February 2022)

Gov.UK (2021b) *Confirmed cases of measles, mumps and rubella in England and Wales: 1996 to 2021*. Available at: www.gov.uk/government/publications/measles-confirmed-cases/confirmed-cases-of-measles-mumps-and-rubella-in-england-and-wales-2012-to-2013 (Accessed 20th June 2022)

Gov.UK (2021c) *United Kingdom food security report 2021: appendix*. Available at: https://www.gov.uk/government/statistics/united-kingdom-food-security-report-2021/united-kingdom-food-security-report-2021-appendix (Accessed 21st June 2022)

Gov.UK (2022) *Make an HACCP food plan.* Available at: https://www.gov.uk/food-safety-hazard-analysis (Accessed 20th June 2022)

Health and Safety Executive (2012) *Working with substances hazardous to health. A brief guide to COSHH.* Available at: https://www.hse.gov.uk/pubns/indg136.pdf (Accessed 21st June 2022)

Health and Safety Executive (2013) *Reporting accidents and incidents at work.* Available at: https://www.hse.gov.uk/pubns/indg453.pdf (Accessed 21st June 2022)

Health and Safety Executive (2015) *Management of health and safety in the workplace.* Available at: https://www.hse.gov.uk/statistics/pdf/oshman.pdf?pdf=oshman (Accessed 21st June 2022)

Health and Safety Executive (2021) *Kind of accident statistics in Great Britain, 2021.* Available at: https://www.hse.gov.uk/statistics/causinj/kinds-of-accident.pdf (Accessed 21st June 2022)

Health and Safety Executive (2022) *Managing risks and risk assessment at work.* Available at: https://www.hse.gov.uk/simple-health-safety/risk/steps-needed-to-manage-risk.htm#article (Accessed 21st June 2022)

Houston, D.M., Lloyd, K., Drysdale, S. and Farmer, M. (2001) 'The benefits of uncertainty: changes in women's perceptions of the cervical screening programme as a consequence of screening errors by Kent and Canterbury NHS Trust', *Psychology, Health and Medicine*, 6(2), pp. 107–113

Massat, N.J., Dibden, A., Parmar, D., Cuzick, J., Sasieni, P.D. and Duffy, S.W. (2016) 'Impact of screening on breast cancer mortality: the UK program 20 years on', *Cancer Epidemiology Biomarkers and Prevention*, 25(3), pp. 455–462

NHS (2018) *Cyclospora.* Available at: https://www.nhs.uk/conditions/cyclospora (Accessed 21st June 2022)

NHS (2021a) *Food poisoning.* Available at: https://www.nhs.uk/conditions/food-poisoning (Accessed 21st June 2022)

NHS (2021b) *NHS screening.* Available at: https://www.nhs.uk/conditions/nhs-screening (Accessed 7th June 2022)

NHS Digital (2020) *Breast screening programme, England 2018–19.* Available at: https://digital.nhs.uk/data-and-information/publications/statistical/breast-screening-programme/england—2018-19 (Accessed 7th May 2022)

O'Leary, M.C., Harding, O., Fisher, L. and Cowden, J. (2009) 'A continuous common-source outbreak of campylobacteriosis associated with to the preparation of chicken liver paté', *Epidemiology and Infection*, 137(3), pp. 383–388

Our World in Data (2022) *Cumulative confirmed COVID-19 deaths.* Available at: https://ourworldindata.org/explorers/coronavirus-data-explorer?facet=none&pickerSort=-desc&pickerMetric=total_deaths&Metric=Confirmed+deaths&Interval=Cumulative&Relative+to+Population=false&Color+by+test+positivity=false&country=USA~ITA~-CAN~DEU~GBR~FRA~JPN~OWID_WRL (Accessed 5th February 2022)

Oxford Vaccine Group (2020) *Vaccine knowledge project: measles.* Available at: https://vk.ovg.ox.ac.uk/vk/measles (Accessed 7th February 2022)

Pan American Health Organization/World Health Organization (2020) *Understanding the infodemic and misinformation in the fight against COVID-19.* Available at: https://iris.paho.org/bitstream/handle/10665.2/52052/Factsheet-infodemic_eng.pdf (Accessed 21st June 2022)

Pennington, H. (2014) 'E. coli 0157 outbreaks in the United Kingdom: past, present, and future', *Infection and Drug Resistance*, 7, pp. 211–222

Perin, J., Mulick, A., Yeung, D. *et al.* (2022) 'Global, regional, and national causes of under-5 mortality in 2000–19; an updated systematic analysis with implications for sustainable development goals', *Lancet Child and Adolescent Health*, 6(2), pp. 106–115

Public Health England (2014) *Communicable disease outbreak management. Operational guidance.* Available at: https://assets.publishing.service.gov.uk/government/uploads/system/uploads/attachment_data/file/343723/12_8_2014_CD_Outbreak_Guidance_REandCT_2__2_.pdf (Accessed 16th June 2022)

Public Health England (2021) *NHS population screening: information for trans and non-binary people.* Available at: https://www.gov.uk/government/publications/nhs-population-screening-information-for-transgender-people/nhs-population-screening-information-for-trans-people#cervical-screening (Accessed 21st June 2022)

Public Health England and Chartered Institute of Environmental Health (2020) *Recommendations for the public health management of gastrointestinal infections 2019.* Available at: https://assets.publishing.service.gov.uk/government/uploads/system/uploads/attachment_data/file/861382/management_of_gastrointestinal_infections.pdf (Accessed 21st June 2022)

Public Health Scotland (2021) *Scottish cervical screening programme statistics. Annual update to 31 March 2021.* Available at: https://publichealthscotland.scot/publications/scottish-cervical-screening-programme-statistics/scottish-cervical-screening-programme-statistics-annual-update-to-31-march-2021 (Accessed 21st June 2022)

Public Health Wales (2021) *Measles.* Available at: www.wales.nhs.uk/sites3/page.cfm?orgId=457&pid=25444 (Accessed 21st June 2022)

Roser, M. and Ritchie, H. (2021) 'Burden of disease', *Our World in Data.* Available at: https://ourworldindata.org/burden-of-disease (Accessed 10th February 2022)

Rubin, G.J., Smith, L.E., Melendez-Torres, G.J. and Yardley, L. (2020a) 'Improving adherence to "test, trace and isolate"', *Journal of the Royal Society of Medicine*, 113(9), pp. 335–338

Rubin, G.J., Webster, R., Amlot, R., Carter, H., Weston, D. and Wessely (2020b) 'Public responses to the Salisbury Novichok incident: a cross-sectional survey of anxiety, anger, uncertainty, perceived risk and avoidance behaviour in the local community', *BMJ Open*, 10(9) doi:10.1136/bmjopen-2019-036071

UK Health Security Agency (2019) *Measles in England.* Available at: https://ukhsa.blog.gov.uk/2019/08/19/measles-in-england (Accessed 21st June 2022)

UK National Screening Committee (2015) *Criteria for appraising the viability, effectiveness and appropriateness of a screening programme.* Available at: https://www.gov.uk/government/publications/evidence-review-criteria-national-screening-programmes/criteria-for-appraising-the-viability-effectiveness-and-appropriateness-of-a-screening-programme (Accessed 9th February 2022)

UK National Screening Committee (2022) *Adult screening programme. Prostate cancer.* Available at: https://view-health-screening-recommendations.service.gov.uk/prostate-cancer (Accessed 21st June 2022)

Wilson, J.M.G. and Jungner, G. (1968) *Principles and practice of screening for disease.* Geneva: World Health Organization

Wiltshire Police Federation (2019) 'Novichok team is up for world class policing award', *Wiltshire Times.* Available at: https://www.polfed.org/wilts/news/2019/novichok-team-is-up-for-world-class-policing-award/ (Accessed 21st June 2022)

World Health Organization (2001) 'News. Science vs "scaremongering" over measles-mumps-rubella vaccine', *Bulletin of the World Health Organization*, 79(3). Available at: https://scielosp.org/pdf/bwho/v79n3/v79n3a23.pdf (Accessed 21st June 2022)

World Health Organization (2016) *1986 to 2016 Chernobyl at 30.* Available at: https://cdn.who.int/media/docs/default-source/documents/publications/1986-2016-chernobyl-at-30476d83ab-985d-416f-b936-576b0c0ca17f.pdf?sfvrsn=434dbe67_1&download=true (Accessed 21st June 2022)

World Health Organization (2021) *Antimicrobial resistance.* Available at: https://www.who.int/news-room/fact-sheets/detail/antimicrobial-resistance (Accessed 21st June 2022)

World Health Organization (2022) *How do vaccines work?* Available at: https://www.who.int/news-room/feature-stories/detail/how-do-vaccines-work (Accessed 21st June 2022)

World Nuclear Association (2021) *Chernobyl accident 1986.* Available at: http://www.world-nuclear.org/information-library/safety-and-security/safety-of-plants/chernobyl-accident.aspx (Accessed 21st June 2022)

Worldometer (2022) *Countries where COVID-19 has spread.* Available at: https://www.worldometers.info/coronavirus/countries-where-coronavirus-has-spread (Accessed 5th February 2022)

11 Arts and health

Trish (Patricia) Vella-Burrows and Christina Davies

Key points

- Introduction
- Arts and health
- History of arts and health
- The arts and their contribution to health
- Performing arts: music, singing and health in community settings
- Online, digital and electronic arts: radio and community health promotion
- Visual arts, design and craft: visual arts in a mental health hospital setting
- The future of arts and health
- Summary

Introduction

In this chapter we introduce the field of arts and health. We explain how arts engagement takes place across the health continuum, led by a diverse range of practitioners working in a wide range of environments. The relevance of the arts for people's health can be traced back to our ancient ancestors. Today, the arts and health field has accumulated over 30 years of evidence to support the rationale for the use of the arts in disease prevention, health promotion and healthcare. This chapter details some of this evidence and includes UK and international examples. We conclude by reflecting on some of the challenges for the future of arts and health.

Arts and health

To understand the concept of 'arts and health', it is first important to understand what is meant by 'the arts' and 'arts engagement'.

The arts and arts engagement

The arts can be defined by five art forms:

- performing arts
- visual arts, design and craft
- community and cultural festivals
- literature
- online, digital and electronic arts

(Davies *et al.*, 2012)

DOI: 10.4324/9780367823696-13

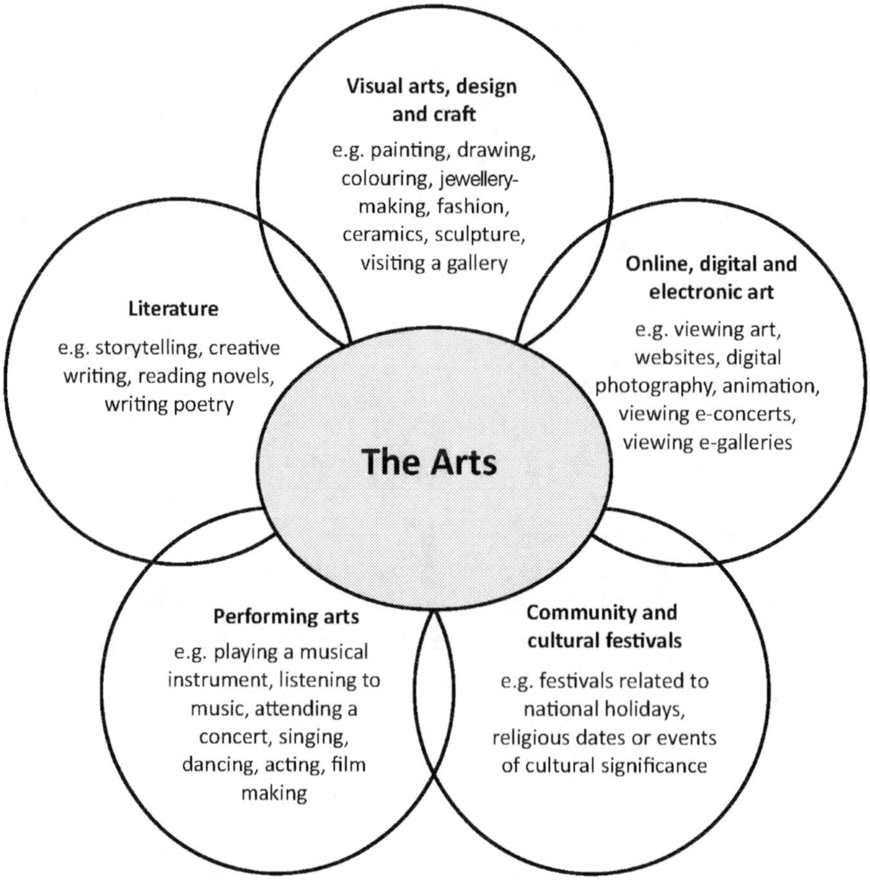

Figure 11.1 Five art forms with examples

Source: Adapted from Davies *et al.*, 2012, p. 208

Figure 11.1 illustrates these five art forms and provides examples of the activities within each.

'Arts engagement' is an umbrella term that encompasses the various ways in which people interact with the arts such as making, performing, attending, listening or viewing art (Archibald and Kitson, 2019; Davies and Pescud, 2020). Art engagement occurs on a continuum from active engagement to receptive engagement.

- Active engagement includes overtly or directly making, performing or creating art as a professional, amateur or hobby artist, e.g. performing in a concert as a musician, singer or dancer; drawing or painting as a visual artist; creative writing or story telling as an author
- Receptive engagement includes experiencing, attending, listening or viewing art as a professional, amateur or hobby artist, e.g. attending a concert or festival as part of an audience or online-audience, listening to music, visiting an art gallery or reading a novel

(Davies *et al.*, 2012; Davies and Pescud, 2020)

Arts engagement occurs in a variety of settings including but not limited to, the home, community centres, schools, workplaces, places of worship, prisons, detention centres, aged care, hospitals, museums, theatres, concert halls, art galleries and in outside settings such as parks, streets and coastal environments (Davies and Pescud, 2020; Vella-Burrows *et al.*, 2014).

There are three main types of arts engagement.

- 'Recreational arts engagement' is something that community members do as part of their everyday life for enjoyment, entertainment, as a social activity or as a hobby
- 'Art therapy' is a form of psychotherapy that involves a therapeutic relationship between a therapist, e.g. an art, music or dance therapist, and a client/patient who works with a creative medium for remedial or diagnostic purposes (ANZACATA, 2022)
- 'Arts interventions' are organised efforts to promote specific behaviours or to change attitudes towards unhealthy habits with the intention of improving physical, mental and social health

Recreational arts engagement, art therapy and arts interventions have a place in maintaining and improving the health and wellbeing of the general population and specific groups within the population (SCHCM, 2014).

Arts and health

The term 'arts and health' describes the practice of applying the arts across the health continuum, meaning it spans end of life, illness, health and optimal wellness. It includes the direct application of the arts with the intention of maintaining or improving health. Arts and health may be for the whole population or for specific target groups such as young people engaging in art classes to increase their mental wellbeing or older adults living with Parkinson's who sing in a group to improve vocal health and mental wellbeing (Irons *et al.*, 2020; Wydenbach and Vella-Burrows, 2020). The impact of arts and health practice may be linked to

- direct and deliberate health-related outcomes such as changes in arts and health policies or practice, increased referrals for art therapy or new arts interventions, e.g. residents of a care home, who are at risk of falling, taking part in a 'dance for falls-prevention' programme to improve their posture, balance and muscle strength (Yan *et al.*, 2018)
- unintentional health-related outcomes such as engaging in recreational arts without the intention to improve health, e.g. a person who attends an art class to learn how to paint and finds the class increases their happiness, relaxation and social interaction with others

Thinking point:

> Consider the art that you do in your everyday life. Do you listen to music, go to the cinema, sing, dance, paint, draw, read a book? Think about the setting in which this occurs e.g. the home, on the way to work, at university or in the workplace. What impact does engaging with the arts have on your wellbeing?

The breadth of arts and health activities requires a diverse and cross-sector workforce. In the UK this includes, but is not limited to, the

- arts and cultural sector, e.g. artists, musicians, dancers, actors and arts organisations
- education sector, e.g. teachers and researchers
- health sector, e.g. nurses, doctors, social prescribers, care co-ordinators, psychologists, psychotherapists, and arts, music, speech and language, occupational and physio therapists
- voluntary sector, e.g. charities associated with the arts, arts and health, religion or community service
- government sector, e.g. policymakers, district and county councils, unitary authorities and national governments

In the UK, useful sources of support for practitioners, researchers and policymakers include:

- Wales Arts Health and Wellbeing Network
- Arts Culture Health and Wellbeing Scotland
- Arts Care, Northern Ireland
- London Arts and Health
- Arts for Health at Manchester Metropolitan University

'Arts and health' refers to the application of the arts for the purpose of preventing disease, maintaining or improving the health of people.

History of arts and health

The arts exist in every society (Morriss-Kay, 2010) and have always played an important part in human health and communication. In the Blombos Cave in South Africa, a 73,000-year-old ochre crayon drawing is thought to be one of the earliest examples of symbolic communication (Henshilwood *et al.*, 2018). In the Grotte du Pech Merle, France, cave paintings and musical instruments, dated as being 45,000 years old, suggest that communities congregated to engage in music and dance (Mithen, 2005). There are several theories about the purpose of the arts for our ancient ancestors. For example, the arts

- were vital for the survival of the species, e.g. activating effective and life-maintaining, communication such as infant-parent bonding, coordinating hunting and war strategies
- helped homo sapiens to make sense of the physical and emotional world
- helped to navigate complex social interactions as communities grew in number
- marked out individual, community and cultural territories
- were used for adornment, e.g. body paint, jewellery, trinkets and homes
- grew as a by-product of homo sapiens' skill and creative development, and served to improve health and wellbeing

(Mithen, 2005; Morley, 2013; Pinker, 1997)

Table 11.1 Examples of pivotal works in the arts and health field, 1996 to 2021

Author and date	Title	Description
Bygren *et al.* (1996)	Attendance at cultural events, reading books or periodicals, and making music or singing in a choir as determinants for survival	First large-scale study to investigate the influence of arts engagements on survival.
Matarasso (1997)	Use or ornament? The social impact of participation in the arts	First large-scale UK study to explore the social impacts of participation in the arts.
Department for Culture Media and Sport (1999)	Policy action team 10: the contribution of sport and the arts	PAT10 suggested that participation in the arts and sport could contribute to neighbourhood renewal.
Smith (2002)	Spend (slightly) less on health and more on the arts	Suggested diverting 0.5% of the healthcare budget to the arts would improve the health of people in Britain.
Staricoff (2004)	Arts in health: a review of the medical literature	Review of the medical literature on the impact of arts and humanities in healthcare. A response to PAT10.
Windsor (2005)	Your health and the arts: a study of the association between arts engagement and health	UK population-based survey of the associations between arts engagement, health and illness. A response to PAT10.
Arts Council England (2007)	UK Arts, health and wellbeing framework	UK framework to promote the integration of the arts into mainstream health strategy and policymaking; and to increase, and effectively deploy, resources for arts and health initiatives, through funding, quality assurance of artists' work and advocacy.
White (2009)	Arts development in community health: a social tonic	The book considers how and why arts in community health evolved and the characteristics and challenges of practice.
Clift *et al.* (2009b)	Arts and health	Launch of an international journal for arts and health research, policy and practice
Clift and Camic (2016)	Oxford textbook of creative arts, health and wellbeing	First arts and health textbook to provide a comprehensive account of the role of the arts in addressing public health needs.
Davies *et al.* (2016)	The art of being mentally healthy	Quantified the arts-mental wellbeing relationship, e.g. two hours of arts engagement per week was found to be associated with good mental wellbeing.
All-party parliamentary group on arts, health and wellbeing (2017)	UK parliamentary inquiry	Inquiry found the arts can help to keep people well, aid recovery and support longer lives better lived. They can help to meet major challenges facing health and social care systems including saving money.
Fancourt and Finn (2019)	What is the evidence on the role of the arts in improving health and wellbeing?	Scoping review for the World Health Organization (Europe) on the role of the arts in improving health.
Davies and Pescud (2020)	The arts and creative industries in health promotion	Systematic review of the impact of the arts on public health.
Corbin *et al.* (2021)	Arts and health promotion. Tools and bridges for practice, research and social transformation	The textbook provides a comprehensive account of the role of the arts for health promotion.

The use of the arts in health and wellbeing has a lengthy history. For example, ancient Greek philosophers, including Aristotle, prescribed calming flute music for patients experiencing mania and music played on the dulcimer for patients with depression (Dobrzyńska *et al.*, 2006). During the middle-ages, art was used in hospitals to enhance the hospital environment (Clift *et al.*, 2009a) and later Florence Nightingale, who revolutionised hospital architecture and design, recognised that the arts could provide spiritual and emotional nourishment to aid healing. Nightingale wrote,

> "Little as we know about the way in which we are affected by form, by colour, and light, we do know this, that they have an actual physical effect ... [and] are actual means of recovery."
>
> (Nightingale, 1860, p. 37)

Over the last 25 years, publications and research studies have promoted the use of the arts in the health field. Some of these are listed in Table 11.1.

> *The arts exist in every society and have always played an important part in human health. In the last 25 years, the field of arts and health, and research demonstating its value, has been growing.*

The arts and their contribution to health

From a theoretical perspective, the field of arts and health contributes to disease prevention and salutogenesis within a biopsychosocial understanding of health across the whole health continuum.

- Disease prevention means the arts contribute to deterring deterioration in health (see Chapter 7). Activities may be designed as primary prevention, secondary prevention or tertiary prevention (Figure 11.2)
- Salutogenesis means the arts contribute to supporting and improving people's quality of life towards optimal wellness (Antonovsky, 1987; Mittelmark and Bauer, 2017) (see Chapter 7)
- The biopsychosocial model of health (Engel, 1977) suggests health is a holistic concept, comprising biological, social and psychological dimensions (see Chapter 1)
- The health continuum spans death, illness, health and optimal wellness (see Chapter 7)

The Healthy Arts Framework (Table 11.2) emerged from an investigation into the relationship between arts engagement and population health outcomes among Australian adults (Davies *et al.*, 2014). The data from semi-structured interviews were analysed and seven primary outcome themes emerged. These were mental health, social health, physical health, economic factors, knowledge, art and identity. Physical, social and mental outcomes were classified as 'health outcomes', ways in which engaging with the arts (arts engagement) affected people's health. Art, knowledge, identity and economic outcomes were classified as being determinants of health or

Health

Good health		Health problems
wellness, wellbeing		disease, disorders, distress

Primary prevention	**Secondary prevention**	**Tertiary prevention**
preventing the development of a health problem by reducing risks and enhancing protection	early detection of a health problem and preventing or reversing its progression	managing a health problem to maximise healthy living and prevent further deterioration
Active arts engagement e.g. taking part in a weekly *creative writing class* at a community centre to learn how to *write* short stories, as a way of relaxing and gaining social interaction with others	**Active arts engagement** e.g. people with mild depression *acting* in a *community play* about mental health to raise awareness of symptoms, avenues for help and reduce stigma	**Active arts engagement** e.g. people with chronic disease *singing* in a *choir* as part of their pulmonary rehabilitation
Receptive arts engagement e.g. people *watching a documentary* about how a family gave up junk food and moved towards healthier eating	**Receptive arts engagement** e.g. *reading a biography* about someone who has type 2 diabetes and the changes they need to make to their health-related behaviours	**Receptive arts engagement** e.g. patients in hospital *listening* to *music* as part of their rehabilitation following a stroke to stimulate various parts of the brain

Figure 11.2 Arts engagement across primary, secondary and tertiary prevention

'health determinant outcomes', meaning these related to the context of people's lives and factors which influence their health. Some of the outcomes were negative and some were positive.

Thinking point:

> Consider how introducing the arts into a setting, such as the home, a hospital or workplace, could improve a person's physical, mental and social wellbeing.

A recent international review of journal articles from the UK, Australia, New Zealand, Canada, the United States of America, Norway, the Netherlands, Germany, Denmark and South Africa, published between 2015 and 2019 ($n = 56$ articles), examined the relationship between the arts, health and health behaviours. The authors found 'strong evidence' for the impact of arts engagement on people's mental wellbeing and 'moderate to strong evidence' for its impact on their social health. This compares to the evidence for healthy eating, physical activity, preventing tobacco use and preventing harm from alcohol use which was rated as 'emerging' or 'low evidence' (Davies and Pescud, 2020). We will describe the impact of three art forms on health:

- performing arts: music, singing and health in community settings
- online, digital and electronic arts: radio and community health promotion
- visual arts, design and craft: visual arts in a mental health hospital setting

Table 11.2 Healthy arts framework

Outcome themes		Outcomes	
		Positive	*Negative*
Health outcomes	Mental health	Happiness, confidence, self-esteem, enjoyment, pleasure, reduced stress, relaxation, self-expression, self-reflection, achievement, satisfaction, feeling respected and valued, compliments, recognition, energy, motivation, creation of good memories, more resilient to poor mental health.	Frustration, criticism, nervousness, anxiety, overwhelmed, confronting, disappointment, emotionally draining, 'arty' stigma, unwanted responsibility.
	Social health	Less isolated, increased network broadens ideas and beliefs, more community minded; feel more 'worldly and cultured', form of entertainment, social occasion, enjoyment in giving/receiving art, shared social experiences, enhances community connection, bridging and bonding social capital.	
	Physical health	Walking, standing, warm-ups, performance-based movement, e.g. dance, physiological benefits.	Injury, pain, tiredness as many events at night, unhealthy behaviours at some events, e.g. smoking or binge drinking, some art materials are toxic/poisonous if not used correctly.
Health determinant outcomes	Knowledge	Intellectual stimulation, increased knowledge and skills, e.g. business, communication, literacy, teamwork, problem-solving, social skills.	
	Identity	Gives life more meaning, enhances connection to self.	
	Economic	Saves money by creating art for self and others, source of income, career opportunities.	Expensive, earn a low income from art.
	Art specific	Creativity, art skills, non-competitive, participation, arts appreciation, interaction with artists and arts organisations, supports artists and arts organisations.	Time consuming.

Source: Adapted from Davies *et al.*, 2014, p. 6.

The arts contribute to disease prevention and salutogenesis within a holistic understanding of health. Engaging with the arts influences health and the determinants of health.

Performing arts: music, singing and health in community settings

Music involves a composition of silence and organised sounds, including vocal and instrumental sounds. Music also contains important elements such as loudness, melody, rhythm, pitch, duration and harmony. The positive effects of engaging with music and singing in the general population and specific groups include improved mental wellbeing, for example happiness and enhanced memory; enriched social health, for example reduced social isolation and better connection to others; and positive physical outcomes, for example pain reduction and improved lung function (Davies and Pescud, 2020; Skingley *et al.*, 2014; 2020; Skingley and Vella-Burrows, 2010; Unadkat *et al.*, 2016).

The positive effects of listening to music are often associated with:

- increased serotonin, which is linked to feeling good and creative thinking
- increased dopamine, which is linked to feeling pleasure, being alert and enhancing focus and concentration
- the regulation of cortisol and reduction of adrenaline which influence stress and anxiety levels

(Baixauli, 2017; Ferreri *et al.*, 2019; Finn and Fancourt, 2018; Helsing *et al.*, 2016; Mavridis, 2015)

Singing as part of a community group has been found to:

- synchronise singers' heart rates, reduce cortisol and increase oxytocin. These influence stress and anxiety levels as well as strengthening social bonding and group cooperation
- stimulate antibody Immunoglobulin A (IgA) which improves people's immunity to disease

(Finn and Fancourt, 2018; Grape *et al.*, 2002; Kreutz *et al.*, 2004; Vickhoff *et al.*, 2013)

These findings reflect singers' own perceptions of the impact of group singing, including self-reported feelings of stress reduction and improved mood, motivation, attention, sense of achievement, cognitive function, social connectedness and a sense of belonging (Clift and Hancox, 2001; Dingle *et al.*, 2021). Some of these findings emerged from the evaluations of BBC Music Day in 2019 (Box 11.1) and singing groups for people with chronic obstructive airways disease (Box 11.2).

Box 11.1 BBC Music Day, 2019

On September 26th 2019, the annual BBC Music Day took place with events and broadcasts spread across a week. These comprised more than 800 projects broadcast on television, radio, online and social media platforms. Across the UK, events included local radio stations, live music, Get Singing events, Music and Dementia events and the launch of the BBC Music Memories website. Music Day ambassadors comprised a selection of musicians, representing a wide genre of music, who made appearances at several events.

Evaluation of the project

The Day was evaluated by examining the ambassadors' comments about their involvement in the project (Vella-Burrows *et al.*, 2019). These provided a record of some of the health-related impacts and were grouped into four themes.

Reduced negative feelings and stress

Many ambassadors spoke about music helping with life stressors and negative feelings. Nina Nesbitt, a singer and songwriter who took the lead with the Get Singing initiative in schools, referred to music as a 'form of expression and therapy'. Singer and music producer, Naughty Boy, said that music helped him to overcome the challenges of today's 'fast paced world',and allowed him to focus and concentrate. He said, "The power of music helps me to forget about the world."

Emotional expression

Ambassadors spoke of music enabling emotional expression. For example, Scottish singer and songwriter Tom Walker, Happy Mondays' singer Rowetta and pop singer Freya Ridings spoke about music being cathartic and healing.

Motivation and achievement

Most of the Music Day ambassadors spoke of a drive to create and perform music. Nina Nesbitt referred to music as an opportunity to create good change. Rapper, Professor Green spoke of how creating and performing music engendered a unique sense of fulfilment. Soprano singer, Lesley Garrett, talked about music's ability to help her make sense of the world. She said, "It's my identity … my reason for being here … my mission."

Social connectedness

Professor Green, a Mancunian rapper; Aitch, from the band Keane; Nile Rogers, an American singer/songwriter/producer; and Ray BLK, a singer and songwriter, all referred to music transcending cultural divisions. It united, bonded and connected people, and it was a vehicle through which life experiences could be shared. Several comments spoke of social connectedness being essential to overall wellbeing.

Conclusion

It is recognised that the mechanisms that underpin the relationship between music and wellbeing are complex and multi-faceted, and the experiences of both active and receptive engagement are by their nature subjective. Within this context, the evaluation of BBC Music Day provided evidence that music has a positive impact at an individual and societal level.

(Source: BBC, 2019a, 2019b)

Box 11.2 Singing for breathing

Chronic obstructive pulmonary disease (COPD) is an umbrella term for a group of incurable lung diseases, such as bronchitis and emphysema, which are characterised by inflamed, damaged and narrowed airways. It is most often seen among smokers. People complain of increasing breathlessness and often experience wheezing, a chesty cough and frequent chest infections. Over time, it can prevent people from engaging in their everyday activities leading to a loss of independence and isolation.

Six singing groups were set up in Kent and led by experienced singing facilitators who received five days of specialised training. Ninety-seven individuals
with diagnosed COPD, and an average age of 69.5 years, participated in weekly
singing across ten months, with breaks for Christmas and Easter. Each singing session lasted for one hour, beginning with 20 minutes of relaxation, work
on posture, breathing and vocal exercises. This was followed by 40 minutes of
singing a wide repertoire of new and familiar songs which was adjusted according to participants' interests. People learnt 'by ear' and many songs were per-
formed without any accompaniment. The participants completed a breathing
test to measure their air flow (spirometry), and a questionnaire at the start, mid-
way and at the end. Questions were asked about their levels of breathlessness,
quality of life, mobility, self-care, usual activities, discomfort/pain, depression
and anxiety. At the start, participants' breathing tests showed a range of COPD
severity: 15% mild, 45% moderate, 30% severe and 10% very severe.

Evaluation of the project

At the end, the average results of the breathing tests demonstrated improvements in breathing. Most participants reported their breathing had improved
because the singing group had

- helped with learning about breathing, e.g. breath control, muscle control,
  understanding breathing and techniques for everyday activities
- promoted relaxation
- improved posture
- provided a 'good workout'
- opened the lungs and increased lung capacity
- made physiotherapy easier
- provided distraction and helped with concentration
- helped to prevent feelings of panic and hyperventilation

A large number reported other improvements in physical health such as having
more energy, increased mobility and better vocal capacity. There were 91 'comments' that referred to enjoyment or fun. The perceived psychological benefits
of the singing groups included they

- lifted the spirits
- boosted confidence and provided a sense of achievement
- promoted general mental/emotional wellbeing
- provided an 'adrenaline buzz'
- promoted a positive attitude and countered feeling low
- helped with relaxation
- helped with coping with the illness
- reduced depression and/or anxiety
- encouraged self-help

There were 110 'comments' about how the singing groups had provided positive
social benefits such as facilitating friendships, social interaction, camaraderie
and meeting others who understood and cared.

Conclusion

The researchers do not claim that every individual benefitted in every way from the singing groups but, for most participants, singing was perceived as acceptable, and beneficial for their breathing and general physical, psychological and social wellbeing.

(Source: Skingley *et al.*, 2014)

Online, digital and electronic arts: radio and community health promotion

Over 30 years ago, the World Health Organization's *Ottawa Charter for Health Promotion* emphasised the right of all citizens of the world to have access to health-related information, life skills and opportunities for making healthy choices (WHO, 1986). Today, such information is widely available via mass media and digital technology. There have been several Cochrane reviews that have investigated the role of mass media in encouraging positive health behaviours. For example, health messages delivered via radio broadcasts have shown a moderate to high-level impact among disadvantaged populations. These include reducing the transmission of human immunodeficiency virus (HIV) (Medeossi *et al.*, 2014), improving sanitation and hygiene (Bamani *et al.*, 2013) and improving child health (Sarrassat *et al.*, 2018). The likely reasons for their success include the low cost of radio equipment; the ability of radio broadcasting to reach remote populations and to focus on local health priorities using local language; and the receptive engagement of the listener. These factors, and the relatively low production and distribution costs, are also appealing to public service broadcasters that serve low-income populations (Skuse, 2004). Some of these findings are illustrated in Box 11.3.

Box 11.3 *Promesas y Traiciones* (Promises and betrayals)

Promesas y Traiciones was a 48-episode radio novella broadcast as part of a variety show by a Spanish-language radio station in the American state of Alabama. A novella is a work of dramatic, narrative fiction similar to a soap opera. The novella was aimed at the Hispanic population who suffer disproportionately from cardiovascular disease, cancer, diabetes, obesity and liver failure. Around a quarter of Hispanic adults, aged 18 to 64, live below the poverty line with poor access to health-related information and treatment. The project was underpinned by Bandura's social learning theory and aimed to

- enhance community engagement
- increase knowledge about prevention (e.g. healthy eating), risk factors for disease and disease symptoms

Developing the radio novella

Twenty-four local Hispanic people took part in a series of story-writing workshops which aimed to explore how they perceived and dealt with health problems. The emerging story lines were centred on an anonymous Hispanic family, the consequences of healthy and unhealthy behaviours and the challenges of changing behaviour. The novella was co-produced, directed, acted by, broadcast and evaluated by the 24 participants with the support of a script writer, diabetes health educator, personnel from social services, two radio station executives and a Hispanic professor of theatre. During the broadcasts, health professionals were available to answer questions from listeners.

Evaluation of the project

Community engagement

To evaluate community engagement, researchers analysed the audio and written records of all workshops; the numbers of listeners to the novella; audio recordings of listeners' on-air health-related questions and the health professionals' responses; and audio recordings of participants' discussions about the content of the episodes including their cultural appropriateness and understanding of the embedded health messages. The data was placed on the radio station's website and shared with the county health department.

Healthy eating

One example of the health behaviours of interest to the researchers was healthy eating. Healthy eating was assessed by asking participants to report their consumption of fried foods, sweet drinks, fruit and vegetables at the start and end of the intervention. The novella included the character of an overweight mother with diabetes who ate several empanadas (fried meat pies) despite protests from her daughter. Later, the mother suffered a heart attack. The evaluation showed eating fried foods between four to seven days per week decreased from 41.6% to 22.6%, while those eating at least two portions of fruit and vegetables increased from 32.2% to 45.1%. The research also showed that the participants' confidence in their ability to avoid fatty food increased.

Conclusion

Overall, the project created a sense of community ownership and excitement. The participants provided highly relevant and powerful material to inform the characters and a plot that resonated with radio listeners who showed a high level of interest in the health topics. Longer-term, there was increased interest in community-based health-related work among the participants, creative partners such as writers, the radio station owners and other radio producers of entertainment-education. There have been further creative outputs including an interactive website and social media platform, and the distribution of merchandise such as water bottles and lunch bags. The challenges for the project related to navigating local county politics, health services and building community trust. Trust was achieved by keeping dialogues open and considering all opinions and ideas. Limited resources and a low project budget were overcome by word-of-mouth advertising, contributions from volunteers and the radio station, and the support of other not-for-profit organisations. The researchers concluded, "The production of a radio drama using the entertainment-education approach was a unique way to address health disparities among the local Hispanic population" (Frazier *et al.*, p. 6).

(Source: Frazier *et al.*, 2012; Kohler *et al.*, 2012)

Visual arts, design and craft: visual arts in a mental health hospital setting

In a healthcare setting, arts engagement for both in-patients and out-patients can have psychological benefits, such as feelings of happiness; social benefits such as forming new friendships, and physical benefits such as reduced heart rate, blood pressure and pain reduction (Chlan, 1998; Chlan *et al.*, 2000; Davies *et al.*, 2021; Good, 1996; Nilsson *et al.*, 2003; Staricoff, 2004) (see Chapter 15). In intensive-care units and among patients with cancer, cardiovascular disease and those undergoing rehabilitation, arts activities have been found to improve patients' perceptions of the hospital environment, as well as reducing their length of stay in hospital (Chlan, 1998; Davies *et al.*, 2021; Selle and Silverman, 2017; Staricoff, 2004). In a hospital setting, visual arts, design and craft activities, events and interventions that increase patient mood and patient-staff interactions have the potential to positively impact care if these mood changes result in improved patient engagement in their treatment and enhance the hospital environment (Davies, 2016) (Box 11.4).

Box 11.4 The Creative Arts Pilot Project

The Ursula Frayne Unit, at St John of God Mt Lawley Hospital in Western Australia, is a 12-bed ward for patients aged 65 and over who are experiencing poor mental health. This includes episodes of grief, loss, depression, bipolar affective disorder, schizophrenia, drug and alcohol dependency, anxiety, psychosis and dementia. The average length of stay in the unit is 49 days. Although patients are offered an extensive programme of care and therapy, it was noticed by staff that there were periods in the day when patients became isolated and bored.

As an Australian leader in arts and health practice, St John of God Health Care Group's Arts and Health Philosophy and Framework is to actively engage patients in their care as creative makers to support health, healing and recovery (Pearson, 2014). The Creative Arts Pilot Project was developed at Mt Lawley Hospital and aimed to support patient wellbeing, foster artistic interest and expand patients' artistic skills by providing visual arts opportunities.

The Creative Arts Pilot Project ran once a week, on Saturday mornings, for three months. The 12 stand-alone sessions provided patients with the opportunity to create art works with a resident artist (not an art therapist). Participation was voluntary and patients could attend as many sessions as they wished. Each session had a particular focus, e.g. felt making, wrapping, printing, solar dying, ink drawing, Shibori, painting, origami, terrarium making, card making, drawing and collage. The artist provided art materials, instructions and encouragement. Patients had the freedom to be guided by their own interests, to continue with an arts activity from a previous week and to continue with their artwork during the week, if they chose to. The artist worked collaboratively with hospital staff, including the resident occupational therapist who also had access to the art materials.

Evaluation of the project

During the course of the project, 23 patients were admitted to the unit, of which 19 took part in the Creative Arts Pilot Project. The number of patients attending each session varied from week to week, with an average of six patients per session. Factors which affected attendance included the patients' health, confidence and interest, as well as other events happening at the same time such as family visits and a football grand finale. The hospital commissioned the University of Western Australia to evaluate the project via survey and qualitative feedback from the patients who participated in the project ($n = 16$); hospital staff and visitors who observed the project ($n = 20$), and key stakeholders who were involved in the design, implementation and delivery of the project (e.g. hospital staff, the artist, executive staff, communications staff, $n = 10$). The evaluation was voluntary, was approved by two ethics committees and included the informed consent of each patient and guardian.

Patients

Most patients indicated they enjoyed the art classes, even though most did not have any arts-related hobbies and had not previously made art with an artist before. Taking part in the project improved their mood and they liked making art with others on the ward (the artist, other patients and hospital staff). Significantly more patients felt happy immediately after taking part in an art session (88% happy, $p < 0.01$) compared with their pre-project baseline (56% happy) and before each art session (59% happy).

> "It makes a big difference. It brings things out of people instead of them sitting in their rooms … It's been a great help to me."
>
> (male patient)

For many patients, the project was an opportunity to learn a new skill, acquire new knowledge and be introduced to a new positive pastime that they could continue to do once they left the ward. Most patients agreed the hospital should continue to run art classes.

> "We did some wonderful work."
>
> (female patient)

Hospital staff and visitors

Staff and visitors observed that after taking part in the project patients seemed happier, that the project appeared to be enjoyable, it taught new skills and it was a positive social experience for patients, staff and visitors.

> "The atmosphere changed. The environment changed as the patients' art works [were] displayed around the ward and around the hospital, creating a sense of community and belongingness." (hospital staff)

Staff and visitors suggested the project was an opportunity to be creative; to develop an interest in the arts as a hobby; and to develop and express ideas. Most thought the project supported the patients' health, healing and recovery and was a positive pastime in a hospital setting. All agreed the project enhanced the hospital environment and should be continued.

> "I would like to see this project continue. I think the patients, caregivers and artist have so much more to offer and we have only just touched the surface." (hospital staff)

Stakeholders

Stakeholders indicated that the project had a positive impact on patients, staff, visitors and the views of the general community (via the mainstream media and social media). They thought the project was well planned, resourced and well run. Stakeholders thought the project should be continued and the art sessions should be expanded to other wards throughout the hospital, for example in oncology, rehabilitation and long-term care.

Conclusions

This study highlights the value, acceptability and positive impact of providing older adult patients with the choice to engage in a recreational, visual arts project while receiving mental health treatment in hospital. The Creative Arts Pilot Project evaluation found that participation in the pilot was a positive social experience and elicited a positive and statistically significant increase in patient mood. Overall, the hospital effectively delivered an arts programme to older adult patients that was enjoyable, supported patient wellbeing, developed art skills and enhanced the hospital environment. The positive impact of the pilot study on patients, staff, service delivery and community engagement was formally recognised and resulted in the pilot becoming a core hospital programme, available nationally, that is now called 'cARTwheels'.

(Source: Davies, 2016)

Research shows that different art forms can have a positive impact on health.

The future of arts and health

To better integrate the arts into mainstream public health and healthcare policy and practice, there is a need to challenge the dominance of the reductionist approach which characterises the medical model of health and illness. By using both qualitative and quantitative methodologies to measure and evaluate the effects of arts engagement on health, we can continue to enhance the evidence base (Daykin *et al.*, 2017; Davies and Pescud, 2020). To expand the use of arts to promote and maintain health, there is a need to inform and educate public health, clinical, social care and healthcare students and staff about the current and emerging evidence, as well as the practical methods, activities and interventions that are relevant to, and can be easily integrated into, their modes of practice. Finally, there is also a need for better integrated arts-based health policies which recognise that the arts can promote and maintain health, aid recovery, and add value to the health system as both a method and setting from which to promote health (APPGAHW, 2017; Davies and Pescud, 2020).

Summary

This chapter has

- described the arts, arts engagement and the field of arts and health
- illustrated how arts and health takes place in many settings across the health continuum
- provided examples of the evidence that demonstrates how the arts contribute to prevention, health promotion and healthcare
- provided examples of the impact of the arts on different dimensions of health
- outlined the challenges for arts and health to fulfil its potential

Further reading

Clift, S. and Camic, P. (eds) (2016) *Oxford textbook of creative arts, health and wellbeing: international perspectives on practice, policy and research.* Oxford: Oxford University Press

Corbin, J., Sanmartino, M., Hennessy, E.A. and Urke, H.B. (eds) (2021) *Arts and health promotion. Tools and bridges for practice, research and social transformation.* Cham: Springer

White, M. (2009) *Arts development in community health: a social tonic.* Oxford: Radcliffe

Useful websites

Culture, Health and Wellbeing Alliance. Available at: https://www.culturehealthandwellbeing.org.uk

Health Arts Research Centre (University of Northern British Columbia). Available at: https://healtharts.ca

Repository for Arts and Heath. Available at: https://www.artshealthresources.org.uk

References

All-party parliamentary group on arts, health and wellbeing (2017) *Creative health: the arts for health and wellbeing (Short Report).* Available at: https://www.culturehealthandwellbeing. org.uk/appg-inquiry (Accessed 18th April 2022)

Antonovsky, A. (1987) *Unravelling the mysteries of health. How people manage stress and stay well.* San Francisco: Jossey-Bass

Archibald, M. and Kitson, A. (2019) 'Using the arts for awareness, communication and knowledge translation in older adulthood: a scoping review', *Arts and Health*, 12(2), pp. 99–115

Arts Council England (2007) *Arts, health and wellbeing.* London: Arts Council England

Australian, New Zealand and Asian Creative Arts Therapies Association (2022) *About creative arts therapies.* Available at: https://www.anzacata.org/About-CAT (Accessed 18th April 2022)

Baixauli, E. (2017) 'Happiness: role of dopamine and serotonin on mood and negative emotions', *Open Access Emergency Medicine*, 7(2) doi:10.4172/2165-7548/1000350

Bamani, S., Toubali, E., Diarra, S. *et al.* (2013) 'Enhancing community knowledge and health behaviors to eliminate blinding trachoma in Mali using radio messaging as a strategy', *Health Education Research*, 28(2), pp. 360–370

British Broadcasting Corporation (2019a) *BBC music day 2019 ambassadors.* Available at: https://www.bbc.co.uk/programmes/articles/3qBPGMX1lqZpTwXrDKB1ld7/bbc-music-day-2019-ambassadors (Accessed 8th June 2022)

British Broadcasting Corporation (2019b) *BBC music day. For the love of music.* Available at: https://www.bbc.co.uk/events/e2gfbp (Accessed 18th April 2022)

Bygren, L.O., Konlaan, B.B. and Johansson, S.E. (1996) 'Attendance at cultural events, reading books or periodicals, and making music or singing in a choir as determinants for survival: Swedish interview survey of living conditions', *BMJ*, 313(7072), pp. 1577–1580

Chlan, L. (1998) 'Effectiveness of a music therapy intervention on relaxation and anxiety for patients receiving ventilatory assistance', *Heart and Lung*, 27(3), pp. 169–176

Chlan, L., Evans, D., Greenleaf, M. and Walker, J. (2000) 'Effects of a single music therapy intervention on anxiety, discomfort, satisfaction, and compliance with screening guidelines in out-patients undergoing flexible sigmoidoscopy', *Gastroenterology Nursing*, 23(4), pp. 148–156

Clift, S. and Camic, P.M. (eds) (2016) *Oxford textbook of creative arts, health, and wellbeing: international perspectives on practice, policy and research*. Oxford, Oxford University Press

Clift, S., Camic, P.M., Chapman, B. *et al.* (2009a) 'The state of arts and health in England', *Arts and Health*, 1(1), pp. 6–35

Clift, S., Camic, P. and Daykin, N. (2009b) 'Editorial. The coming of age for arts and health: what we hope to achieve', *Arts and Health*, 1(1), pp. 3–5

Clift, S. and Hancox, G. (2001) 'The perceived benefits of singing: findings from preliminary surveys of a university college choral society', *Perspectives in Public Health*, 121(4), pp. 248–256

Corbin, J., Sanmartino, M., Hennessy, E.A. and Urke, H.B. (eds) (2021) *Arts and health promotion. Tools and bridges for practice, research and social transformation*. Cham: Springer

Davies, C. (2016) *The impact and effectiveness of the 2015 St John of God health cCare creative arts pilot project*. Perth: The University of Western Australia

Davies, C., Knuiman, M. and Rosenberg, M. (2016) 'The art of being mentally healthy: a study to quantify the relationship between recreational arts engagement and mental well-being in the general population', *BMC Public Health*, 16(1) doi:10.1186/s12889-015-2672-7

Davies, C.R., Knuiman, M., Wright, P. and Rosenberg, M. (2014) 'The art of being healthy: a qualitative study to develop a thematic framework for understanding the relationship between health and the arts', *BMJ Open*, 4(4) doi:10.1136/bmjopen-2014-004790

Davies, C. and Pescud, M. (2020) *Evidence check. The arts, creative industries and health promotion*. Sax Institute for The Victorian Health Promotion Foundation. Available at: https://www.saxinstitute.org.au/wp-content/uploads/20.12_Evidence-Check_arts-and-health-promotion.pdf (Accessed 18th April 2022)

Davies, C.R., Rosenberg, M., Knuiman, M., Ferguson, R., Pikora, T. and Slatter, N. (2012) 'Defining arts engagement for population-based health research: art forms, activities and level of engagement', *Arts and Health*, 4(3), pp. 203–216

Davies, C.R., Shurdington, J., Murray, K., Slater, L. and Pearson, D. (2021) 'Music for wellness in rehabilitation patients: programme description and evaluation results', *Public Health*, 194, pp. 109–115

Daykin, N., Gray, K., McCree, M. and Willis, J. (2017) 'Creative and credible evaluation for arts, health and well-being: opportunities and challenges of co-production', *Arts and Health: International Journal for Research, Policy and Practice*, 9(2), pp. 123–138

Department for Culture Media and Sport (1999) *Policy action team 10: the contribution of sport and the arts*. Available at: https://www.artshealthresources.org.uk/docs/pat10-policy-action-team-10-report/#:~:text=Produced%20by%20the%20UK%20Department,and%20people%20from%20ethnic%20minorities (Accessed 18th April 2022)

Dingle, G.A., Sharman, L.S., Bauer, Z. *et al.* (2021) 'How do music activities affect health and well-being? A scoping review of studies examining psychosocial mechanisms', *Frontiers in Psychology*, 12 doi:10.3389/fpsyg.2021.713818

Dobrzyńska, E., Cesarz, H., Rymaszewska, A.K. and Kiejna, A. (2006) 'Music therapy – history, definitions and application', *Archives of Psychiatry and Psychotherapy*, 8(1), pp. 47–52

Engel, G.L. (1977) 'The need for a new medical model: a challenge for biomedicine', *Science*, 196(4286), pp. 129–136

Fancourt, D. and Finn, S. (2019) *What is the evidence on the role of the arts in improving health and well-being? A scoping review. Health evidence network synthesis report 67*. Copenhagen: World Health Organization (Europe)

Ferreri, L., Mas-Herrero, E., Zatorre, R.J. *et al.* (2019) 'Dopamine modulates the reward experiences elicited by music', *Proceedings of the National Academy of Sciences of the United States of America*, 116 (9), pp. 3793–3798

Finn, S. and Fancourt, D. (2018) The biological impact of listening to music in clinical and nonclinical settings: a systematic review. *Progress in Brain Research*, 237, pp. 173–200

Frazier, M., Massingale, S., Bowen, M. and Kohler, C. (2012) 'Engaging a community in developing an entertainment-education Spanish-language radio novella aimed at reducing chronic disease risk factors, Alabama, 2010–2011', *Preventing Chronic Disease*, 9 doi:10.5888/pcd9.110344

Good, M. (1996) 'Effects of relaxation and music on post-operative pain: a review', *Journal of Advanced Nursing*, 24(5), pp. 905–914

Grape, C., Sandgren, M., Hansson, L., Ericson, M. and Theorell, T. (2002) 'Does singing promote well-being? An empirical study of professional and amateur signers during a singing lesson', *Integrative Psychological and Behavioural Science*, 38(1), pp. 65–74

Helsing, M., Västfjäll, D., Bjälkebring, P., Juslin, P. and Hartig, T. (2016) 'An experimental field of study of the effects of listening to self-selected music on emotions, stress, and cortisol levels', *Music and Medicine*, 8(4), pp. 187–198

Henshilwood, C.S., D'errico, F., van Niekerk, K.L., Dayet, L., Queffelec, A. and Pollarolo, L. (2018) 'An abstract drawing from the 73,000-year-old levels at Blombos Cave, South Africa', *Nature*, 562, pp. 115–118

Irons, J.Y., Hancox, G., Vella-Burrows, T., Han, E., Chong, H., Sheffield, D. and Stewart, D.E. (2020) 'Group singing improves quality of life for people with Parkinson's: an international study', *Aging and Mental Health*, 25(4), pp. 650–656

Kohler, C.L., Frazier, M., Bowen, M., Massingale, S. and Hunter, E. (2012) 'A Spanish language radio drama for obesity and tobacco prevention', *Proceedings of the 140th American Public Health Association Annual Meeting and Exposition 2012. Prevention and Wellness across the Life Span. San Francisco.* Washington: American Public Health Association

Kreutz, G., Bongard, S., Rohrmann, S., Hodapp, V. and Grebe, D. (2004) 'Effect of choir singing or listening on secretory immunoglobulin A, cortisol and emotional state', *Journal of Behavioural Medicine*, 27(6), pp. 623–635

Matarasso, F. (1997) *Use or ornament? The social impact of participation in the arts.* Stroud: Comedia

Mavridis, I.N. (2015) 'Music and the nucleus accumbens', *Surgical and Radiologic Anatomy*, 37(2), pp. 121–125

Medeossi, B., Stadler, J. and Delany-Moretlwe, S. (2014) '"I heard about this study on the radio": using community radio to strengthen good participatory practice in HIV prevention trials', *BMC Public Health*, 14(876) doi:10.1186/1471-2458-14-876 (Accessed 18th April 2022)

Mithen, S. (2005) *The singing neanderthals: the origins of music, language, mind and body.* London: W&N

Mittelmark, M. and Bauer, G. (2017) 'The meanings of salutogenesis', in Mittelmark, M., Sagy, S., Eriksson, M., Bauer, G.F., Pelikan, J.M., Lindstrom, B. and Espnes, G.A. (eds) *The handbook of salutogenesis.* Switzerland: Springer, pp. 7–13

Morley, I. (2013) *The prehistory of music: human evolution, archaeology, and the origins of musicality.* Oxford: Oxford University Press

Morriss-Kay, G.M. (2010) 'The evolution of human artistic creativity', *Journal of Anatomy*, 216(2), pp. 158–176

Nightingale, F. (1860) *Notes on nursing. What it is, and what it is not.* New York: D. Appleton and Company

Nilsson, U., Rawal, N. and Unosson, M. (2003) 'A comparison of intra-operative or post-operative exposure to music – a controlled trial of the effects on postoperative pain', *Anaesthesia*, 58(7), pp. 684–711

Pinker, S. (1997) *How the mind works.* New York: W.W. Norton

Pearson, D. (2014) *St John of God health care arts and health philosophy and framework.* Perth: St John of God Health Care

Sarrassat, S., Meda, N., Badolo, H. *et al.* (2018) 'Effect of a mass radio campaign on family behaviours and child survival in Burkina Faso: a repeated cross-sectional, cluster-randomised trial', *The Lancet Global Health*, 6(3) doi:10.1016/S2214-109X(18)30004-4

Selle, E.W. and Silverman, M.J. (2017) 'A randomized feasibility study on the effects of music therapy in the form of patient-preferred live music on mood and pain in patients on a cardiovascular unit', *Arts and Health*, 9(3), pp. 213–223

Skingley, A., Billam, D., Clarke, D. *et al.* (2020) 'Carers create: carer perspectives of a creative programme for people with dementia and their carers on the relationship within the (carer and cared-for) dyad', *Dementia*, 20(4), pp. 1319–1335

Skingley, A., Page, S., Clift, S., Morrison, I., Coulton, S., Treadwell, P., Vella-Burrows, T., Salisbury, I. and Shipton, M. (2014) '"Singing for breathing": participants' perceptions of a group singing programme for people with COPD', *Arts and Health*, 6(1), pp. 59–74

Skingley, A. and Vella-Burrows, T. (2010) 'Therapeutic effects of music and singing for older people', *Nursing Standard*, 24(19), pp. 35–41

Skuse, A. (2004) *Radio broadcasting for health: a decision maker's guide.* Department for International Development. Available at: https://pdf4pro.com/cdn/icd-report-radio-broadcasting-for-health-a-decision-356484.pdf (Accessed 18th April 2022)

Smith, R. (2002) 'Spend (slightly) less on health and more on the arts', *BMJ*, 325(7378), pp. 1432–1433

Standing Council on Health and Cultural Ministers (2014) *National arts and health framework.* Department of Communications and the Arts, Australian Government. Available at: https://www.artshealthresources.org.uk/wp-content/uploads/2019/03/2014-National-Arts-and-Health-Framework.pdf (Accessed 18th April 2022)

Staricoff, R. (2004) *Arts in health: a review of the medical literature.* London: Arts Council England

Unadkat, S., Camic, P.M. and Vella-Burrows, T. (2016) 'Understanding the experience of group singing for couples where one partner has a diagnosis of dementia', *Gerontologist*, 57(3), pp. 469–478

Vella-Burrows, T., Ewbank, N., Gilbert, R., Forrester, M. and Barnes, J. (2019) *Music and health: a short review of research and practice for BBC music day 2019.* Available at: www.artshealthresources.org.uk/docs/music-and-health-a-short-review-of-research-and-practice (Accessed 20th April 2022)

Vella-Burrows, T., Ewbank, N., Mills, S., Shipton, M., Clift, S. and Gray, F. (2014) *Cultural value and social capital: investigating social capital, health and wellbeing impacts in three coastal towns undergoing culture-led regeneration.* Available at: https://www.artshealthresources.org.uk/wp-content/uploads/2017/01/2014-Vella-Burrows-Cultural-value-and-social-capital-report.pdf (Accessed 2nd May 2022)

Vickhoff, B., Malmgren, H., Aström, R. *et al.* (2013) 'Music structure determines heart rate variability of singers', *Frontiers in Psychology*, 4(344) doi:10.3389/fpsyg.2013.00334

White, M. (2009) *Arts development in community health: a social tonic.* Oxford: Radcliffe

Windsor, J. (2005) *Your health and the arts: a study of the association between arts engagement and health.* Arts Council England. Available at: https://www.artshealthresources.org.uk/docs/your-health-and-the-arts-a-study-of-the-association-between-arts-engagement-and-health (Accessed 18th April 2022)

World Health Organization (1986) *The Ottawa charter for health promotion, 1986.* Available at: https://www.euro.who.int/en/publications/policy-documents/ottawa-charter-for-health-promotion,-1986 (Accessed 18th April 2022)

Wydenbach, N. and Vella-Burrows, T. (2020) *Singing for people with Parkinson's.* Oxford: Compton Publishing Ltd

Yan, A.F., Cobley, S., Chan, C. *et al.* (2018) 'The effectiveness of dance interventions on physical health outcomes compared to other forms of physical activity: a systematic review and meta-analysis', *Sports Medicine*, 48(4), pp. 933–951

Part III

Tackling priorities for health promotion and public health

12 Tackling tobacco, alcohol and drugs

Sally Robinson

Key points

- Introduction
- Models of substance use
- International guidance
- UK principles for tackling tobacco, alcohol and drugs
- Health promotion interventions to reduce substance-related harm
- Summary

Introduction

This chapter explains how the UK tackles the substances tobacco, alcohol and drugs in ways that seek to prevent harm. It describes three models of understanding and approaching substance use: the moral, medical and social models. The chapter outlines examples of international guidance and conventions that influence how countries, including the UK, approach preventing substance-related harm. It identifies the eight common principles which the four nations of the UK share within their policies. The chapter ends with examples of substance-related interventions that enact the preventive, educational, empowerment and social change models of health promotion.

Models of substance use

The use of tobacco, alcohol and drugs, collectively called substances, can cause a range of physical, psychological and social harms to health, including the potential for users to become dependent and acquire a range of diseases that cause early death. These are examined in the companion book to this one, *Priorities for Health Promotion and Public Health* (Robinson, 2021a). Substances are produced, marketed, distributed and sold by powerful international organisations such as the alcohol, tobacco and pharmaceutical industries as well as drug traffickers. How a society thinks about substance use, and the approaches it takes to prevent related harm, reflect its history and culture. It also reflects the dominant models of health and illness in that society. Models of health and illness are about how people understand health and illness. What causes health? What causes illness?

- In the traditional model, illness is caused by an imbalance within a person or an imbalance between the person and the metaphysical environment. The latter is called 'personalistic' and it includes becoming ill due to a supernatural force or sin

DOI: 10.4324/9780367823696-15

- In the medical model, illness is caused by a malfunction in the body or a germ
- In the social model, illness is caused by the social, economic and physical environment which influences people's psychology, biology and health-related behaviours

(Robinson, 2021b)

Here, we describe three models of substance use: the moral model, the medical model and the social model.

Moral model

The moral model of substance use is based on the belief that the act of substance use is morally wrong, a sin. It sits within the traditional (personalistic) model of health and illness (Robinson, 2021b). Dependency occurs in morally weak individuals; it is a character fault. People need guidance to resist temptation and/or threats of punishment to keep the moral code. The moral model underpins the criminal justice approach to substance use; rather than sin, it identifies crime. Holland (2020) explains how the belief in something being immoral leads to it being made illegal, and illegality leads to it being perceived as immoral. He writes,

> "... possessing a drug is illegal because buying it is morally wrong; buying it is morally wrong because it provides funding for organised criminal gangs; it provides funding for organised criminal gangs because they control the market for that drug ... because it is illegal to possess it."

(p. 3)

Some of the questions that emerge from this model concern who decides the moral code, to what degree a moral-based approach reduces harms and whether what is defined as legal or illegal is correct.

Moral model in the UK

The moral model is most clearly seen in how UK law classifies drugs (Table 12.1). The Misuse of Drugs Act 1971 and the Psychoactive Substances Act 2016 outline penalties for producing, possessing or supplying

- Class A drugs which include crack cocaine, MDMA (ecstasy), heroin, methadone, LSD, magic mushrooms and methamphetamine

Table 12.1 UK drug penalties

Class of drug	Penalty for possession	Penalty for production and supply
A	Maximum 7 years in prison and/or unlimited fine	Maximum of life imprison and/or unlimited fine
B	Maximum 5 years in prison and/or unlimited fine	Maximum of 14 years in prison and/or unlimited fine
C	Maximum 2 years in prison and/or unlimited fine (excludes anabolic steroids)	Maximum of 14 years in prison and/or unlimited fine or both
Temporary class drugs	None, but police can take away	Maximum of 14 years in prison and/or unlimited fine
Psychoactive substances	None, unless the person is in prison	Maximum of 7 years in prison and/or unlimited fine

Source: Adapted from Gov.UK (2021a).

- Class B drugs which include amphetamines, barbiturates, cannabis, codeine, ketamine, synthetic cannabinoids and synthetic cathinones
- Class C drugs which include anabolic steroids, benzodiazepines, gamma-hydroxybutyrate (BGHB) and khat

and

- producing or supplying a psychoactive substance or carrying it with the intention of supplying another

(Legislation.gov.uk, 1971; 2016a)

Some policymakers are recommending that drug laws, particularly those relating to personal possession, should be decriminalised (APPG, 2021; HSCC, 2019). In September 2021, the Lord Advocate of Scotland announced that possession of Class A drugs may be considered for a Recorded Police Warning instead of prosecution (COPFS, 2021). This brought Class A drugs into line with Class B and C in Scotland. In effect, it was a significant move towards decriminalising drugs in Scotland.

Medical model

The medical model of substance use focusses on the effects of using substances on the body. The aim is to remove, reduce, treat or cure the potential or actual harm caused by tobacco, alcohol and drugs. Medical research uses the scientific method, meaning it examines whether a cause produces an observed, universal effect in humans. It may focus on genes, biochemical changes or the brain. People need care and treatment to fix their body and achieve an 'absence of disease'. Sometimes life-long abstinence may be advocated as the only cure. Dependency is a disease for which the person is not held responsible. The search for a purely biological cause of substance dependency is ongoing, but it is becoming more commonly understood as a biopsychosocial condition. For example, Heilig and colleagues (2021) explain how neurons in each person's brain develop in response to their experiences. They hold memories. This unique neuronal network drives how people make choices and respond to situations, such as being offered an alcoholic drink. Harmful levels of substance use seem to interfere with the neurons that govern decision-making, which leads to choosing the substance over another option. They report,

> "… pre-existing vulnerabilities and persistent drug use lead to a vicious circle of substantive disruptions in the brain that impair and undermine choice capacities for adaptive behaviour, but do not annihilate them."

(Heilig *et al.*, 2021, p. 1720)

Epidemiologists study substance use across populations and identify the risk factors that increase the chances of dependence and other substance-related harms to health. People's behaviours, such as binge drinking or injecting, are established as important risk factors, so medical experts try to persuade people to change behaviour. The direction of travel remains towards an 'absence of disease', but those working with a medical model, and others, recognise that this is not always realistic. Some people will always engage in potentially health harming substance use regardless of evidence, expert advice or the law. This has led to the acceptance of an incremental approach. The term 'harm reduction' is a *process* which has a specific meaning associated

Box 12.1 Biopsychosocial: drug, set and setting model

The 'drug, set and setting' model considers the person as a biological, psychological and social being. The impact of a substance is the result of the

Drug – its pharmacological properties
Set – the personal physical and psychological characteristics of the person
Setting – the physical and social environment in which the substance is taken

(Source: Zinberg, 1986)

with the empowerment model of health promotion, discussed later in this chapter. Recently, policymakers have begun to use the phrase more loosely to encompass any policy, programme or practice that leads to the *outcome* of reduced substance-related harm. In this chapter, we make the distinction clear by referring to 'reducing harmful outcomes' or 'harm minimisation' when referring to *outcomes*.

Medical model in the UK

The UK population's health is protected by *The Misuse of Drugs Regulations 2001* which govern how professionals, such as pharmacists, store, prescribe, administer and keep records of controlled (illegal) drugs used for medical purposes (Legislation.gov.uk, 2001). In the medical model, examples of harm minimisation in the UK include

- nicotine replacement medicines and nicotine-containing e-cigarettes (ENDS) can help with tobacco cessation
- opiate substitution therapy, e.g. prescribing oral methadone as a substitute for heroin reduces risks associated with heroin and the way it is taken
- needle and syringe exchange services provide sterile equipment to prevent the transmission of viruses such as hepatitis C (Figure 12.1)

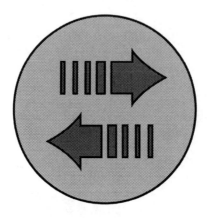

Figure 12.1 The UK national needle exchange symbol

- take-home naloxone, a medicine which reverses an opioid overdose, can be prescribed for people whose lives may be at risk through dependency
- proposals for the introduction of drug consumption rooms. These are rooms where individuals can use drugs in a clean and safe environment. They not only minimise harm for individuals but reduce the number of discarded needles in the community
- residential rehabilitation services to support those with dependencies

(APPG, 2021; H.M. Government, 2021; HSCC, 2019; PHE, 2019)

Social model

The social model of substance use recognises that people's use of tobacco, alcohol and/or drugs is not always a free choice. Some people become dependent on addictive substances and others are harmed by other people's use. The social determinants of health include the physical and social environment and the distribution of power, money and resources (WHO, 2010a; 2021a). The power, money and resources of alcohol, tobacco and drugs manufacturers are used to produce, market and sell their products to achieve the cultural normalisation of substance use. Mosher and Akins (2021) outline five social theories of substance use.

- 'Social control theories' refer to a group of sociological theories which argue people need to integrate and conform to the accepted norms of society to maintain social harmony. Although substance use is a natural behaviour, it also weakens the bonds that hold society together. Dependency represents social failure, which increases the likelihood of the behaviour being seen as something requiring social control, perhaps legal or moral controls
- 'Strain theory' suggests stresses within society, such as loss, economic hardship or confrontation, increase the chances of people turning to substances to deal with the strain. The substances may provide physiological benefits such as relaxation or provide psychological coping behaviours
- 'Social learning theory' has its origins in psychology and suggests substance use is a learned behaviour from others, especially those who are role models with whom the user identifies. The behaviour is encouraged if the user receives, and then begins to anticipate, positive feedback from the substance, other people and the wider social setting
- 'Social conflict theory' focusses on inequalities in power in society. The powerful control the laws, politics, media and other channels of influence, while others become marginalised and relatively powerless. Some argue that substance-related laws disproportionately penalise those with least power such as ethnic minorities and the poor (Lassiter and Spivey, 2018). Others argue this is one reason why international and UK drugs laws are out of date and not fit for purpose (GCDP, 2019; Holland, 2020)
- 'Life course approach' seeks to understand the key social risk factors that influence people's experience of substance use and its health consequences across their lifetimes. It considers the impact of the accumulation of substance use over time, and identifies the critical periods and life events that encourage or discourage some people to embark on a trajectory towards dependency while others never begin or disembark. For example, adverse childhood experiences, unemployment and trauma in adulthood are known risk factors for developing dependency (HCSAC, 2019)

Unlike the moral and medical models, the social model incorporates the idea that lay/non-professional people are experts in their own health and their own substance use. The inclusion of their insight and experience has led to a more holistic understanding of substance use, peer support, innovations in prevention and treatment, and important contributions to cultural and political debates about how substance use is perceived and tackled (Denis-Lalonde *et al.*, 2019; DoH, 2021; HCSAC, 2019).

Social model in the UK

UK law does not make alcohol or tobacco illegal substances, but it does use both legal and other social approaches to reduce the harmful outcomes associated with using alcohol and tobacco. The UK's tobacco control legislation comprises the *Standardised Packaging of Tobacco Products Regulations 2015* and *Tobacco and Related Products Regulations 2016*. The latter is currently under review (Gov.UK, 2021b). Examples of UK law and tobacco include

- manufacturers and importers of tobacco products must pay duty (tax) to the UK Government
- manufacturers and suppliers of tobacco products and e-cigarettes must comply with packaging and labelling regulations
- a maximum limit of 10 mg tar, 1 mg nicotine and 10 mg carbon monoxide per cigarette
- no smoking in private vehicles carrying children under 18
- advertising of all tobacco products is banned
- advertising of e-cigarettes containing nicotine (ENDS) is banned in the press, television, radio and online
- a producer of a novel tobacco product must notify the Secretary of State and provide the required details

(Gov.UK, 2021c; Legislation.gov.uk,2014; 2021)

Examples of UK law and alcohol include

- banning the sale of alcohol to someone under 18
- penalties for drinking alcohol or carrying open containers of alcohol on public transport in London
- per 100 ml, legal drink drive limits in England, Wales and Northern Ireland are 35 mg breath and 80 mg blood
- per 100 ml, legal drink drive limits in Scotland are 22 mg breath and 50 mg blood
- specified quantities of alcohol that can be served in glasses, bottles and boxes
- minimum unit pricing of alcoholic drinks

(Drinkaware, 2021; Gov.UK, 2021d; 2021e; Woodhouse, 2020)

Examples of UK law and drugs include

- The Modern Slavery Act 2015 protects those who are forced into drug trafficking against their will
- The Policing and Crime Act 2009 can be cited to prevent gang-related drug dealing activities
- The Anti-social Behaviour Crime and Policing Act 2014 enables local agencies to respond to anti-social behaviour, including closing premises

(The Crown Prosecution Service, 2018)

Non-legislative, social approaches to reducing substance-related harmful outcomes include

- the provision of universal smoking cessation services, free and accessible to the whole population through the National Health Service
- voluntary extensions of smoke free environments
- voluntary agreements with the alcohol industry
- encouraging sales of low and no alcohol drinks
- enabling local communities to have a say in alcohol licensing decisions
- encouraging the health service, local authorities, the police, local agencies and businesses to decide the maximum number of alcohol-selling venues in an area
- aiming to reduce health inequalities by providing extra substance-related support to areas of deprivation and vulnerable communities such as prisoners and those with mental health problems
- support for social housing and safe spaces for people struggling with dependency
- including the public and a wide range of stakeholders in the development of substance-related policies

(APPG, 2021; DH, 2017; DHSSPS, 2012; H.M. Government, 2012;2021; HSCC, 2019; Scottish Government, 2018a; Welsh Government, 2017)

Models of substance use describe how a society views substance use and they influence its approach to preventing substance-related harm. The UK adopts a combination of the moral, medical and social models.

Box 12.2 Historical overview of tackling alcohol, drug and tobacco use in the United States of America and the United Kingdom

The origins of the temperance movement lay in a book written by the American physician Dr Rush in 1790. Alcohol caused intemperance in people, and they needed to move towards temperance. The clergy, concerned that excess alcohol consumption prevented people from fully serving God, supported the movement and preached about taking alcohol in moderation. The movement spread to the UK, and by the mid-1830s the message in both countries shifted towards abstinence and people were encouraged to sign 'the pledge' to remain teetotal. By the early 20th century, the temperance movement became a strong political force in America culminating in Prohibition (1920–1933), a ban on the production, transport and sale of alcohol. The British Beer and Pub Association argued against similar legislation being introduced in the UK with their anti-American campaign citing the protection of British liberties, fears for unemployment and insisting beer was a food, a tonic and better than tea. American Prohibition led to an environment in which alcohol-related crime flourished leading to a black market and many deaths. In 1933, Congress repealed Prohibition in favour of regulation and taxes, partly to fund the recovery from the Great Depression. The UK sought to control the alcohol trade, reduce the alcoholic strength of drinks and the social impacts of drinking such as reducing pub opening hours; while taking a medical approach towards individuals with alcohol problems and seeing alcoholism as a disease.

During the 1840s, imports of opioids to both countries increased. Opium was widely used as a 'cure all' even for babies in the form of laudanum, and drug dependence rose. In the UK, both penal and medical forms of control were introduced in the 1920s. The Dangerous Drugs Act 1920 made it an offence to sell substances such as opioids and cocaine without a medical prescription. In 1926, it was recommended that individuals who were dependent on drugs, and their attempts to withdraw had failed, could be prescribed a maintenance dosage. In the UK, 'drug addiction' was seen as a disease and drug users as a social concern. This contrasted to America, where the expression 'war on drugs' emerged during the Second World War and legal measures to fine and imprison criminal drug sellers were increased. By the early 1970s, American presidents were declaring drugs to be 'public enemy number one'. Drug users continued to be treated as criminals, but there was some interest in developing treatments for problems related to prescribed/legal drug use. During the 1980s, drugs such as cocaine became much stronger and the association between drug injecting and acquiring the fatal HIV/AIDS multiplied the stigma and fear of drugs in both countries. Nancy Reagan, wife of the president, started her 'Just Say No' campaign. She described drugs as having, "No moral middle ground. Indifference is not an option" (p. 36). American cries for tougher law enforcement, criminalisation and abstinence grew, while in the UK the Advisory Council on the Misuse of Drugs argued that HIV was a greater threat to the population's health than drug misuse. Harm reduction, pioneered by volunteers, included educating drug users about safe injecting and needle exchange schemes. These became accepted alongside other harm minimisation and law enforcement measures.

Tobacco smoking had a different trajectory. Although individual doctors had long identified tobacco as causing disease, it was the accumulation of the epidemiological evidence by the 1950s that led to tobacco smoking becoming a population-based public health issue and anti-smoking warnings emerged in both countries. Research turned to the psychosocial determinants of substance use. A greater understanding of the reasons why people used substances, and the factors which increased their risk of dependency and other harms, led to the doors of the tobacco, alcohol and illegal drugs producers as causes of social disorder, crime and ill health. This led to more holistic, up-stream, population-based approaches to substance-related disease prevention.

Today, UK government policy includes a range of harm minimisation strategies for tobacco, alcohol and drugs alongside treatment services and a criminal justice approach comprising laws, penalties and imprisonment. The United States of America has one of the highest imprisonment rates for illegal drug use in the world, and there is a growing movement calling for more harm minimisation and treatment services. Meanwhile, alcohol and tobacco, which are legal, cause significantly more ill health and deaths in both countries than illegal drugs.

(Source: Lassiter and Spivey, 2018; Mold, 2018;
Peacock *et al.*, 2018; UWL, 2017)

International guidance

The UK participates in international initiatives which influence how it tackles substance use. The word 'control' refers to government control of substances through policies, including laws. The UK government is committed to the United Nations' *2030 Agenda for Sustainable Development* which set goals to address climate change, reduce poverty and deprivation, improve education, health and economic growth, and reduce inequalities by 2030 (UN, 2015). 'Sustainable Development Goal (SDG) 3: Ensure healthy lives and promote well-being for all at all ages' includes

- SDG 3.5 Strengthen the prevention and treatment of substance abuse, including narcotic drug abuse and harmful use of alcohol
- SDG 3a Strengthen the implementation of the World Health Organization Framework Convention on Tobacco Control in all countries, as appropriate

(UN, 2021)

Tobacco control

The *World Health Organization Framework Convention on Tobacco Control* is an international treaty created in 2003. It directs a coordinated international movement to counter the powerful tobacco industry and the consequences of its health-damaging products across the world. In 2008, new tobacco and nicotine products, which include e-cigarettes (ENDS and ENNDS) and heated tobacco products (HTPs), were incorporated into the framework. The UK signed in 2004, and today it is endorsed by member states who represent 90% of the world's population (WHO, 2021b). It seeks to meet the MPOWER measures.

- Monitoring tobacco use
- Protecting people from tobacco smoke
- Offer help to quit tobacco use
- Warning about the dangers of tobacco
- Enforcing tobacco advertising, promotion and sponsorship bans
- Raising taxes on tobacco

Alcohol control

The World Health Organization's *Global Strategy to Reduce the Harmful Use of Alcohol* was initiated in 2010 (WHO, 2010b). The World Health Organization formally ratified its *Global Alcohol Action Plan 2022 to 2030 to strengthen the effective implementation of the Global Strategy* in January 2022 (WHO, 2022). There are six key areas for proposed action.

- Action area 1: Implementation of high-impact strategies and interventions
  This includes five policy options and interventions (SAFER)
  - strengthen restrictions on alcohol availability
  - advance and enforce drink-driving countermeasures
  - facilitate access to screening, brief interventions and treatment
  - enforce bans or comprehensive restrictions on alcohol advertising, sponsorship and promotion
  - raise prices on alcohol through excise taxes and other pricing policies
- Action area 2: Advocacy, awareness and commitment
  Raise awareness and educate about alcohol-related harm, using various communication channels, with decision-makers and the public. This includes preventing the initiation of drinking among children, preventing drinking among pregnant women and providing protection from the pressures to drink.

- Action area 3: Partnership, dialogue and coordination
  National and regional intersectoral coordination between health, finance, transport, culture, sport, law etc. to strengthen alcohol control measures.

- Action area 4: Technical support and capacity building
  Countries need to create, enforce and sustain policies and legislation based on the best scientific evidence.

- Action area 5: Knowledge production and information systems
  International collaboration and research are needed to improve knowledge and understanding about alcohol-related harm.

- Action area 6: Resource mobilisation
  Adequate resources need to be mobilised at all levels to develop, implement and monitor alcohol policies. These include funding and human resources such as workforce capacity and international cooperation and partnerships.

Drug control

International treaties include the *Single Convention on Narcotic Drugs 1961*, the *Convention on Psychotropic Substances 1971* and the *Convention against Illicit Traffic in Narcotic Drugs and Psychotropic Substances 1988*. Within the parameters of these agreements, governments set out how drugs are to be imported/exported, sold, kept, prescribed, recorded, administered and destroyed in ways that benefit society while keeping people safe. Each country balances the drug's value to medical care against potential concerns about dependency or social harms and develops its own laws (Gallagher *et al.*, 2020). The Global Commission on Drug Policy, which includes former heads of states from across Europe and the Americas, is calling for the treaties to be revised and replaced with a better international, coordinated drugs policy which supports sustainable development, human rights, inclusive communities and people's health and wellbeing (GCDP, 2020). They argue that the distinction between legal and illegal substances means the alcohol, tobacco and pharmaceutical industries thrive on their considerable profits; organised crime and corruption is endemic; public health suffers and prisons are overcrowded (GCDP, 2019). The distinction is based on historical culture, politics, prejudice and power, and needs to be urgently revised. The Commission's five pathways for reform are

- put health and community safety first
- ensure access to essential medicines and pain control
- end the criminalisation and incarceration of people who use drugs
- refocus enforcement responses to drug trafficking and organised crime
- regulate drug markets to put governments in control

(GCDP, 2014)

The World Health Organization's *International Standards on Drug Use Prevention* (WHO/UNODC, 2018) summarises the characteristics of an effective drug prevention system. These are

- a range of interventions and policies based on evidence. These need to
  - support children and youth, particularly at critical transition periods in their life course
  - be both universal, for the population, and targeted at groups who are at risk

- address factors within individuals that make them vulnerable to risky behaviours and enhance their resilience
- remove environmental factors which encourage risky behaviours and support substance-free environments
- reach the population through multiple settings such as the workplace, families, communities and schools

- a supportive policy and regulatory framework. This would

  - be a health-centred system of drug control; one that includes a reduction in the supply of drugs, a reduction in drug dependence, treatment and support for dependence and the prevention of the wider health and social consequences of drug use
  - understand and treat drug use disorders as health conditions resulting from biopsychosocial factors rather than reasons for punishment
  - be linked to national public health strategies which operate across the life course and recognise that effectiveness can be reduced by social inequalities
  - recognise that programmes are likely to be more effective if supported by national regulation and standards

- a strong basis of research and scientific evidence. This would include

  - robust data gathering to gain an accurate understanding of the current situation, for example how many are using substances and who is most vulnerable
  - evaluations of the effectiveness, and where possible the cost effectiveness, of policies and interventions, and identify what is needed
  - dissemination of the evidence through peer-reviewed, published literature

- different sectors involved at different levels. This means

  - a national prevention system requiring coordinated input from many sectors, e.g. education, criminal justice, health, universities, welfare and the voluntary and private sector
  - a strong lead and coordinating agency for the national programme

- a strong infrastructure of the delivery system. This includes

  - adequate financial support
  - training and education for policymakers and practitioners
  - technical assistance
  - academic and research expertise

- Sustainability. This necessitates

  - medium and long-term investment to ensure sustainability

International goals, frameworks, action plans, treaties and standards influence how many governments approach substance use.

UK principles for tackling tobacco, alcohol and drugs

A review of current tobacco, alcohol and drugs policies, and reports presented by parliamentary committees, suggest there is broad agreement across the four nations of the UK about how they tackle substance use. The following eight principles are common

(APPG, 2021; DH, 2017; DHSSPS, 2012; DoH, 2018; H.M. Government, 2012; 2021; HSCC, 2019; Khan, 2022; Scottish Government, 2018a; 2018b; Welsh Government, 2017, 2021).

Universal and targeted approaches

Policies aim is to support the whole population as well as targeting those seen as vulnerable or at risk; for example pregnant women, children and young people, those with mental disorders, prisoners and those who already have a substance use concern. This is often linked to the wider goal of reducing inequalities in health.

Early intervention

There is a strong focus on protection and primary prevention for the young. This includes the antenatal period, children, families and schools.

Life course approach

There are interventions for the antenatal period, infancy, children, teenagers, adults and older people.

Law enforcement, treatment and prevention

A combination of legislation, healthcare and health promotion measures. These include using the law and other formal directives to change policies; change taxes and licences; invest in new treatments, care, rehabilitation, support, information, education and make changes to the social and physical environment.

Partnerships, multi-sectoral and multi-agency approaches

There is an emphasis on partnership working across government departments; sectors such as health, education and police; public, private and voluntary sectors; local communities, stakeholders, service users and substance users.

Reducing harmful outcomes

Policies include harm minimisation measures which include safer alternatives, behaviours and healthier environments for individuals and communities.

Protection from commercial interests

All nations include developing public policies, including legislation, codes of practice and voluntary agreements to limit the supply, demand and impact of tobacco, alcohol and drugs on the public's health.

Data collection and monitoring

There is support for ongoing research to collect and analyse the data on which to evaluate how effective strategies have been, and to plan forward with the appropriate funding.

Thinking point:

> Consider the relationship between the UK principles and international guidance.

> *The UK's approach towards preventing substance-related harm is characterised by eight common principles which are shared by the four nations.*

Health promotion interventions to reduce substance-related harm

Health promotion comprises communications which encourage health-related learning (health education) complemented by policies which help 'healthy choices to become easier choices'. This is discussed in Chapters 7 and 8. Here we provide examples of health promotion interventions that seek to reduce potential substance-related harm (Table 12.2). These include health warnings, mass media campaigns, brief opportunistic interventions, substance-related education, harm reduction, mutual aid and social change.

Health warnings

Health warnings reflect the preventive model of health promotion. They inform the public about potential health dangers associated with a product, process or experience. Based on health-related evidence, warnings seek to provide information that persuades the user to take care, be restrained or to abstain. The user is responsible for

Table 12.2 Health promotion interventions to reduce substance-related harm

Health promotion model	Preventive	Educational	Empowerment	Social change
Characteristics of model	Expert-led and persuasive.	Educator-led.	Person/ community-led.	Focussed upstream on the underlying structural causes of poor health.
	Based on medical or epidemiological evidence.	Based on a range of holistic health-related evidence.	Based on sharing insights about own health.	Based on making the healthy choice the easier choice.
	Comprises one-way instruction or training.	Comprises discussion, facilitation, enablement.	Comprises facilitation, empathy and active learning.	Comprises policies, regulations, rules, directives and laws.
	Anticipates compliance with treatment or new behaviour.	Anticipates active questioning, reflection and decision-making.	Anticipates reflection, skills and action.	Anticipates compliance.
	Aims for absence of disease.	Aims for autonomy and informed choice.	Aims for autonomy and empowerment.	Aims for healthier physical/social/ cultural environments: healthy settings.
Examples of health promotion interventions	Health warnings. Mass media campaigns. Brief opportunistic interventions.	Substance-related education. Mutual aid.	Harm reduction.	Laws. Policies. Cultural and environmental change.

their choices, purchases, level of engagement and consequences. Traditionally, health warnings did little more than raise awareness at best and/or fear which caused defensiveness, avoidance, defiance and denial at worst (Boshoff and Toerien, 2017; Shen, 2015). Recent research acknowledges that some emotional engagement, including fear, can enhance information processing when complemented by information about positive, healthier actions and consequences (Tannenbaum *et al.*, 2015). Graphic pictures, rather than text, further enhance the impact (Brewer *et al.*, 2019; Clarke *et al.*, 2020; Pang *et al.*, 2021). In summary, recent research shows that prominent, well-designed, accurate, comprehensive, graphic and rotated warnings can

- increase the chances of a consumer noticing and attending to the message
- encourage key messages to accumulate in the consumers' minds
- deepen consumers' engagement with the message
- counteract consumers' own minimisation of risks
- encourage feelings of fear
- encourage conversations with others about the warnings
- effectively communicate risks of second-hand smoke
- enhance motivation to reduce alcohol use
- encourage intentions to quit tobacco
- contribute to deterring young people from engaging with tobacco products
                        (Brewer *et al.*, 2019; Hobin *et al.*, 2020; WHO, 2021b)

The World Health Organization (2021b; 2022) is encouraging all countries to use health warnings to protect the public from the health harms caused by alcohol, tobacco and the nicotine in e-cigarettes (ENDS). These may be placed within advertising, on products or packaging, or at the point of sale. The World Health Organization argues health warnings are well supported by the public, relatively cheap for governments and contribute to young people's awareness of the negative health consequences associated with tobacco and alcohol, as well as deterring young people from engaging with smoking and smokeless tobacco products.

Tobacco

Health warning labels on cigarette packets were introduced in 1966, initially in the United States of America. Despite the tobacco industry undermining and delaying progress at every stage, their appearance, content and placement have developed from

- vague health warnings on the side of packets, e.g. "Caution cigarette smoking may be hazardous to your health" (USA)

  to

- smoking as a clear health hazard, associated with specific diseases, e.g. "Warning: cigarette smoking can cause lung cancer and heart diseases" (Iceland)

  to

- stronger and more visible messages on the front of packets, e.g. "Smoking is a main cause of cancer, diseases of the lung, and diseases of the heart and the arteries" (Saudi Arabia)

  to

Table 12.3 Health warnings on cigarette packets across the world, 2021

Country	Average space coverage at front and rear of packet	Does the law mandate health warnings?	Number of health warnings approved by law	Do health warnings describe harmful effect of tobacco use on health?	Do health warnings rotate?	Are health warnings written in principal language of the country?	Do health warnings include photographic or graphic images?
Australia	83%	Yes	14	Yes	Yes	Yes	Yes
China	35%	Yes	3	Yes	Yes	Yes	No
Congo	30%	No	–	No	Yes	Yes	No
Germany	65%	Yes	15	Yes	Yes	Yes	Yes
India	85%	Yes	1 'tobacco causes cancer'	Yes	Yes	Yes	Yes
Mozambique	28%	No	0	No	No	Yes	No
Peru	50%	Yes	12	Yes	Yes	Yes	Yes
Saudi Arabia	65%	Yes	4	Yes	Yes	Yes	Yes
UK	65%	Yes	14	Yes	Yes	Yes	Yes
United States of America	50%	Yes	11	Yes	Yes	Yes	Yes

Source: World Health Organization (2021b).

- rotating detailed health messages on the front of packets, e.g. "Smokers run an increased risk of heart attacks and certain diseases of the arteries" (Sweden)

  to

- graphic health warnings, pictures on the front and back of packets, e.g. images of black lungs or a diseased heart (Iceland)

(Hiilamo *et al.*, 2014)

Today, about half the world's population is exposed to health warnings on the packaging of tobacco products, and stronger graphic warnings are more prevalent among high-income (69%) than low-income countries (24%) (WHO, 2021b) (Table 12.3) (Figure 12.2). In the UK, the *Tobacco and Related Products Regulations 2016* set out requirements for health warnings on e-cigarettes (ENDS) and on all tobacco products including cigarettes, hand rolling tobacco, cigars, water pipe tobacco, herbal smoking products, smokeless tobacco and novel tobacco products which include heated tobacco products (HTPs), with penalties including fines and imprisonment for non-compliance (Legislation.gov.uk, 2016b; 2021). Health warnings on products for sale in Northern Ireland must comply with the European Union requirements. Under discussion, are recommendations to extend the use of health warnings to inside packaging and directly onto individual cigarettes and cigarette papers (APPG, 2021).

Alcohol

About 50 countries have health warnings on containers of alcohol, but the UK is not one of them (WHO, 2021c) (Table 12.4). These include warnings about cancer, drink driving, risks when operating machinery, under-age drinking and pregnancy risks.

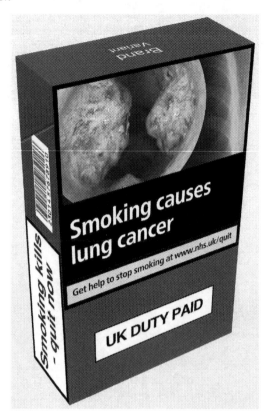

Figure 12.2 Example of health warnings on a packet of cigarettes

Source: Wee Creative for Action on Smoking and Health. Pack conforms with 2021 GB regulations

Table 12.4 Health warnings and alcohol across the world, 2016

Country	Health warning labels on alcohol advertising	Health warning labels on alcohol containers	Health warnings about alcohol and pregnancy	Health warnings about drink-driving
Australia	No	No	No	No
China	No	No	No	No
Congo	No	No	No	No
Germany	No	No	No	No
India	Yes	Yes	No	No
Mozambique	Yes	Yes	No	No
Peru	Yes	Yes	Yes	Yes
Saudi Arabia	No data	No data	No data	No data
UK	No	No	No	No
United States of America	No	Yes	Yes	Yes

Source: World Health Organization (2021d).

Recent research with the British public suggests health warnings would be generally accepted (AHAUK, 2018; RSPH, 2018). Young drinkers and those from lower socio-economic groups were most in favour of messages about drink driving and pregnancy harms. The researchers proposed these harms could be illustrated by a pictogram on the front label. However, the alcohol industry is using all its power to deter governments from increased regulation, including warning labels (O'Brien *et al.*, 2018).

Mass media campaigns

Simple mass media campaigns are designed to raise awareness of a health-related concern, communicate a key message and, sometimes, induce an emotional response. They normally reflect a preventive model of health promotion. Anti-tobacco mass media campaigns are strongly advocated by the World Health Organization (2021b). They are expensive but can reach large populations and are most effective when well-designed, repeated at least every two years, use television, use graphic images and are disseminated across a range of communication channels. Those campaigns which are augmented by warnings, supportive e-mails, tracking apps, support services such as smoking cessation and encourage temporary abstinence as a cultural norm seem to have a greater impact on people's behaviour (De Visser, 2019; PHE, 2020; WHO 2021b) because they not only reflect a preventive model, but aspects of the social change model as well. Examples include the UK's Stoptober campaign, which encourages smokers to quit in October (Figure 12.3), and the Better Health: Quit Smoking campaign; as well as Dry January, which encourages abstinence from alcohol for one month each year.

Brief opportunistic interventions

Brief conversations about a person's substance use tend to reflect the preventive model of health promotion. For example, the Northern Ireland Government suggests brief opportunistic advice may comprise a healthcare professional encouraging someone in

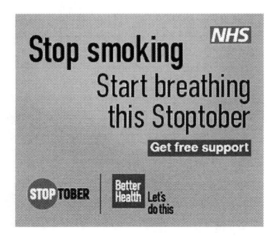

Figure 12.3 Stoptober 2021

Source: Department of Health and Social Care, 2021. Reproduced under the terms of the Open Government Licence v.3.0

an attempt to quit smoking tobacco or motivating them to consider quitting. It takes about five to 10 minutes and could include

- a brief assessment of the person's commitment to quit
- advice to stop
- referral to cessation services
- offering nicotine replacement therapy
- providing written information

(DHSSPS, 2012, p. 61)

The Scottish Government defines an alcohol brief intervention as,

> "... a short, structured conversation about alcohol consumption with an individual that seeks in a non-confrontational way to motivate and support them to think about or plan a change in their drinking behaviour."
>
> (Scottish Government, 2018a, p. 38)

Substance-related education

Substance-related education, which reflects the educational model of health promotion, is that which achieves learning such as a shift in awareness, the acquisition of knowledge, thinking, reflecting, clarifying values, developing skills, and making informed decisions which may, or may not, match advice from medical 'experts'. Substance-related education is commonly seen in schools, colleges and universities. An example of education for the public includes the UK's *Low Risk Drinking Guidelines* (DH, 2016) (Box 12.3) which state,

> "Government has a responsibility to ensure this information is provided for the public in a clear and open way, so they can make informed choices."
>
> (p. 3)

Box 12.3 Weekly drinking guidelines

"The Chief Medical Officers' guideline for both men and women is that:

- To keep health risks from alcohol to a low level, it is safest not to drink more than 14 units a week on a regular basis.
- If you regularly drink as much as 14 units per week, it is best to spread your drinking evenly over 3 or more days. If you have one or two heavy drinking episodes a week, you increase your risks of death from long-term illness and from accidents and injuries.
- The risk of developing a range of health problems (including cancers of the mouth, throat and breast) increases the more you drink on a regular basis.
- If you wish to cut down the amount you drink, a good way to help achieve this is to have several drink-free days each week."

(Source: DH, 2016, p. 4. Reproduced under the terms of the Open Government Licence v.3.0)

The National Health Service's smoking cessation services adopt an educational model. They are open to people who have yet to decide whether they wish to quit smoking and include

- listening to people's experience of smoking and any attempts they have made to quit in the past
- a breath test to provide information about the amount of carbon monoxide in their body
- time to talk and consider options
- if the person decides to try to quit, the adviser works with them on an action plan
- the person listens to information about forms of nicotine-replacement therapy and chooses whether to use it
- there is ongoing support from the adviser
- if the person relapses, there is no judgement

(NHS, 2018)

Harm reduction

The origins of harm reduction evolved during the 1980s in recognition that abstinence was not a realistic goal for those with a substance dependence. The shockingly high death rate associated with intravenous drug use spreading HIV/AIDS forced a cultural rethink in some countries, including the UK, led by those who injected drugs trying to protect their friends. Needle exchange initiatives, to provide clean needles, and the prescribing of methadone as an alternative to injecting heroin became more socially and politically acceptable (Friedman *et al.*, 2007). Laverack (2014) places harm reduction firmly within a humanistic, person-centred approach to health and the empowerment model of health promotion, arguing it is about working with people, collaborating on their terms and in their context. Empowerment means giving the power to the individual, in a counselling context, or to a support group of peers, so that they may direct their own learning and choices and put them into action. Harm reduction means providing a safe, secure space where all individuals are welcomed, equal and can remain anonymous within a non-judgemental ethos. Denis-Lalonde and colleagues (2019) carried out a detailed analysis of literature and concluded that harm reduction has seven key attributes. It

- focusses on the harms of using the substance. This means reducing the harms but not necessarily the use, such as changing the pattern of use or the way a substance is administered
- includes the participation of people. Those who use the substance are involved in the planning and delivery of the harm reduction programme. A high value is placed on peer support and empowerment
- promotes human rights. A person has the right to be treated with dignity and respect regardless of their substance use
- takes a public health approach. Harm reduction could or should be part of a multi-agency, intersectoral approach to disease prevention and health promotion across communities and populations

- values neutrality and non-judgement. Taking a neutral, non-judgemental approach towards those who engage in substance use has its origins in Carl Rogers' core conditions, which are central to a humanistic and empowering approach to health education (see Chapter 7)
- is practical and pragmatic. The aim is to reduce the immediate and tangible harms, and some extend this to the harms associated with criminalisation
- encourages innovation and adaptability. Harm reduction strategies should be flexible, dynamic, responsive to need and have a minimum requirement for involving substance users in the process

The authors recorded some of the positive outcomes associated with a harm reduction approach in the context of drugs. It

- increased knowledge about how to avoid negative outcomes
- enhanced skills in self-care and the care of others
- connected people to treatment and rehabilitation services
- lowered personal risks
- supported the reintegration of users into the community
- reduced the spread of disease
- reduced overdoses
- saved lives
- improved environments
- reduced public expenses
- helped some to achieve abstinence

They also noted that harm reduction facilitators created alliances which led to innovations in research and practice, and enabled front-line workers to access people who were of concern, at-risk and hard to reach through other routes. The authors conclude harm reduction approaches have the potential to reduce stigma and normalise the non-problematic use of substances.

Mutual aid

Mutual aid organisations are peer support groups which aim to be welcoming, safe, secure, equal and anonymous. Unlike harm reduction with its emphasis on self-care and acceptance of a person's choices, here the emphasis is on self-help and the aim is abstinence. Organisations offer support and direction with becoming substance free and staying substance free by using the educational model of health promotion. They include Narcotics Anonymous (NA), Cocaine Anonymous (CA) (Box 12.4) and Alcoholics Anonymous (AA), which are based on the 12-step philosophy developed during the 1930s, and SMART Recovery, which includes cognitive behavioural therapy techniques, an emphasis on self-management and individuals' recovery journeys. There is evidence to show these groups can support recovery from dependence and they are recommended within mainstream UK drug and alcohol services (PHE, 2018).

Box 12.4 Cocaine Anonymous

"Cocaine Anonymous is a Fellowship of men and women who share their experience, strength and hope with each other that they may solve their common problem and help others recover from their addiction. The best way to reach someone is to speak to them on a common level. The members of C.A. are all recovering addicts who maintain their individual sobriety by working with others. We come from various social, ethnic, economic, and religious backgrounds, but what we have in common is addiction.

The only requirement for membership is a desire to stop using cocaine and all other mind-altering substances. Anyone who wants to stop using cocaine and all other mind-altering substances (including alcohol and other drugs) is welcome.

There are no dues or fees for membership; we are fully self-supporting through our own contributions. We do ask for voluntary contributions at meetings to cover expenses such as coffee, rent, literature and services to help those who are still suffering. However, newcomers need not feel obligated to contribute. We do not accept donations from organizations or individuals outside the Fellowship.

We are not allied with any sect, denomination, politics, organization or institution. In order to maintain our integrity and avoid any possible complications, we are not affiliated with any outside organization. Although C.A. is a spiritual program, we do not align ourselves with any religion. Our members are free to define their spirituality as they see fit. Our individual members may have opinions of their own, but C.A. as a whole has no opinion on outside issues. We are not affiliated with any rehabs, recovery houses or hospitals, but many do refer their patients to Cocaine Anonymous to maintain their sobriety.

Our primary purpose is to stay free from cocaine and all other mind-altering substances and to help others achieve the same freedom. The only purpose of Cocaine Anonymous is to offer recovery to individuals who are suffering from addiction. Our experience has shown that the most effective way to attain and maintain sobriety is to work with others suffering from the same malady.

We use the Twelve-Step recovery program because it has already been proven that the Twelve-Step recovery program works. The Steps of C.A. are adapted from the original Twelve Steps of Alcoholics Anonymous."

(Source: Cocaine Anonymous, 2021. Reproduced with permission from Cocaine Anonymous World Services, Inc.)

Social change

The social change model of health promotion concerns those legal and social approaches to reducing the harmful outcomes of substances discussed in the social model of substance use, above. They include policies to protect the population from health-harming commercial interests and help to make healthy choices easier choices. For example,

- alcohol, tobacco and drugs laws
- policies which curb the power and the health harming impacts of substance-related industries
- increased taxes and prices

- increasing the age at which substances can be legally purchased
- policies to create and fund health, education, voluntary and other local and national substance-related services
- policies to make environments/settings substance-free or substance-safe
- interventions, such as campaigns that seek to normalise a substance-free or substance-safe culture

Health promotion interventions to tackle substance-related harm reflect the preventive, educational, empowerment and social change models.

Summary

This chapter has

- described three models of substance use and their application within the UK
- outlined substance-related international conventions and guidance which influence the UK
- identified eight common principles for reducing substance-related harms shared across the four nations of the UK
- provided examples of health promotion interventions that span the four health promotion models

Further reading

Gispen, M.E. and Toebes, B (eds) *Human rights and tobacco control.* Cheltenham: Edward Elgar
Rassool, G.H. (2018) *Alcohol and drug misuse. A guide for health and social care professionals.* 2nd edn. London: Routledge

Useful websites

Action on Smoking and Health. Available at: https://ash.org.uk
Institute of Alcohol Studies. Available at: www.ias.org.uk
National Institute for Health and Care Excellence: lifestyle and wellbeing. Available at: www.nice.org.uk/guidance/lifestyle-and-wellbeing

References

Alcohol Health Alliance UK (2018) *How we drink, what we think.* Available at: https://ahauk.org/wp-content/uploads/2018/11/AHA_How-we-drink-what-we-think_2018_FINAL.pdf (Accessed 9th June 2022)
All Party Parliamentary Group on Smoking and Health (2021) *Delivering a smokefree 2030: the all party parliamentary group on smoking and health recommendations for the tobacco control plan 2021.* London: APPG on Smoking and Health
Boshoff, C. and Toerien, L. (2017) 'Subconscious responses to fear-appeal health warnings: an exploratory study of cigarette packaging', *South African Journal of Economic and Management Sciences,* 20(1) doi:10.4102/sajems.v20i1.1630
Brewer, N.T., Parada, H., Hall, M.G., Boynton, M.H., Noar, S.M. and Ribisl, K.M. (2019) 'Understanding why pictorial cigarette pack warnings increase quit attempts', *Annals of Behavioural Medicine,* 53(3), pp. 232–243

Clarke, N., Pechey, E., Kosīte, D., König, L.M., Mantzari, E., Blackwell, A.K.M., Marteau, T.M. and Hollands, G.J. (2020) 'Impact of health warning labels on selection and consumption of food and alcohol products: systematic review with meta-analysis', *Health Psychology Review*, July doi:10.1080/17437199.2020.1780147

Cocaine Anonymous (2021) *What is C.A.?* Available at: https://ca.org/literature/what-is-ca (Accessed 9th June 2022)

Cocaine Anonymous UK (2021) *What is cocaine anonymous?* Available at: https://cocaineanonymous.org.uk/what-is-cocaine-anonymous (Accessed 10th June 2022)

Crown Office and Procurator Fiscal Service (2021) *Lord advocate statement on diversion from prosecution*. Available at: https://www.copfs.gov.uk/media-site-news-from-copfs/1983-lord-advocate-statement-on-diversion-from-prosecution (Accessed 9th June 2022)

De Visser, R. (2019) *Dry January. Evaluation of dry January 2019*. Available at: https://alcohol-change.org.uk/publication/dry-january-evaluation-2019 (Accessed 9th June 2022)

Denis-Lalonde, D., Lind, C. and Estefan, A. (2019) 'Beyond the buzzword: a concept analysis of harm reduction', *Research and Theory for Nursing Practice: An International Journal*, 33(4), pp. 310–323

Department of Health (2016) *UK chief medical officers' low drinking guidelines*. Available at: https://assets.publishing.service.gov.uk/government/uploads/system/uploads/attachment_data/file/545937/UK_CMOs__report.pdf (Accessed 8th June 2022)

Department of Health (2017) *Towards a smokefree generation. A tobacco control plan for England*. Available at: https://assets.publishing.service.gov.uk/government/uploads/system/uploads/attachment_data/file/630217/Towards_a_Smoke_free_Generation_-_A_Tobacco_Control_Plan_for_England_2017-2022__2_.pdf (Accessed 8th June 2022)

Department of Health (2018) *New strategic direction for alcohol and drugs. Phase 2. Final review October 2018*. Available at: https://www.health-ni.gov.uk/sites/default/files/publications/health/NSD%20PHASE%202%20Final%20Review%20-%20October%202018_0.pdf (Accessed 10th June 2022)

Department of Health (2021) *Making life better. Preventing harm and empowering recovery: a strategic framework to tackle the harm from substance use. A consultation document*. Available at: https://www.health-ni.gov.uk/sites/default/files/consultations/health/doh-sus-consultation.pdf (Accessed 8th June 2022)

Department of Health and Social Care (2021) *Stoptober 2021*. Available at: https://campaignresources.phe.gov.uk/resources/campaigns/126-stoptober-2021/resources (Accessed 7th December 2021)

Department of Health, Social Services and Public Safety (2012) *Ten-year tobacco control strategy for Northern Ireland*. Available at: https://www.health-ni.gov.uk/sites/default/files/publications/health/tobacco-control-10-year-strategy.pdf (Accessed 8th June 2022)

Drinkaware (2021) *Alcohol and the law*. Available at: www.drinkaware.co.uk/facts/alcohol-and-the-law (Accessed 9th June 2022)

Friedman, S.R., de Jong, W., Rossi, D., Touzé, G., Rockwell, R., Des Jarlais, D.C. and Elovich, R. (2007) 'Harm reduction theory: users culture, micro-social indigenous harm reduction and the self-organization and outside-organizing of users' groups', *International Journal of Drug Policy*, 18(2), pp. 107–117

Gallagher, C.T., Atik, S.K., Isse, L. and Mann, S.K. (2020) 'Doctor or drug dealer? International legal provisions for the legitimate handling of drugs of abuse', *Drug Science, Policy and Law*, 6 doi:10.1177/2050324519900070

Global Commission on Drug Policy (2014) *Taking control: pathways to drug policies that work*. Available at: https://www.globalcommissionondrugs.org/wp-content/uploads/2016/03/GCDP_2014_taking-control_EN.pdf (Accessed 6th June 2022)

Global Commission on Drug Policy (2019) *Classification of psychoactive substances. When science was left behind*. Available at: https://www.drugsandalcohol.ie/30714/1/2019Report_EN_web.pdf (Accessed 9th June 2022)

Global Commission on Drug Policy (2020) *Enforcement of drug laws. Refocusing on organized crime elites.* Available at: https://www.globalcommissionondrugs.org/wp-content/uploads/2020/06/2020report_EN_web_100620.pdf (Accessed 8th June 2022)

Gov.UK (2021a) *Drugs penalties.* Available at: https://www.gov.uk/penalties-drug-possession-dealing (Accessed 9th June 2022)

Gov.UK (2021b) *Tobacco products duty.* Available at: www.gov.uk/guidance/tobacco-products-duty (Accessed 9th June 2022)

Gov.UK (2021c) *Weights and measures: the law.* Available at: www.gov.uk/weights-measures-and-packaging-the-law/specified-quantities (Accessed 9th June 2022)

Gov.UK (2021d) *Food labelling and packaging.* Available at: https://www.gov.uk/food-labelling-and-packaging/food-labelling-what-you-must-show (Accessed 9th June 2022)

Gov.UK (2021e) *The tobacco and related products regulations 2016.* Available at: https://www.legislation.gov.uk/uksi/2016/507/contents (Accessed 9th June 2022)

Health and Social Care Committee (2019) *Drug policy. First report of session 2019.* London: House of Commons Available at: https://publications.parliament.uk/pa/cm201919/cmselect/cmhealth/143/143.pdf (Accessed June 9th 2022)

Heilig, M., MacKillop, J., Martinez, D., Rehm, J., Leggio, L. and Vanderschuren, L.J.M.J. (2021) 'Addiction as a brain disease revised: why it still matters, and the need for consilience', *Neuropsychopharmacology*, 46(10), pp. 1715–1723

Hiilamo, H., Crosbie, E. and Glantz, S.A. (2014) 'The evolution of health warning labels on cigarette packs: the role of precedents, and tobacco industry strategies to block diffusion', *Tobacco Control*, 23(1) doi:10.1136/tobaccocontrol-2012-050541

H.M. Government (2012) *The government's alcohol strategy.* London: The Stationery Office

H.M. Government (2021) *From harm to hope. A 10-year drugs plan to cut crime and save lives.* Available at: https://www.gov.uk/government/publications/from-harm-to-hope-a-10-year-drugs-plan-to-cut-crime-and-save-lives (Accessed 8th June 2022)

Hobin, E., Schoueri-Mychasiw, N., Weerasinghe, A., Vallance, K., Hammond, D., Greenfield, T.K., McGavock, Paradis, C. and Stockwell, T. (2020) 'Effects of strengthening alcohol labels on attention, message processing, and perceived effectiveness: a quasi-experimental study in Yukon, Canada', *International Journal of Drug Policy*, 77(1) doi:10.1016/j.drugpo.2020.102666

Holland, A. (2020) 'An ethical analysis of UK drug policy as an example of a criminal justice approach to drugs: a commentary on the short film Putting UK Drug Policy into Focus', *Harm Reduction Journal*, 17(97) doi:10.1186/s12954-020-00434-8

House of Commons Scottish Affairs Committee (2019) *Problem drug use in Scotland. First report of session 2019.* Available at: https://publications.parliament.uk/pa/cm201919/cmselect/cmscotaf/44/44.pdf (Accessed 9th June 2022)

Khan, J. (2022) *The Khan review: making smoking obsolete.* Available at: https://assets.publishing.service.gov.uk/government/uploads/system/uploads/attachment_data/file/1081366/khan-review-making-smoking-obsolete.pdf (Accessed 9th June 2022)

Lassiter, P.S. and Spivey, M.S. (2018) 'Historical perspectives and the moral model', in Lassiter, P.S. and Culbreth, J.R. (eds) *Theory and practice of addiction counselling.* London: Sage, pp. 27–46

Laverack, G. (2014) *The pocket guide to health promotion.* Maidenhead: Open University Press

Legislation.gov.uk (1971) *Misuse of drugs act 1971.* Available at: https://www.legislation.gov.uk/ukpga/1971/38/contents (Accessed 9th June 2022)

Legislation.gov.uk (2001) *The misuse of drugs regulations 2001.* Available at: https://www.legislation.gov.uk/uksi/2001/3998/contents/made (Accessed 9th June 2022)

Legislation.gov.uk (2014) *Children and families act 2014.* Available at: www.legislation.gov.uk/ukpga/2014/6/contents/enacted (Accessed 9th June 2022)

Legislation.gov.uk (2016a) *Psychoactive substances act 2016.* Available at: https://www.legislation.gov.uk/ukpga/2016/2/contents/enacted (Accessed 9th June 2022)

Legislation.gov.uk (2016b) *The tobacco and related products regulations 2016.* Available at: https://www.legislation.gov.uk/uksi/2016/507/contents/made (Accessed 7th June 2022)

Legislation.gov.uk (2021) *The tobacco and related products regulations 2016.* Available at www. legislation.gov.uk/uksi/2016/507/contents (Accessed 9th June 2022)

Mold, A. (2018) 'Framing drug and alcohol use as a public health problem in Britain: past and present', *Nordic Studies on Alcohol and Drugs*, 35(2), pp. 93–99.

Mosher, C.J. and Akins, S. (2021) *Drugs and drug policy. The control of consciousness alteration.* 3rd edn. London: Sage

National Health Service (2018) *NHS stop smoking services help you quit.* Available at: https:// www.nhs.uk/live-well/quit-smoking/nhs-stop-smoking-services-help-you-quit (Accessed 9th June 2022)

O'Brien, P., Gleeson, D., Room, R. and Wilkinson, C. (2018) 'Commentary on "communicating messages about drinking": using the "big legal guns" to block alcohol health warning labels', *Alcohol and Alcoholism*, 53(3), pp. 333–336

Pang, B., Slaeme, P., Seydel, T., Jeawon, K., Knox, K. and Rundle-Thiele, S. (2021) 'The effectiveness of graphic health warnings on tobacco products: a systematic review on perceived harm and quit intentions', *BMC Public Health*, 21(884) doi:10.1186/s12889-021-10810-z

Peacock, A., Leung, J., Larney, A., *et al.* (2018) 'Global statistics on alcohol, tobacco and illicit drug use: 2017 status report', *Addiction*, 113(10), pp. 1905–1926

Public Health England (2018) *Mutual aid toolkit for alcohol and drug misuse treatment.* Available at: https://www.gov.uk/government/publications/mutual-aid-toolkit-for-alcohol-and-drug-misuse-treatment (Accessed 9th June 2022)

Public Health England (2019) *Health matters: stopping smoking – what works?* Available at: https://www.gov.uk/government/publications/health-matters-stopping-smoking-what-works/health-matters-stopping-smoking-what-works (Accessed 8th June 2022)

Public Health England (2020) *Stoptober 2019 campaign evaluation.* Available at: https:// assets.publishing.service.gov.uk/government/uploads/system/uploads/attachment_data/ file/992284/Stoptober_2019_Evaluation.pdf (Accessed 9th June 2022)

Robinson, S. (ed) (2021a) *Priorities for health promotion and public health. Explaining the evidence for disease prevention and health promotion.* London: Routledge

Robinson, S. (2021b) 'Social context of health and illness', in Robinson, S. (ed) *Priorities for health promotion and public health. Explaining the evidence for disease prevention and health promotion.* London: Routledge, pp. 3–33

Royal Society for Public Health (2018) *Labelling the point. Towards better alcohol information.* Available at: https://www.rsph.org.uk/static/uploaded/4ae31b49-c4d7-4355-ad94a660aba36108. pdf (Accessed 8th June 2022)

Scottish Government (2018a) *Alcohol framework 2018: preventing harm.* Edinburgh: The Scottish Government

Scottish Government (2018b) *Raising Scotland's tobacco-free generation. Our tobacco control plan 2018.* Edinburgh: The Scottish Government

Shen, L. (2015) 'Antecedents to psychological reactance: the impact of threat, message frame, and choice', *Health Communication*, 30(10), pp. 975–985

Tannenbaum, M.B., Hepler, J., Zimmerman, R.S., Saul, L., Jacobs, S., Wilson, K. and Albarracin, D. (2015) 'Appealing to fear: a meta-analysis of fear appeal effectiveness theories', *Psychological Bulletin*, 141(6), pp. 1178–1204

The Crown Prosecution Service (2018) *'County lines': typology.* Available at: https://view. officeapps.live.com/op/view.aspx?src=https%3A%2F%2Fwww.cps.gov.uk%2Fsites%2Fdefault%2Ffiles%2Fdocuments%2Flegal_guidance%2FCounty-Lines-typology.docx&wd-Origin=BROWSELINK (Accessed 9th June 2022)

United Nations (2015) *Transforming our world: the 2030 agenda for sustainable development.* Available at: https://sdgs.un.org/2030agenda (Accessed 9th June 2022)

United Nations (2021) *Global indicator framework for the sustainable development goals and targets of the 2030 agenda for sustainable development.* Available at: https://unstats.un.org/ sdgs/indicators/Global%20Indicator%20Framework%20after%202021%20refinement_Eng.pdf (Accessed 9th June 2022)

University of Warwick Library (2017) *"Rob you of your beer": the British fight against prohibition.* Available at: https://warwick.ac.uk/services/library/mrc/archives_online/exhibitions/prohibition (Accessed 8th June 2022)

Welsh Government (2017) *Tobacco control delivery plan for Wales 2017–2020.* Available at: https://gov.wales/sites/default/files/publications/2017-11/tobacco-control-delivery-plan-for-wales-2017-to-2020.pdf (Accessed 8th June 2022)

Welsh Government (2021) *Substance misuse delivery plan 2019–2022.* https://gov.wales/sites/default/files/publications/2021-01/substance-misuse-delivery-plan-2019-to-2022.pdf (Accessed 9th June 2022)

Woodhouse, J. (2020) *Alcohol: minimum pricing. Briefing paper 5021.* Available at: https://researchbriefings.files.parliament.uk/documents/SN05021/SN05021.pdf (Accessed 9th June 2022)

World Health Organization (2010a) *A conceptual framework for action on the social determinants of health.* Geneva: World Health Organization

World Health Organization (2010b) *Global strategy to reduce the harmful use of alcohol.* Geneva: World Health Organization

World Health Organization (2021a) *Social determinants of health.* Available at: https://www.who.int/health-topics/social-determinants-of-health#tab=tab_1 (Accessed 8th June 2022)

World Health Organization (2021b) *WHO report on the global tobacco epidemic 2021: addressing new and emerging products.* Available at: https://www.who.int/teams/health-promotion/tobacco-control/global-tobacco-report-2021 (Accessed 23rd August 2021)

World Health Organization (2021c) *Global health observatory.* Available at: https://www.who.int/data/gho/data/indicators (Accessed 24th August 2021)

World Health Organization (2021d) *Global health observatory. Health warning labels on alcohol containers.* Available at: https://www.who.int/data/gho/data/indicators/indicator-details/GHO/health-warning-labels-on-alcohol-containers (Accessed 23rd August 2021)

World Health Organization (2022) *Political declaration of the third high-level meeting of the general assembly on the prevention and control of non-communicable diseases. Appendix 1: draft action plan (2022–2030) to effectively implement the global strategy to reduce the harmful use of alcohol as a public health priority.* Available at: https://apps.who.int/gb/ebwha/pdf_files/EB150/B150_7Add1-en.pdf (Accessed 25th May 2022)

World Health Organization/United Nations Office on Drugs and Crime (2018) *International standards on drug use prevention.* 2nd edn. Available at: https://www.globalcommissionondrugs.org/wp-content/uploads/2020/06/2020report_EN_web_100620.pdf (Accessed 8th September 2021)

Zinberg, N. (1986) *Drug, set and setting: basis for controlled intoxicant use.* London: Yale University Press

13 Tackling overweight

Sally Robinson

Key points

- Introduction
- Excess body fat and health
- Energy balance
- Energy imbalance
- Eating to lose weight
- Monitoring and the microbiome
- Obesogenic environment
- Principles for tackling overweight
- Summary

Introduction

We begin this chapter by outlining metabolism and a scientific truth: we gain body fat if we consume more calories than the body uses for living and movement. The chapter examines why tackling overweight is more complex than the 'calories in: calories out' equation implies. We discuss genes, physical activity, sedentary behaviour and factors which encourage the overconsumption of calories. We explain why some weight loss dieting practices are unhealthy and counterproductive while others are healthy and successful. We include the importance of a Mediterranean-style diet, the microbiome and the obesogenic environment. The chapter presents evidence-based principles for tackling overweight in individuals and populations.

Excess body fat and health

We use the terms 'overweight' or 'obese' to imply an individual is carrying excess body fat for health. It is common to calculate an individual's weight to height ratio, their body mass index (BMI), and if it is above the 'normal weight' range of 18.5 to 24.99 (WHO, 2021) to conclude they need to lose weight, or more precisely, lose excess body fat. This is simplistic for many reasons including BMI

- is designed to be used with populations not individuals
- someone may have a high BMI due to being well muscled
- it does not indicate the location of the body fat, which is known to be important

(Nuttall, 2015)

DOI: 10.4324/9780367823696-16

Body shape, particularly waist circumference or a combination of BMI with waist circumference, are better indicators of whether a population or an individual may be at an increased risk of disease and early death (Christakoudi *et al.*, 2020; Ross *et al.*, 2020). Although excess fat under the skin is strongly linked to many diseases, visceral fat which surrounds and infiltrates the vital organs in the abdomen producing an 'apple' body shape is even more concerning. An individual's waist should be less than half their height. The current 'obesity epidemic' is a public health priority because excess body fat is associated with an increased risk of developing

- chronic low-grade inflammation
- cardiovascular disease, including atherosclerosis and high blood pressure
- insulin resistance and type 2 diabetes
- metabolic syndrome
- non-alcoholic fatty liver disease
- cancer
- death from COVID-19 coronavirus
- musculoskeletal conditions such as osteoarthritis and joint pain
- poor physical functioning of the body
- social disadvantage
- psychological distress

(Robinson, 2021a)

Energy balance

We measure the energy, the fuel, that our bodies use for living and moving in kilocalories (Kcals). We also measure the energy contained within foods and drinks in kilocalories. In everyday language, we shorten this to 'calories'. If we

- consume the same number of calories that the body uses, we are in energy balance (Figure 13.1)
- consume fewer calories than the body uses, we lose body fat
- consume more calories than the body uses, we gain body fat

Inside the body, this 'calories in: calories out' mechanistic model can be explained by understanding metabolism.

- Digestion is the breaking down of food and drink into carbohydrates, proteins and fats, and then into small molecules such as glucose, amino acids and fatty acids, as they pass through the gastro-intestinal tract (Figure 13.2)
- Absorption refers to these small molecules being absorbed into the bloodstream

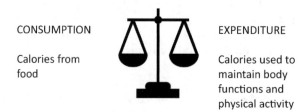

CONSUMPTION

Calories from food

EXPENDITURE

Calories used to maintain body functions and physical activity

Figure 13.1 Energy balance

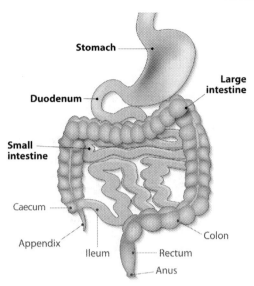

Figure 13.2 Gastrointestinal tract
Source: Designua/Shutterstock.com

- Metabolism is made up of catabolism and anabolism
  - Catabolism is the process of breaking down food and drink into small molecules. Some of the small molecules are broken down to release energy, the body's fuel, which we measure in calories
  - Anabolism means that the body changes the chemistry of small molecules to make bigger molecules, perhaps skin or hair cells

For example, digestion changes proteins into amino acids (catabolism). The amino acids pass out of the small intestine, across the wall and into the nearby capillaries which carry blood. The blood takes the amino acids to cells where they use calories (energy) to form chains of amino acids. These chains make up the proteins that the body needs, such as those for making hair (anabolism). Metabolic rate is the speed at which the body is 'breaking down', catabolism, and 'building up', anabolism.

The number of calories used in a typical day to fuel metabolism is the body's total energy expenditure (TEE). When people speak of 'speeding up' their metabolism, it means their body is using more calories per day; they have a higher TEE. When people speak of 'slowing down' their metabolism, it means their body is using fewer calories per day, they have a lower TEE. An invidual's TEE is influenced by their diet-induced thermogenesis (DIT), their basal metabolic rate (BMR) and their physical activity level (PAL).

- Diet induced thermogenesis (DIT) means the calories used to digest and absorb food. Over a day, thermogenesis needs about five to 10% of all the calories the body uses (TEE)
- Basal metabolic rate (BMR) is the speed of the body's basal metabolism. Basal metabolism refers to keeping the body alive, allowing the body to function and

repair while we are resting, awake and fasting. Age, sex, illness, body size and body composition affects people's BMR. For example, being older, female, having a body composition of low muscle and higher fat, and a smaller body size are each associated with a slightly lower BMR. At times of growth, pregnancy and lactation, the BMR rises as more calories are needed. Over a day, BMR needs about 45% to 70% of all the calories the body uses (TEE)

- Physical activity level (PAL) is the number of calories we need to support physical activities including standing, sitting, walking, running and jumping. We can calculate how many calories are being used for an activity by dividing a person's TEE by their BMR over a minute or an hour.

(UN/WHO/FAO, 2004)

In a research laboratory, we can measure how many calories an individual uses in one day (TEE) by multiplying the calories used for their BMR by the calories used for activity (PAL) and adding a small estimated number of calories for DIT.

TEE = BMR × PAL + DIT estimate

If we

- consume the same number of calories that the body uses to support its metabolism, we are in energy balance. We neither lose nor gain body fat
- consume fewer calories than the body uses to support its metabolism, we lose body fat
- consume more calories than the body uses to support its metabolism, we gain body fat

We can encourage a population to maintain its weight, neither increase nor decrease body fat, by recommending they consume the same number of calories, called the population estimated average requirement (EAR) for calories, as they use on an average day.

If we want the population to

- stay the same average weight, the EAR will match the average number of calories the population uses to support metabolism
- gain weight, on average, the EAR will be a higher number of calories than the population uses to support metabolism
- lose weight, on average, the EAR will be a lower number of calories than the population uses to support metabolism

Table 13.1 shows the average recommended number of calories that healthy men and women in the UK, who undertake average levels of physical activity, need to consume each day for good health. In making these recommendations, the Scientific Advisory Committee on Nutrition (2012) considered concerns about rising overweight and obesity in the population, so the EAR is a slightly lower number of calories than the population uses to support metabolism.

Table 13.1 Estimated average requirements for energy

Age	Men (kcals)	Women (kcals)
19–24 years	2,772	2,175
25–34 years	2,749	2,175
35–44 years	2,629	2,103
45–54 years	2,581	2,103
55–64 years	2,581	2,079
65–74 years	2,342	1,912
75+ years	2,294	1,840

Source: Adapted from SACN (2012, p. 85).

Pregnancy and lactation

Energy balance during pregnancy and after birth needs to factor in the calories needed to help the baby to grow to a healthy weight by birth and to meet the mother's energy needs during pregnancy, birth and for breastfeeding. Normally, in the UK, most pregnant women are monitored by midwives who tailor their advice to individual need. Obesity, that is very high levels of body fat, can present serious risks to both mother and baby, including death (Knight *et al.*, 2020), but losing weight in pregnancy is never recommended and it is best if a woman is a healthier weight before becoming pregnant. Most women need to consume extra calories, that is 191 kcals per day, only in the final stage of pregnancy, during weeks 27 to 40 (SACN, 2012). After birth, a mother's calorie needs will vary as her body composition changes and according to her infant's need for breast milk.

We stay in energy balance when we expend the same number of calories as we consume.

Energy imbalance

We tip the balance into consuming more calories than we are using and gaining body fat by consuming more calories, decreasing physical activity, increasing sedentary behaviour and decreasing the body's muscle mass (Figure 13.3). We tip the balance into consuming fewer calories than we are using and losing body fat by consuming fewer calories, increasing physical activity, decreasing sedentary behaviour and increasing the body's muscle mass (Figure 13.4). However, as we shall see throughout this chapter

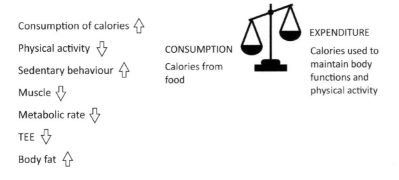

Figure 13.3 Energy imbalance and gaining body fat

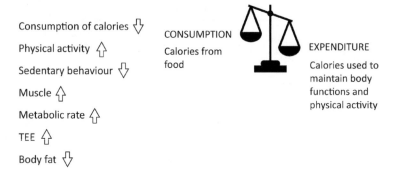

Consumption of calories ⇩

Physical activity ⇧

Sedentary behaviour ⇩

Muscle ⇧

Metabolic rate ⇧

TEE ⇧

Body fat ⇩

CONSUMPTION
Calories from food

EXPENDITURE
Calories used to maintain body functions and physical activity

Figure 13.4 Energy imbalance and losing body fat

the 'calories in: calories out' model is much more complex than a simple equation in 'real life', because humans are biopsychosocial beings, we are neither machines nor identical.

Genes

Genes are inherited from an individual's parents and are influenced by the individual's environment. Genes influence every human trait and behaviour. Between 30% and 70% of body fat is associated with inherited genes. For example, genes can influence appetite, abdominal/visceral fat and total body fat (Yeo, 2017). People do not start their life's journey with their body fat from an equal place.

Fat cells

Adults have a constant number of fat cells. Most fat cells are adipocytes. They are like little bags whose job is to fill with fat, store it and, when needed, empty it out. Spalding and colleagues (2008) found an obese child adds new fat cells at twice the rate of a lean child and the number of fat cells in a person's body is fixed by their early 20s. Obese adults have many more fat cells than lean adults, while the proportion of new cells that replenish old ones is the same. Even when adults lose a lot of weight, the number of fat cells remains constant. When adults gain weight, they increase the volume of fat inside their fat cells and when they lose weight, the fat cells shrink but they do not disappear and nor does their innate urge to refill. As people age, the fat cells' ability to empty their fat decreases (Arner *et al.*, 2019). If older people do not reduce their calorie intake accordingly or do not increase physical activity which can enhance the functioning of fat cells, they will gain weight. In summary, current research suggests

- the propensity for overweight and obesity in adulthood is determined by weight and the number of fat cells that develop during childhood and adolescence
- a reason for why overweight children are more likely to become overweight adults compared to others
- explains why older people tend to gain weight
- helps to explain why many overweight adults find it hard to lose weight

Some inherited genes and higher body fat in childhood seem to encourage greater body fat in adulthood which is then exacerbated with age.

Expending calories: sedentary behaviour and physical activity

The number of calories used by the body mostly depends on how much and for how long the body moves (PAL), and how much of it is composed of muscle mass, which increases BMR. Table 13.2 shows how sedentary people in the UK use fewer calories than those who are moderately active, across all age ranges and both sexes. Sedentary behaviour means lying, sitting or reclining while we are awake and it includes driving a car, watching television or computer screens, desk-based work and regular use of a wheelchair (WHO, 2020). Physical activity includes standing, walking, running and so forth. We are becoming an increasingly sedentary and less active population (Sheppard, 2021). Table 13.2 also shows fewer calories being used as people age. This is because people become more sedentary with age, especially after the age of 50 when the body develops a higher proportion of body fat and less muscle mass, and so uses fewer calories (Westerterp, 2013). The World Health Organization (2020) reports there is a wealth of evidence showing the health benefits of reducing sedentary behaviour and increasing physical activity, not least for the prevention of cardiovascular disease. In adults, the relationship between sedentary behaviour and gaining excess body fat, and between physical activity and losing excess body fat, is less clear. There is

- no clear evidence of an association between sedentary behaviour and increased body fat
- some evidence that physical activity may be helpful when trying to lose body fat
- stronger evidence that physical activity can help to prevent adults gaining excess body fat

(WHO, 2020)

Table 13.2 Comparison of calorie expenditure between sedentary behaviour and moderate activity

	Age (years)	Sedentary (PAL 1.49) kcals	Moderately active (PAL 1:78) kcals
Men	19–24	2,532	3,009
	25–34	2,508	3,009
	35–44	2,388	2,866
	45–54	2,365	2,818
	55–64	2,365	2,818
	65–74	2,150	2,556
	75+	2,102	2,508
Women	19–24	2,006	2,388
	25–34	1,982	2,388
	35–44	1,935	2,317
	45–54	1,911	2,293
	55–64	1,887	2,269
	65–74	1,744	2,078
	75+	1,672	2,006

Source: Adapted from SACN (2012, p. 61).

Table 13.3 UK Physical Activity Guidelines

Adults (19–64 years)	150 minutes of moderate-intensity activity OR 75 minutes of vigorous activity per week Muscle strengthening activities on two days per week Break up long periods of being sedentary with light intensity activity or standing
Older adults (65 years and over)	150 minutes of moderate-intensity aerobic activity per week If already active, add 75 minutes of vigorous (or vigorous and moderate) activity per week Include weight bearing activities Break up long periods of being sedentary with light activity or standing
Disabled adults	150 minutes of moderate-intensity activity per week Keep active on each day of the week Include strength and balance activities on two days per week

Where someone is unable to meet these recommendations, they should aim to be as physically active as their abilities allow. Some may start by doing small amounts and increasing frequency and duration over time.

Source: DHSC (2019).

In the UK, all adults are encouraged to meet the UK Physical Activity Guidelines (Table 13.3). Those with health conditions, which may include severe obesity, are encouraged to seek medical advice (PHE, 2020).

Food and activity

When someone eats carbohydrates, that is foods and drinks which contain sugars and starches, some are quickly broken down and the molecules are released into the blood stream. The rest is stored in the form of glycogen in the muscles and liver. Glycogen is like a petrol pump, ready to deliver fuel when needed. When we are active, we break down the glycogen into smaller molecules which releases the calories, the fuel, for that activity. People who are very active, such as sports professionals, are careful to eat a regular supply of carbohydrates so they can physically perform well. Wholegrains and starchy carbohydrates, and fruit and vegetables, are much healthier and sustain longer performance than sugary products (Table 13.4). Women in late pregnancy are also

Table 13.4 Carbohydrates

Carbohydrates		
Simple carbohydrates	*Complex carbohydrates*	
Sugars	*Starches with low dietary fibre*	*Starches with high dietary fibre*
Sugar (all types/all colours) Honey Syrup Malt	White flour White rice Cornflour White pasta	Wholegrains Wholemeal flour Wholemeal bread Jacket potatoes Brown rice Oats Barley

encouraged to eat more wholegrains, fruit and vegetables to increase their calories and to help sustain their energy levels.

The molecules from all food and drink, which includes fats, carbohydrates and proteins, that are neither needed to keep the body healthy and in good repair nor needed to top up the glycogen levels, will either be excreted or stored in the body's fat cells. This is body fat. When we are active, to obtain the fuel we need, we first break down glycogen and when this is used, we start to break down, use and lose body fat.

Individual differences in energy expenditure

Individuals with similar daily lifestyles, consuming the same number of calories, may use more or fewer calories because of differences in their metabolism (DIT + BMR + PAL). Individuals may be more sedentary for a range of reasons including illness, upbringing, home environment, enjoyment of sedentary activities, lack of support with physical activities and environmental concerns such as safety (Rawlings *et al.*, 2019). Current research suggests some people are highly motivated to be physically active because they have cannabinoid type 1 receptors which gives them an activity-induced 'high' similar to cannabis. Others have fewer receptors and find activity more disagreeable (Muguruza *et al.*, 2019; Siebers *et al.*, 2021).

> *Physical activity can help to prevent weight gain and aid weight loss but, alone, it will not lead to significant weight loss.*

Consuming calories

The number of calories we consume is the sum of the 'amount' we consume and 'what' we consume. Both are influenced by 'why' we consume.

Portion sizes

The larger the portion size, the greater the number of calories it will contain. Many foods and drinks are sold in large portions, which we begin to see as 'normal'. The British Nutrition Foundation (2021) provides a comprehensive list of recommended portion sizes (Table 13.5).

Calorie density of nutrients

All foods and drinks contain combinations of the nutrients: carbohydrate, protein and fat. All are needed by the body and all contain calories, but not equal calories.

One gram of carbohydrate contains 3.75 kcals
One gram of protein contains 4 kcals
One gram of fat contains 9 kcals

Box 13.1 shows how we calculate the number of calories in food and drink. That which contains a high proportion of calorie-dense fat will be high in calories.

Table 13.5 Examples of recommended portion sizes

Eatwell Guide	Recommended portions per day	Examples of foods	Portions
Potatoes, bread, rice, pasta and other starchy carbohydrates	3–4 portions	Muesli Wholemeal bread Cooked pasta Baked potato	About 3 handfuls Medium roll 2 hands cupped together Size of a person's fist
Beans, pulses, fish, eggs, meat and other protein	2–3 portions	Roast chicken Lentils, beans and other pulses	About 2.5 slices About 6 dessert spoons
Dairy and alternatives	2–3 portions	Semi-skimmed milk on cereal Hard cheese	About half a glass About the size of two thumbs
Fruit and vegetables	At least 5 portions	Apple Large broccoli spears Cooked carrots, peas, sweetcorn	medium 2 3 heaped serving spoons
Unsaturated oils and spreads	Small amounts	Olive/vegetable oil	1 teaspoon
Treats (foods high in fat, salt and/or sugar)	Eat less often and in small amounts	Chocolate Crisps	4 squares One small bag

Source: BNF (2021).

Mindless and mindful eating

We are more likely to mindlessly consume excess calories when being sedentary, especially when sitting watching television or other screen content, compared to driving or being in social situations. Ogden and colleagues (2013) carried out research which suggests

- the screens distract people from hunger. It breaks the 'eating as a response to hunger' relationship
- we are distracted but not distracted enough, in the way that driving takes up concentration, to challenge the effort required to eat
- mindless eating happens in places where we are not watched or hindered by concerns about what others may think/social stigma

Mindful eating is about conscious eating in the moment. Some mindful instructions may include

- avoid television or other screens when eating
- sit down to eat
- serve the recommended portion sizes
- have an open mind
- be patient
- have no judgement
- trust in yourself, notice your own personal responses to the food

---

Box 13.1 Counting calories in crunchy nut peanut butter

The label shows that 100 grams of crunchy peanut butter contains

- carbohydrates 11.6 g
- protein 29.6 g
- fat 46 g

Multiply the grams by the calories per gram

- carbohydrate 11.6 g × 3.75 kcals = 43.5 kcals
- protein 29.6 g × 4 kcals = 118.4 kcals
- fat 46 g × 9 kcals = 414 kcals

43.5 kcals + 118.4 kcals + 414 kcals = 575.9 kcals (round up to 576 kcals)
100 grams of crunchy peanut butter contains 576 kcals

$$\frac{43.5 \times 100}{576} = 7.5\% \text{ of the total calories are coming from carbohydrates}$$

$$\frac{118.4 \times 100}{576} = 20.5\% \text{ of the total calories are coming from proteins}$$

$$\frac{414 \times 100}{576} = 71.8\% \text{ of the total calories are coming from fat}$$

If we eat a large spoonful (25 g) of peanut butter, we will be eating 114 kcals.

$$\frac{576 \text{ kcals}}{100 \text{ g}} \times 25 \text{ g} = 114 \text{ kcals}$$

- have no goal other than focussing on the present eating experience
- accept the moment, it is what it is
- let go of past experiences around the food or eating

(Nelson, 2017)

Emotional eating

Emotional eating is where an individual consumes food and drink as a way to manage difficult emotions rather than to satisfy hunger. Eating food may provide a temporary distraction, a way to avoid the feelings; it may feel like compensation for difficult feelings (Box 13.2). Some adults learn these attitudes and behaviours from childhood. Food, such as sweets, becomes associated with rewards and achievement, a sign of having pleased an adult. Adults may offer food, such as chocolate, as a means of keeping a child quiet or content. They may also offer food as a way of showing love, perhaps a way of trying to make up for the absence of a parent. Feeding children when they are not hungry teaches them that food is not about hunger and it may desensitise their ability to even know when they are hungry or not (Birch, 1991). If we eat when we are not hungry, we are likely to consume more calories than we need.

Box 13.2 Emotional eating as compulsive eating

"I remember the first time I ate compulsively. I was seventeen years old … sitting at the breakfast table with my American roommate and our German landlords … I feel that I am about to remember something and then, unaccountably, I am moved to tears. But I do not cry. I say nothing, I look furtively around me, then, I am eating. My hand is reaching out. And the movement, even in the first moments, seems driven and compulsive. I am not hungry. I had pushed away my plate moments before. But my hand is reaching and I know that I am reaching for something that has been lost. I hope for much from the food that is on the table before me but suddenly it seems to me that nothing will ever still this hunger – an immense implacable craving that I do not remember having felt before … everyone laughs and I am mortified … I am blushing … I MUST go on eating … I stuff the two rolls in my pocket … I begin running. And as I run I eat … I catch a glimpse of myself in … a store window … astonishment that the body I see … is … very slender when I imagine that it is terribly fat …, I don't … wait, I can't wait, I can't bear waiting … and I know exactly what I am doing when I suddenly dart forward, grab the plate [of sausage] and run … a sudden sense of release … urgently dipping the sausage into the mustard, stuffing large chunks of it into my mouth. And then I am crying …"

(Source: Chernin, 1981, pp. 5–7)

With high levels of unwanted stress, some people eat less, while others eat more. This is called the stress eating paradox (Stone and Brownell, 1994). From the viewpoint of biology, it makes sense for the adult to eat less. The highly stressed body is one that is ready for 'fight, flight or freeze'. The heart rate, blood pressure and breathing increases as cortisol and adrenalin surge through the body. Yet for many, and for women more than men, it seems stress prompts greater eating. One explanation is that the learned behaviour of swallowing food to 'swallow' difficult emotions overrides the body's natural response. Susie Orbach (1978) argues that women often describe food as a comforter and yet women are discouraged from eating freely in a society that promotes slimness and self-control around food. It is mostly women who describe having 'good days' and 'bad days' around food. Food may automatically remind women, and men, of their weight and size, which they struggle to control in accordance with cultural expectations about acceptable body sizes (Chernin, 1986; VanKim *et al.*, 2016; Williams and Annandale, 2018).

We may consume excess calories by eating large portions of calorie-dense food and drink, we may consume mindlessly and we may eat for emotional reasons.

Eating to lose weight

Healthy weight loss means,

"… cutting your overall calories by at least one-quarter and reducing your intake of high-sugar foods and saturated fat."

(Harvie and Howell, 2013, p. 12)

This might sound simple, but it is not.

Mediterranean diet

The first step for anyone wishing to lose weight is to reduce processed foods including high fat and sugar snacks because these add calories and have poor nutritional value. The Mediterranean diet is a healthy diet, and the UK's Eatwell Guide (PHE, 2018) (Figure 13.5) and the flexitarian planetary health diet (EAT, 2019) are variations of it. A healthy diet includes

- plenty of fruit, vegetables, nuts, legumes/pulses and wholegrains
- small to moderate amounts of fish/oily fish, poultry, eggs, lean meat and lowfat dairy products such as cheese and yoghurt
- unsaturated oil
- minimal or no processed meat, sugary foods or high fat snacks
- fluid such as water, tea, coffee or sugar free drinks

Dietary fibre

Healthy diets include plenty of dietary fibre found in wholegrains, oats, barley, rye, wheat, brown rice, pulses, fruit and vegetables. Dietary fibre is not digested in the small intestine, unlike all other food and drink. It remains unchanged until it reaches the colon. There, it loses water and is finally excreted. UK adults are recommended to eat 30 grams per day, but they are eating about 19 grams (NatCen *et al.*, 2020). In addition to preventing diseases, plenty of dietary fibre

- helps people to feel full by distending the stomach. This deters people from over-consuming at a mealtime
- boosts the microbiome, the microorganisms in the intestine which help to deter the accumulation of body fat

(Davis, 2017; Robinson, 2021b)

Dieting health warning

People who have medical conditions, are pregnant or breast feeding, the under 18s, those who need help with drug or alcohol use and those undergoing medical treatment need to check with a healthcare professional before starting any weight loss diet, other than a healthy Mediterranean-style diet with recommended portion sizes.

Continuous dieting/continuous energy restriction

Continuous dieting means restricting calories (energy) every day, such as consuming 1,000 kcals per day until a goal weight is achieved.

- A low calorie diet is one that provides between 800 and 1600 kcals per day
- A very low calorie diet is one that provides less than 800 kcals per day

(NICE, 2014)

Diets of 810 to 850 kcals per day have been used, under medical supervision, for short time periods for obese people who have additional health conditions. They are successful at rapid, short-term weight loss, which have enabled people to be fit for surgery and to reverse type 2 diabetes (Jebb *et al.*, 2017; Lean *et al.*, 2019). Rapid weight loss is

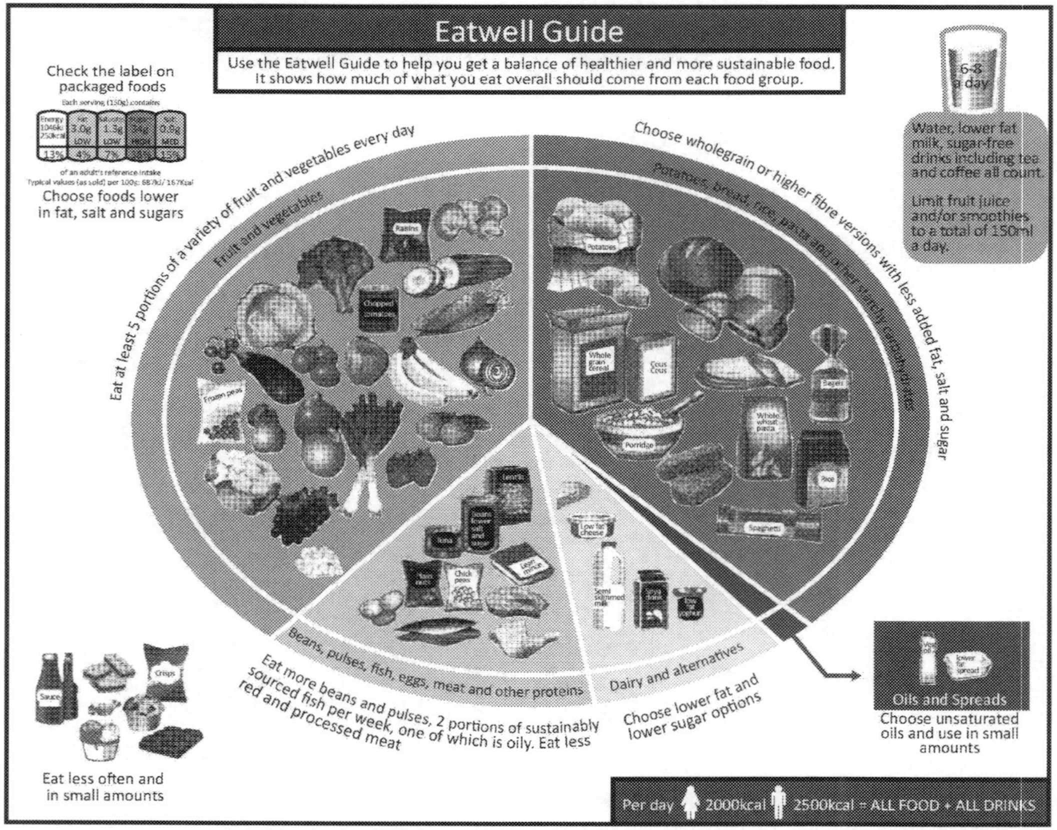

Figure 13.5 Eatwell Guide

Source: PHE (2018) in association with the Welsh Government, Food Standards Scotland and the Food Standards Agency in Northern Ireland (2018, p. 5). Reproduced under the terms of the Open Government Licence v3 and with permission from Taylor Francis.

motivating but eating less than about 1,000 calories per day continuously puts people at risk of nutritional deficiencies and they are likely to go into preservation mode, which means they will regain this weight loss (NICE, 2014).

Starvation and preservation

When we consume very little food and drink, the body is starving and it goes into preservation mode. It needs fuel to keep alive. Initially it searches for glucose in the blood stream, and then glucose from the glycogen that is stored in the liver and muscles. When the glycogen is depleted, it turns to breaking down the fat in the body's adipose tissue, producing ketones which can be used as fuel. This is ketosis. After about a week, the body starts to consume its own self, its protein, such as that which makes up muscles, organs and tissues. Protein is broken down into amino acids, from which glucose can be made and then fuel. The body is in a distressed state, muscle is lost, weight is dropping fast and metabolic rate slows down so that the body can conserve what it has. The body now requires less fuel (fewer calories) to keep going than before the undereating started. Weight loss is halted. The only way to keep losing weight is further starvation, which eventually leads to death. This process is accelerated when accompanied by physical activity.

Yo-yo dieting

For people whose bodies have entered preservation mode, it can feel frustrating that weight loss has stopped. Even if they continue to consume a very low calorie diet, it becomes very difficult to lose any more weight. If, perhaps due to hunger, lethargy, boredom or misery, they consume slightly more calories they will gain weight because their metabolic rate is so low. In time, they find themselves back to their original weight. Starting the cycle again is called yo-yo dieting (Figure 13.6).

We need to reduce calories in a way that reduces body fat but preserves muscle to maintain metabolic rate.

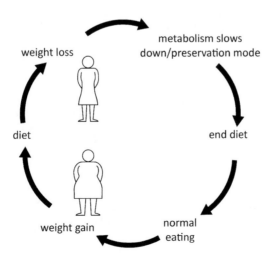

Figure 13.6 Yo-yo dieting

Psychology of continuous dieting

Peter Herman and Janet Polivy (1991) invited female students to take part in an experiment about the taste of ice cream. One group was asked to drink one milk shake (210 ml), another group was asked to drink two milk shakes (420 ml) and the third group had no milk shake. Afterwards, in a private room, each student was given a large bowl of weighed ice cream and told they could eat as much as they wanted. At the end of the experiment, all the students completed a questionnaire which allowed the researchers to identify who were dieters and who were non-dieters, and the remaining ice cream was weighed. The non-dieters ate less ice cream after one milk shake compared to those who drank none, and they ate less after two milk shakes compared to those who drank one or none (Figure 13.7). This suggests that they compensated for their prior consumption. Conversely, dieters ate more ice cream following milk shake than when they had none.

Non-dieters may eat when they feel hungry and when food is available and tasty. Dieting is about controlling one's eating, food denial, resolving to ignore delicious offerings and to stick to a regime. When someone or something undermines that resolve, such as a researcher asking them to drink a milk shake and help with a piece of research, or being given a cake for their birthday, or a crisis happens, they are temporarily released from their abstinence. Having broken their resolve, what we might call the 'what the heck' response, the temptation is to continue to enjoy the moment and indulge. Tomorrow, fuelled by guilt, self-control will be re-asserted and the diet will start again. This is another type of emotional eating, where emotions not hunger are in control. Eating disorders take these elements of rigid control and denial of food to an extreme level. Anorexia nervosa takes it to starvation, and bulimia nervosa includes periods of disinhibited eating on a grand scale, known as binge eating.

Herman and Polivy (1991) argue that continuous daily dieting is unnatural and, over time, the natural rhythm of eating in response to hunger becomes distorted. The calories eaten at moments of disinhibition may outweigh those that were denied

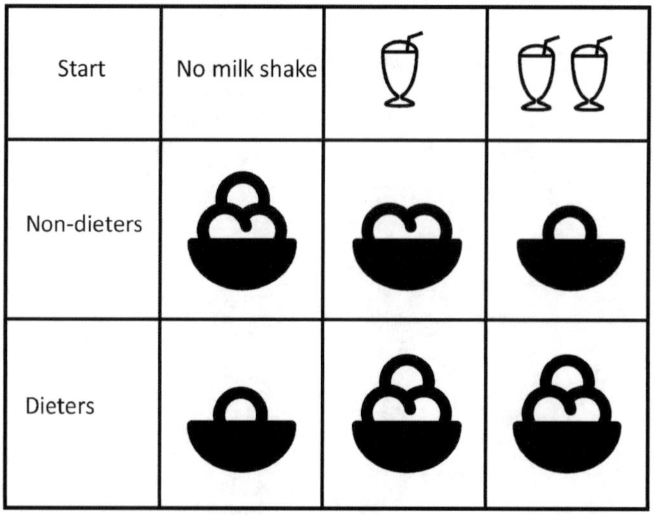

Figure 13.7 Ice cream consumption in dieters and non-dieters

before that point. Food denial is all the harder in a context of plentiful, cheap, food designed by food technologists to be tasty and tempting without the inconvenience of cutlery. The psychological impact of continuous dieting may contribute to yo-yo dieting, and the banning of favourite foods can be self-defeating, as it only makes them more attractive.

Fad diets

A fad diet is any weight loss diet that is not substantially based around a Mediterranean diet, with its emphasis on variety and plant-based foods. Fad diets are often based on pseudo-science and promises of fast weight loss. Some recent examples include blood type diets, the detox tea/skinny coffee diet, slimming sachets such as 'Slim Me' and the alkaline water diet. Limiting food variety can leave people with nutritional deficiencies and health conditions that cannot always be reversed. Very fast weight loss is starvation by another name.

Meal replacements

Astbury and colleagues. (2019) studied the use of meal replacements such as soups, bars and shakes. Replacing one or more meals or snacks led to weight loss. Greater weight loss was achieved when people were supported by a dietitian, received advice about food choices and undertook 30 minutes of physical activity for five or more days per week.

Total diet replacements

Replacing all meals with a diet product or programme is called 'total diet replacement', and this needs to be viewed with caution. They

- can be expensive
- might include behavioural support
- are convenient and easy
- can become boring
- can be socially isolating
- may not help with transitioning back to normal food
- can be very low in calories, which may encourage fast weight loss leading to later weight gain

Timing of meals

Eating more calories at breakfast and fewer towards the end of the day is associated with weight loss and reduced waist circumference. In one study, over 12 weeks, eating

- 700 kcals for breakfast
- 500 kcals for lunch
- 200 kcals for dinner

led to two and half times more weight loss than eating

- 200 kcals for breakfast
- 500 kcals for lunch
- 700 kcals for dinner

(Jakubowicz *et al.*, 2013)

A Mediterranean-style diet and eating more at the beginning of the day are good starting points for weight loss. Continuous low calorie and fad diets should be avoided.

Fasting

Absolute fasting means consuming no food or drink. Fasting usually includes drinking water or sometimes black tea and coffee. When someone is fasting, they are starving and their body enters preservation mode. Mattson and colleagues (2014) explain how humans' circadian rhythms evolved to the natural light and dark cycle. Eating scarce food was associated with daylight and fasting with night. This diurnal rhythm affected humans' behaviour, physiology and metabolism. Modern life includes artificial light and shift work, encourages plentiful and continuous eating, and shorter times of fasting. It also includes obesity. Many researchers have become interested in the benefits of slightly extending periods of fasting to better mimic the more natural human state.

Overeating and gaining fat damages the body's cells. It causes chronic low-grade inflammation which is associated with the development of cancer, arthritis, type 2 diabetes, cardiovascular disease and neurological diseases (Gupta *et al.*, 2018). When we fast, we give the cells time to recover, cleanse and revive, and inflammation is reduced. Scientists believe that periods of fasting may have a range of health benefits, and short periods of fasting can help with weight loss (Ganesan *et al.*, 2018; Kroeger *et al.*, 2018).

Intermittent fasting

Intermittent fasting is where people are asked to fast or severely restrict their eating for a short period of time and to eat normally for a period. The fasting undertaken by Muslims from sunrise to sunset during the month of Ramadan is a type of intermittent fasting. For weight loss, a diet might instruct fasting for a day and eating normally for six days. Time-restricted feeding is a variant of intermittent fasting. It is where people are asked to shorten the period of eating to a window of, perhaps, eight or 10 hours during the day, and extend the period of fasting to 14 or 16 hours.

Intermittent energy restriction

Intermittent energy restriction is where people greatly reduce the number of calories they consume for some of the week. For example, consuming 800 calories per day for two days in a week and otherwise eating normally.

Which is best for weight loss?

When people have been given the same number of calories, but are asked to follow different dietary regimes, a few studies have reported greater weight loss among those who practised intermittent fasting or intermittent energy restriction compared to those who practised continuous energy restriction (Byrne *et al.*, 2018; Davis *et al.*, 2016; Hutchison *et al.*, 2019). It may be because controlling one's eating for a short period is easier to adhere to. In one study, where people ate a low calorie diet for two days of the week, they had spontaneously reduced their calorie intake on the other five as well (Harvie *et al.*, 2018).

Including short periods of fasting or energy restriction helps with losing weight.

Nutrients, hunger and satiety

Janet Latner and Marlene Schwartz (1999) asked 12 female students at Yale University to drink a liquid lunch on three occasions. They were asked to keep both their breakfasts and exercise level constant for each day. Each liquid lunch contained 450 kcals. The students did not know whether they were given a carbohydrate drink, a protein drink or a drink which was half carbohydrate and half protein (Figure 13.8). They were invited to a buffet dinner at the end of the day.

Thinking point:

Who is going to be most hungry before dinner?
Who is going to eat the most at dinner?

The researchers found

- most hunger before dinner was reported from those who had drank the high carbohydrate lunch
- least hunger before dinner was reported by those who drank the protein lunch
- the hunger of those who drank the protein and carbohydrate mix lay in between
- those who drank the high carbohydrate lunch ate the most at dinner
- those who drank the protein lunch ate the least at dinner
- those who drank the protein and carbohydrate mix ate an amount in between

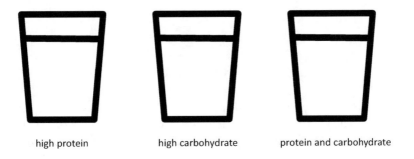

high protein   high carbohydrate   protein and carbohydrate

Figure 13.8 Liquid lunches

There is also some evidence that

- foods or drinks which are, or are perceived to be, more viscous/thicker, solid or heavier seem to encourage people to feel satiated ('feel full')
- food labels that declare the product 'will keep us feeling full for longer' may influence satiety
- supersizing, such as very large buckets of popcorn, can encourage over-eating, but not greater satiety

(Chambers *et al.*, 2015)

When trying to cut down calories, it is useful to know

- protein keeps us feeling satiated for a long time
- protein helps to maintain muscle and therefore metabolism
- fat and carbohydrates are less satiating than protein
- it is easy to eat a lot of calories in a very small portion, when a food is high in fat. This is called the passive overconsumption of calories
- we need some fats, the unsaturated types, for good health
- 'low fat diets' are based around reducing the calorie-dense fat. It is common to replace the calories from fat with calories from carbohydrates. We need to be sure these are not the sugary/low fibre types because sugar and starchy low fibre carbohydrates are absorbed into the blood stream quickly, leading to spikes in glucose followed by insulin which makes people feel weak and hungry
- 'low carbohydrate diets' are based around reducing sugar and the starchy low fibre carbohydrates such as white bread, white rice and pasta, couscous, cornflakes, sugary cereals, instant oat cereals, crisps, biscuits, cakes, mashed potato, chips and crackers. Low carbohydrate diets encourage ketosis, the burning of body fat
- dietary fibre is low in calories. It is not digested. It is filling because it distends the stomach and slows the rate of gastric emptying. It does not cause spikes in insulin
- we need at least five portions of fruit and vegetables per day, or more, for good health and these contain dietary fibre
- good sources of dietary fibre include granary and wholemeal bread, wholemeal pasta, brown rice, oatcakes, porridge, wholemeal cereals and nuts

When trying to reduce calories, it is helpful to understand which nutrients help to enhance or reduce feelings of hunger.

A healthy weight loss diet

The 2-Day Diet was developed by Dr Michelle Harvie, a research dietitian, and Professor Tony Howell, professor of medical oncology (Box 13.3). It includes intermittent energy restriction. All proceeds from their book are donated to the Genesis Breast Cancer Prevention charity.

Box 13.3 The 2-Day Diet

5 days

For 5 days a week, eat a Mediterranean diet including '5 a day' fruit and vegetables, wholegrain carbohydrates, beans, pulses, nuts, eggs, fish, poultry, low-fat dairy and lean meat.

2 days

For 2 days a week, eat

- high protein (4 to–14 servings)
- healthy fats (max 6 servings)
- low-fat dairy (3 servings)
- vegetables (5 servings)
- fruit (1 serving)
- plenty of water, tea, coffee or sugar-free drinks

The number of servings shown here is for men over 12.5 stones and provides 1,100 kcals per day.

(Source: Harvie and Howell, 2013)

Monitoring and the microbiome

Self-monitoring

Regular self-monitoring of diet, activity and weight has been shown to help with weight loss (Burke *et al.*, 2011; Harvey *et al.*, 2019). It may include counting steps using a pedometer, the Active 10 app, keeping a food diary and/or regular weighing.

Microbiome

The microbiome refers to trillions of microorganisms that live in people's gastrointestinal tract. Most of these live in the large intestine, the colon. The majority are bacteria. The number and diversity of microorganisms depend on an individual's genes, physical activity, drugs and diet. These come together to make each person's microbiome unique. The microbiome powerfully affects systems in the body and a large number of widely diverse microorganisms are associated with better health. In addition to influencing immunity, depression, the development of metabolic disease, cardiovascular disease and type 2 diabetes; the microbiome influences energy metabolism, how an individual responds to nutrients, foods and drinks, and their body fat (Le Roy *et al.*, 2019; Valdes *et al.*, 2018).

Physical activity and diet can encourage microbiome diversity (Asnicar *et al.*, 2021; Monda *et al.*, 2017) (Figure 13.9). Those nutrients from the diet which are not absorbed from the small intestine into the bloodstream continue to travel down into the large intestine. Most notably, this includes dietary fibre. This is the diet on which the gut

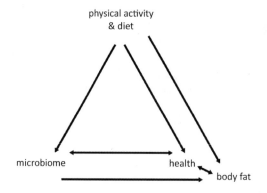

Figure 13.9 The microbiome, health and body fat

microorganisms feed and multiply. Diets which are high in processed foods are associated with a limited range of microorganisms (Spector, 2015). Mediterranean-type diets are associated with protecting widely diverse microbiomes as well those specific microorganisms known to be associated good health (Ghosh *et al.*, 2020; Tsigalou *et al.*, 2021). Intermittent fasting can also stimulate microbiome diversity provided it is within the context of a healthy, varied diet like the Mediterranean diet (Spector, 2015).

A wide diversity of microorganisms is associated with helping to prevent and reduce excess body fat. Individuals defined as being obese have microbiomes of low diversity (Ghosh *et al.*, 2020). One example is the bacteria *Bacteroides* found in high numbers in lean people and low numbers in people defined as obese; with weight loss, these bacteria rise (Ley *et al.*, 2006). When people who are obese adopt a Mediterranean diet, their *Bacteroides* bacteria increase (Haro *et al.*, 2017). The implications of understanding the relationship between diet, activity, an individual's microbiome and body fat means

- we can be confident that a Mediterranean-style diet alongside activity is well suited to preventing weight gain and is the basis for long-term weight loss
- researchers are starting to understand, more than ever before, why individuals respond differently to similar diets, why some regain body fat quickly after weight loss and some seem to remain lean whatever they eat
- we are moving to a time when an individual's diet can be tailored to their individual microbiome in ways that will protect and enhance good health and a healthy weight

A diverse microbiome helps with weight loss, and this can be achieved by a Mediterranean-style diet and physical activity.

Obesogenic environment

The UK has become an obesogenic environment, one where the physical, social and cultural surroundings encourage people to gain excess body fat. We are more sedentary and less physically active because of

- increased motorised transport
- less walking
- sedentary jobs
- more computers/high screen time, online working and shopping

- mechanisation/labour saving devices
- more lifts and escalators
- built environments with limited green spaces, pollution and safety concerns

Simultaneously, we overconsume calories because of more processed/junk/fast food and drink which is

- easy to consume, highly palatable and energy dense
- high fat, high sugar, high salt to make it tasty
- low in protein to encourage hunger and repeat consumption
- highly advertised, widely available and used in food promotions
- cheap, as a proportion of household expenditure
- convenient, e.g. eat immediately or warm in the microwave oven
- limited nutrition labelling

and it has led to social and cultural changes that have encouraged less eating at home and more 'eating on the go'. Current evidence shows

- people who are genetically predisposed to gaining excess body fat are more vulnerable than others to an obesogenic environment
- frequent eating outside the home, for example from cafés, takeaways, vending machines and restaurants is associated with eating more fat in the diet, and greater body fat
- high numbers of fast food outlets in areas of deprivation, where more people of lower socio-economic position live and work, are consistently associated with poor weight management, less physical activity for leisure, high consumption of fast food and high rates of overweight and obesity

(Brandkvist *et al.*, 2019; Townshend and Lake, 2017; Wilkins *et al.*, 2019)

The obesogenic environment disadvantages those in lower socio-economic circumstances and contributes to UK health inequalities, meaning the greater disease and early death among those who have a lower socio-economic position compared to those who have a higher socio-economic position.

The obesogenic environment is the primary reason for the 'obesity epidemic' as it encourages energy imbalance and poor quality diets in everyday life.

Principles for tackling overweight

When tackling overweight, the priority is to address the obesogenic environment because this will support the whole population including those with a genetic predisposition to gain body fat and those living in lower socio-economic circumstances who suffer from the greatest health disadvantage. This is a social change model of health promotion. The following initiatives are being discussed across the UK by governments, local councils, the food and drinks industry and businesses including caterers, but action is far too slow. We need to

- increase green spaces and walkable neighbourhoods
- increase opportunities for 'active travel' e.g. make cycling and scooting safer and easier

Table 13.6 Factors which encourage and discourage excess body fat

Factors which increase chances of accumulating excess body fat and do not help with healthy, long-term weight loss	*Factors which prevent accumulation of excess body fat and can help with healthy, long-term weight loss*
Non-modifiable factors	
Inherit genes which predispose a body to accumulate body fat	Inherit genes which do not predispose a body to accumulate body fat
Older	Younger
Few cannabinoid type 1 receptors	Many cannabinoid type 1 receptors
Number of fat cells inherited from childhood and adolescence	Avoid overweight and obesity in childhood
Calorie expenditure	
More sedentary behaviour/sitting and less physical activity	More physical activity and less sedentary behaviour/sitting
Few psychosocial incentives to be active	Many psychosocial incentives to be active
Calorie consumption	
Consume large portions	Consume recommended portions
Consume many calorie dense foods	Consume few calorie dense foods
Mindlessly eat	Mindfully eat
Emotional eating	Eat when hungry, obtain psychological support for emotional concerns
Do not eat a varied Mediterranean-style diet	Eat a varied Mediterranean-style diet
Eat little dietary fibre	Eat plenty of dietary fibre
Eat few calories continuously, yo-yo diet, fad diets	Incorporate intermittent fasting or intermittent energy restriction
Eat most calories at the end of the day	Eat most calories at the start of the day
Consume low protein, relying on fat and carbohydrates	Consume sufficient protein and dietary fibre through the day
Consume many sugary/starchy-low fibre carbohydrates	Limit consumption of sugary/starchy-low fibre carbohydrates
Frequently eat outside the home	Infrequently eat outside the home
Calorie expenditure and consumption	
Consume more calories than we use for living and moving	Use more calories for living and moving than we consume
No self-monitoring when trying to lose weight	Self-monitor when trying to lose weight
Low diversity microbiome associated with a limited or processed diet and sedentary behaviour	High diversity microbiome associated with a varied, Mediterranean-style diet and physical activity
Obesogenic environment	
Live and work in an obesogenic environment comprising passive travel, sedentary behaviour and wide-spread, cheap, highly advertised processed/fast foods	Live and work in a healthy environment comprising active travel, physical activity and wide-spread, cheap, highly advertised healthy foods
Few foods and drinks have nutrition labels	All foods and drinks have nutrition labels
High numbers of fast food outlets in an area	Few fast food outlets in an area

- improve affordable and accessible physical activity opportunities such as leisure centres, exercise referral schemes and land-based activities such as allotments and woodland skills
- provide standing desks and allow short walking breaks in the workplace
- discourage large portions/supersizing food and drink
- provide a greater range of healthier options for food and drink eaten outside the home

- make healthier options cheaper in all outlets including restaurants
- introduce mandatory nutrition labelling for all food and drink bought and eaten outside the home
- deter price promotions of calorie dense foods and drinks, such as 'two for one' deals
- encourage local councils to adopt planning policies which restrict the opening of new fast food takeaway outlets and encourage healthier alternatives
- provide training for businesses to support staff and customers e.g. smaller portion sizes; increase fruit, vegetables and dietary fibre; include sufficient protein; provide time and facilities to eat
- work with the food industry to reformulate foods and drinks to reduce calories
- levy tax on sugary soft drinks
- restrict advertising for processed, high fat and high sugar foods

While we wait to live and work in a health promoting environment, individuals who wish to lose weight need to be aware of all the factors that may be responsible for their excess body fat (Table 13.6). They need a flexible, personalised, holistic/biopsychosocial approach to weight loss that is based on understanding 'why', not simply 'what', people consume or do. Changes need to easily fit into their wider lifestyle, feel manageable and achievable, while keeping those factors which are important to them so the change can be maintained in the long term. Start with one small step only, because habits are hard to change, and one small step can make an important difference. Practitioners may utilise psychology theories (Chapter 5) with the emphasis on 'change and gain' not 'loss'. They may work with an educational or empowerment model of health promotion (Chapters 7 and 8) and need to keep the individual's personal definition of health to the fore (Chapter 1). In future, although we will be able to describe and enhance each individual's microbiome, and even modify certain genes, the moral imperative and the more effective long-term solution is to change the physical and social environment.

Summary

This chapter has

- explained metabolism, energy balance and imbalance
- described factors which influence calorie expenditure
- explored reasons for overconsuming calories
- examined dietary practices associated with unhealthy and healthy weight loss
- argued why tackling the obesogenic environment is a public health priority
- set out evidence-based principles for tackling overweight

Further reading

Lake, A.A., Townshend, T.G., and Alvanides, S. (2010) *Obesogenic environments. Complexities, perceptions and objective measures.* London: Blackwell

Useful websites

Association for the Study of Obesity. https://aso.org.uk
Obesity UK. https://www.obesityuk.org.uk

References

Arner, P., Bernard, S., Appelsved, L., Fu, K.-Y., Andersson, D.P., Salehpour, M., Thorell, A., Rydén, M. and Spalding, K.L. (2019) 'Adipose lipid turnover and long-term changes in body weight', *Nature Medicine*, 25(9), pp. 1385–1389

Asnicar, F., Berry, S., Valdes, A. *et al.* (2021) 'Microbiome connections with host metabolism and habitual diet from 1,098 deeply phenotyped individuals', *Nature Medicine*, 27(2) doi:10.1038/s41591-020-01183-8

Astbury, N.M., Piernas, C., Hartmann-Boyce, J., Lapworth, S., Aveyard, P. and Jebb, S.A. (2019) 'A systematic review and meta-analysis of the effectiveness of meal replacements for weight loss', *Obesity Reviews*, 20(4), pp. 569–587

Birch, L.L. (1991) 'Obesity and eating disorders: a developmental perspective', *Bulletin of the Psychonomic Society*, 29, pp. 265–272

Brandkvist, M., Bjørngaard, J.H. and Ødegard, R.A. (2019) 'Quantifying the impact of genes on body mass index during the obesity epidemic: longitudinal findings from the HUNT Study', *BMJ*, 366(14067) doi:10.1136/bmj.14067

British Nutrition Foundation (2021) *Get portion wise!* Available at: https://www.nutrition.org.uk/putting-it-into-practice/balancing-the-diet/get-portion-wise (Accessed 10th June 2022)

Burke, L.E., Wang, J. and Sevick, M.A. (2011) 'Self-monitoring in weight loss: a systematic review of the literature', *Journal of the American Dietetic Association*, 111(1), pp. 92–102

Byrne, N.M., Sainsbury, A., King, N.A., Hills, A.P. and Wood, R.E. (2018) 'Intermittent energy restriction improves weight loss efficiency in obese men: the MATADOR study', *International Journal of Obesity*, 42(2), pp. 129–138

Chambers, L., McCrickerd, K. and Yeomans, M.R. (2015) 'Optimising foods for satiety', *Trends in Food Science & Technology*, 41(2015), pp. 149–160

Chernin, K. (1981) *Womansize*. London: The Women's Press

Chernin, K. (1986) *The hungry self*. London: Virago

Christakoudi, S., Konstantinos, K. and Tsilidis, D.C. *et al.* (2020) 'A body shape index (ABSI) achieves better mortality risk stratification than alternative indices of abdominal obesity: results from large European cohort', *Scientific Reports*, 10(14541) doi:10.1038/s41598-020-71302-5

Davis, H.C. (2017) 'Can the gastrointestinal microbiota be modulated by dietary fibre to treat obesity?', *Irish Journal of Medical Science*, 187(2), pp. 393–402

Davis, C.S., Clarke, R.E., Coulter, S.N., Rounsefell, K.N., Walker, R.E., Rauch, C.E., Huggins, C.E. and Ryan, L. (2016) 'Intermittent energy restriction and weight loss: a systematic review', *European Journal of Clinical Nutrition*, 70(3), pp. 292–299

Department of Health and Social Care (2019) *UK chief medical officers' physical activity guidelines*. Department of Health and Social Care/Welsh Government/Department of Health/Scottish Government. Available at: https://assets.publishing.service.gov.uk/government/uploads/system/uploads/attachment_data/file/832868/uk-chief-medical-officers-physical-activity-guidelines.pdf (Accessed 10th June 2022)

EAT (2019) *Healthy diets from sustainable food systems. Food planet earth. Summary report of the EAT-lancet commission*. Available at: https://eatforum.org/content/uploads/2019/01/EAT-Lancet_Commission_Summary_Report.pdf (Accessed 10th June 2022)

Ganesan, K., Habboush, Y. and Sultan, S. (2018) 'Intermittent fasting: the choice for a healthier lifestyle', *Cureus*, 10(7) doi:10.7759/cureus.2947

Ghosh, T.S., Rampelli, S., Jeffrey, I.B. *et al.* (2020) 'Mediterranean diet intervention alters the gut microbiome in older people reducing frailty and improving health status: the NU-AGE 1-year dietary intervention across five European countries', *BMJ*, 69(7), pp. 1218–1228

Gupta, S.C., Kunnumakkara, A.B., Aggarwal, S. and Aggarwal, B.B. (2018) 'Inflammation, a double-edge sword for cancer and other age-related diseases', *Frontiers in Immunology*, 9(2160) doi:10.3389/fimmu.2018.02160

Haro, C., Carcía-Carpintero, S., Rangel-Zúñiga, O.A., Alcalá-Díaz, J.F., Landa, B.B., Clemente, J.C., Pérez-Martínez, P., López-Miranda, J., Pérez-Jiménez, F. and Camargo, A. (2017) 'Consumption of two healthy dietary patterns restored microbiota dysbiosis in obese patients with metabolic dysfunction', *Molecular Nutrition*, 61(12) doi:10.1002/mnfr.201700300

Harvey, J., Howell, A., Morris, J. and Harvie, M. (2018) 'Intermittent energy restriction for weight loss: spontaneous reduction of energy intake on unrestricted days', *Food Science and Nutrition*, 6(1), pp. 674–680

Harvey, J., Krukowski, R., Priest, J. and West, D. (2019) 'Log often, lose more: electronic dietary self-monitoring for weight loss', *Obesity*, 27(3), pp. 380–384

Harvie, M. and Howell, A. (2013) *The 2 day diet*. London: Vermillion

Harvie, M.N., Pegington, M., Mattson, M.P. *et al.* (2011) 'The effects of intermittent or continuous restriction on weight loss and metabolic disease risk markers: a randomised trial in young overweight women', *International Journal of Obesity*, 35(5), pp. 714–727

Herman, C.P. and Polivy, J. (1991) 'Fat is a psychological issue', *New Scientist*, 1795, pp. 41–45

Hutchison, A.T., Liu, B., Wood, R.E., Vincent, A.D., Thompson, C.H., O'Callaghan, N.J.O., Wittert, G.A. and Heilbronn, L.K. (2019) 'Effects of intermittent versus continuous energy intake on insulin sensitivity and metabolic risk in women with overweight', *Obesity*, 27(1), pp. 50–58

Jakubowicz, D., Barnea, M., Wainstein, J. and Froy, O. (2013) 'High caloric intake at breakfast vs. dinner differentially influences weight loss of overweight and obese women', *Obesity*, 21(12), pp. 2504–2512

Jebb, S.A., Astbury, N.M., Tearne, S., Nickless, A. and Aveyard, P. (2017) 'Doctor referral of overweight people to low-energy treatment (DROPLET) in primary care using total diet replacement products: a protocol for a randomised controlled trial', *BMJ Open*, 7 doi:10.1136/bmjopen-2017-016709

Knight, M., Bunch, K., Tuffnell, D., Shakespeare, J., Kotnis, R., Kenyon, S. and Kurinczuk, J.J. (eds) (2020) *Saving lives, improving mothers' care. Lessons learned to inform maternity care from the UK and Ireland confidential enquiries into maternal deaths and morbidity 2016–2018.* Oxford: National Perinatal Epidemiology Unit, University of Oxford

Kroeger, C.M., Trepanowski, J.F., Klempel, M.C., Barnosky, A., Bhutani, S., Gabel, K. and Varady, K.A. (2018) 'Eating behaviour traits of successful weight losers during 12 months of alternate-day fasting: an exploratory analysis of a randomized controlled trial', *Nutrition and Health*, 24(1), pp. 5–10

Latner, J.D. and Schwartz, M. (1999) 'The effects of high-carbohydrate, high-protein or balanced lunch upon later food intake and hunger ratings', *Appetite*, 33(1), pp. 119–128

Le Roy, C.I., Bowyer, R.C.E., Castillo-Fernandez, J.E. *et al.* (2019) 'Dissecting the role of gut microbiota and diet on visceral fat mass accumulation', *Scientific Reports*, 9(1) doi:10.1038/s42598-019-46193-w

Lean, M.E.J., Leslie, W.S., Barnes, A.C. *et al.* (2019) 'Durability of a primary care-led weight-management intervention for remission of type 2 diabetes: 2-year results of the DiRECT open-label cluster-randomised trial', *The Lancet Diabetes & Endocrinology*, 7(5), pp. 344–355

Ley, R.E., Turnbaugh, P.J., Klein, S. and Gordon, J.I. (2006) 'Human gut microbes associated with obesity', *Nature*, 444, pp. 1022–1023

Mattson, M.P., Allison, D.B., Fontana, L. *et al.* (2014) 'Meal frequency and timing in health and disease', *Proceedings of the National Academy of Sciences of the United States of America*, 111(47), pp. 16647–16653

Monda, B., Villano, I. and Messina, A. (2017) 'Exercise modifies the gut microbiota with positive health effects', *Oxidative Medicine and Cellular Longevity*, 2017 doi:10.1155/2017/3831972

Muguruza, C., Redon, B. and Fois, G.R. (2019) 'The motivation for exercise over palatable food is dictated by cannabinoid type-1 receptors', *JCI Insight*, 4(5) doi:10.1172/jci.insight.126190

NatCen Social Research/National Institute of Health Research Cambridge Biomedical Research Centre/Medical Research Council Elsie Widdowson Laboratory (2020) *National diet and nutrition survey. Rolling programme years 9 to 11 (2016/2017 to 2018/2019)*. London: Public Health England

National Institute for Health and Clinical Excellence (2014) *Obesity: identification, assessment and management. Clinical guideline (CG189)*. Available at: https://www.nice.org.uk/guidance/cg189 (Accessed: 10th June 2022)

Nelson, J.B. (2017) 'Mindful eating: the art of presence while you eat', *Diabetes Spectrum*, 30(3), pp. 171–174

Nuttall, F.Q. (2015) 'Body mass index. Obesity, BMI and health: a critical review', *Nutrition Research*, 50(3), pp. 117–128

Ogden, J., Coop, N., Cousins, C., Crump, R., Field, L., Hughes, S. and Woodger, N. (2013) 'Distraction, the desire to eat and food intake: towards an expanded model of mindless eating', *Appetite*, 62, pp. 119–126

Orbach, S. (1978) *Fat is a feminist issue*. London: Arrow Books

Public Health England (2018) *The eatwell guide*. London: Public Health England

Public Health England (2020) *Health matters: physical activity – prevention and management of long-term conditions*. Available at: https://www.gov.uk/government/publications/health-matters-physical-activity/health-matters-physical-activity-prevention-and-management-of-long-term-conditions (Accessed 10th June 2022)

Rawlings, G.H., Williams, R., Clarke, D.J. *et al.* (2019) 'Exploring adults' experiences of sedentary behaviour and participation in non-workplace interventions designed to reduce sedentary behaviour: a thematic synthesis of qualitative studies', *BMC Public Health*, 19(1) doi:10.1186/s12889-019-7365-1

Robinson, S. (2021a) 'Weight', in Robinson, S. (ed) *Priorities for health promotion and public health. Explaining the evidence for disease prevention and health promotion*. London: Routledge, pp. 325–351

Robinson, S. (2021b) 'Diet and health', in Robinson, S. (ed) *Priorities for health promotion and public health. Explaining the evidence for disease prevention and health promotion*. London: Routledge, pp. 200–232

Ross, R., Neeland, I.J. and Yamashita, S. *et al.* (2020) 'Waist circumference as a vital sign in clinical practice: a consensus statement from the IAS and ICCR working group on visceral obesity', *Nature Reviews Endocrinology*, 16(3) doi:10-.1038/s1574-019-0310-7

Scientific Advisory Committee on Nutrition (2012) *Dietary reference values for energy*. London: The Stationery Office

Sheppard, G. (2021) 'Physical inactivity and health', in Robinson, S. (ed) *Priorities for health promotion and public health. Explaining the evidence for disease prevention and health promotion*. London: Routledge, pp. 175–199

Siebers, M., Biedermann, S.V., Bindila, L., Lutz, B. and Fuss, J. (2021) 'Exercise-induced euphoria and anxiolysis do not depend on endogenous opioids in humans', *Psychoneuroendocrinology*, 126 doi:10.1016/j.psyneuen.2021.105173

Spalding, K.L., Arner, E., Westermark, P.O. *et al.* (2008) 'Dynamics of fat cell turnover in humans', *Nature*, 453, pp. 783–787

Spector, T. (2015) *The diet myth*. London: Weidenfeld and Nicolson

Stone, A.A. and Brownell, K.D. (1994) 'The stress-eating paradox: multiple measurements in adult males and females', *Psychology and Health*, 9(6), pp. 425–436

Townshend, T. and Lake, A. (2017) 'Obesogenic environments: current evidence of the built and food environments', *Perspectives in Public Health*, 137(1), pp. 38–44

Tsigalou, C., Paraschaki, A., Karvelas, A., Kantartzi, K., Gagali, K., Tsairidis, D. and Bezirtzoglou, E. (2021) 'Gut microbiome and Mediterranean diet in the context of obesity. Current knowledge, perspectives and potential therapeutic targets', *Metabolism Open*, 9 doi:10.1016/j.metop.2021.100081

United Nations/World Health Organization/Food and Agriculture Organisation (2004) *Human energy requirements. Report of a Joint FAO/WHO/UNU Expert Consultation.* Rome: Food and Agriculture Organization of the United Nations

Valdes, A., Walter, J., Segal, E. and Spector, T.D. (2018) 'Role of the gut microbiota in nutrition and health', *BMJ*, 361(Suppl1), pp. 36–44

VanKim, N., Porta, C.M., Eisenberg, M.E., Neumark-Sztainer, D. and Laska, M.N. (2016) 'Lesbian, gay and bisexual college student perspectives in weight-related behaviours and body image: a qualitative analysis', *Journal of Clinical Nursing*, 25(23/24), pp. 3676–3686

Westerterp, K.R. (2013) 'Physical activity and physical activity induced energy expenditure in humans: measurement, determinants, and effects', *Frontiers in Physiology*, 4(90) doi:10.3389/fphys.2013.00090

Wilkins, E., Radley, D., Morris, M., Hobbs, M., Christensen, A., Marwa, W.L., Morrin, A. and Griffiths, C. (2019) 'A systematic review employing the GeoFERN framework to examine methods, reporting quality and associations between the retail food environment and obesity', *Health and Place*, 57(2019), pp. 186–199

Williams, O. and Annandale, E. (2018) 'Obesity, stigma and reflexive embodiment: feeling the "weight" of expectation', *Health: An Interdisciplinary Journal for the Social Study of Health, Illness and Medicine*, 24(4) doi:10.1177/1363459318812007

World Health Organization (2020) *WHO guidelines on physical activity and sedentary behaviour.* Geneva: World Health Organization

World Health Organization (Europe) (2021) *A healthy lifestyle – WHO recommendations.* Available at: https://www.who.int/europe/news-room/fact-sheets/item/a-healthy-lifestyle—who-recommendations (Accessed 10th June 2022)

Yeo, G.S. (2017) 'Genetics of obesity: can an old dog teach us new tricks?', *Diabetologia*, 60(5), pp. 778–783

Part IV
Promoting health within settings

14 Promoting health in workplaces

Sally Robinson

Key points

- Introduction
- Work-related poor health
- Work environments and health
- Individuals in the workplace
- Healthy workplaces
- Summary

Introduction

We begin this chapter with an overview of the most common work-related health concerns in the UK and describe how occupations contribute to inequalities in health. The chapter explains how the physical and psychosocial work environment can be a powerful influence on workers' health. Workers are individuals who do not enter the workplace with equal health, but their experiences at work can enhance their health or cause it to deteriorate. We describe several examples of how workplaces can protect and promote the health of workers within the wider concept of a healthy workplace.

Work-related poor health

Employment and the quality of work affects people's health, and health affects people's work. Unemployment means being 16 or over, without a job but seeking one; workless means being unemployed or economically inactive perhaps due to retirement, study, sickness or family commitments (PHE, 2018). Waddell and Burton's (2006) review of the evidence concluded work is much better for most people's health than being unemployed or workless. They found that while unemployment is strongly associated with poor mental and physical health, long-standing illness and earlier death; for many

- employment is an important way of obtaining the resources we need for material wellbeing and participation in society
- socio-economic status and employment are the main influences on people's physical and mental health and their life expectancy
- in societies where employment is the norm, work meets important psychological and social needs

DOI: 10.4324/9780367823696-18

- work is central to a person's identity, it provides a social status and a social role
- who are sick and disabled, when their health condition permits, work can be therapeutic, enable recovery and rehabilitation, reduce long-term sickness absence, reduce poverty, enhance quality of life and lead to better health
- work involves both physical and psychosocial risks to health, so the health benefits depend on the nature and quality of work and where it is situated, for example in an area of wealth or deprivation

(Waddell and Burton, 2006)

Workers' health is affected by all the factors that influence health or illness in the general population. Here we focus on work-related poor health, meaning that which is partly caused by working conditions or where work is a factor in exacerbating poor health.

Common work-related deaths, diseases and injuries in the UK

The first global report into work-related poor health (WHO/ILO, 2021) found that in 2016 1.88 million deaths across the world were linked to risks in the workplace. Four-fifths of deaths were due to work-related diseases such as chronic obstructive pulmonary disease and cardiovascular disease. Features of work which were most strongly associated with death were

- long working hours of over 55 hours per week, associated with 744,924 deaths
- air pollution, including gases, fumes and particulates in the air, associated with 450,381 deaths
- work-related injuries, associated with 363,283 deaths

In Great Britain, 1.7 million workers reported ill health in 2020/21 (HSE, 2021a). The main work-related health concerns were stress, depression and anxiety; musculoskeletal disorders, breathing or lung problems and workplace injuries.

Stress, depression and anxiety

In Great Britain, 50% of self-reported work-related illness concerned stress, depression or anxiety in 2020/21 (HSE, 2021a; 2021b). This comprised 822,000 cases. Between 2018 and 2021, these were reported most frequently by those in Public administration/defence/compulsory social security; Human health and social work; and Education industries. Among occupations, the most frequent reports came from health professionals, teaching and other educational professionals and those working in protective and customer services were notably high. The causes included

- workload
- a lack of support
- violence, threats or bullying
- changes at work

The global report concluded that working more than 55 hours per week increased a person's risk of stroke by 35% and their risk of coronary heart disease by 17% when compared to working 35 to 40 hours per week (WHO/ILO, 2021). Workload pressures are revealed through leavism and presenteeism. Leavism means working outside of contracted hours such as after-hours and during holiday entitlement. The UK's *Health and Wellbeing at Work* survey 2021 (CIPD, 2021a) found 70% of respondents had observed leavism. Presenteeism means working when unwell. The survey found 75% of respondents observed presenteeism in the workplace and 77% while working at home over the previous 12 months. Often both leavism and presenteeism co-exist, and the high levels are thought to be related to digital technology, home and work life becoming blurred and it becoming harder to 'switch off'.

Musculoskeletal disorders

About a third (28%) of all self-reported work-related ill-health in Great Britain concerned musculoskeletal conditions such as back, neck or limb disorders in 2020/21 (HSE, 2021a). Of these 0.5 million cases, most were reported by the Construction industry followed by those working in Human health and social work. The causes included

- manual handling
- being in awkward or tiring positions
- key board work or other repetitive actions

Breathing or lung problems

In 2020/21, about 47,000 current workers in Great Britain reported a breathing or lung problem that was either caused or made worse by their work, and about 142,000 people who have *ever* worked reported the same (HSE, 2021c). Work-related asthma and allergic alveolitis can develop quickly, but other lung diseases take time to develop and reflect working conditions of the past. Lung diseases make up about 12,000 of the 13,000 annual deaths related to past work exposures (HSE, 2021a). In 2020/21, the Health and Safety Executive (2021c) reported deaths related to

- chronic obstructive pulmonary disease (34%)
- non-asbestos related lung cancer (23%)
- asbestos-related lung cancer (20%)
- mesothelioma (20%)

The causes of work-related respiratory diseases contracted recently included

- general work environment, e.g. too hot/cold/wet/dry
- dust from stone, cement, concrete and bricks
- airborne materials from manufacturing foam products or spray painting
- air borne materials from soldering, welding or cutting/grinding materials
- dust from cereal grains, flour, animal feed or straw

Workplace injuries

In 2020/21, 142 workers were killed at work in Great Britain, fewer than many other European countries, and 0.4 million workers sustained a non-fatal injury (HSE, 2021a).

These injuries were most frequently reported in the Agriculture, forestry and fishing and Construction industries, followed by Accommodation/food service activities; Manufacturing; and Wholesale/retail trade and repair of motor vehicles industries. The types of injuries included

- slips, trips or falls on the same level
- handling, lifting or carrying
- begin struck by a moving object
- acts of violence
- falls from a height

Occupations and inequalities in health

The Standard Occupational Classification (SOC) for the UK provides a code for each type of job. This classification is used by governments and researchers for surveys about the workforce. Jobs are grouped into occupations. An occupation acts as an indicator of associated education, income and living conditions. The UK National Statistics Socio-economic Classification (NS-SEC) divides these occupations into eight non-hierarchical socio-economic categories (ONS, 2010).

1 Higher managerial, administrative and professional occupations
2 Lower managerial, administrative and professional occupations
3 Intermediate occupations
4 Small employers and own account workers
5 Lower supervisory and technical occupations
6 Semi-routine occupations
7 Routine occupations
8 Never worked and long-term unemployed

Inequalities in work-related deaths

The 2001 Census asked people across the UK to provide the full title of their last main job. From this, Katikireddi and colleagues (2017) were able to code the jobs of a very large sample of the population using the SOC (Table 14.1). Next, they examined mortality rates, that is death rates, in 2011 in England, Wales and Scotland. Taking into account sex and age, they concluded overall death rates (age-standardised all-cause mortality rate per 100,000 person years) across most occupations have improved compared to previous decades, but there was significant inequality. Generally, the higher managerial and professional occupations, that is those in socio-economic categories 1, 2 and 3 had lower death rates than those in routine occupations, but the link between socio-economic category and death was more mixed for those occupations in between. Death rates were up to three times higher for some occupations than others. Men in basic construction work, housekeeping and factory work had the highest death rate, as did women who worked in factories and the garment trade. Scotland had a higher death rate than England and Wales, mostly due to excess deaths among lower skilled occupations such as female cleaners.

Table 14.1 Death rates by occupation in England and Wales, 2001 to 2011

	Men *(mean mortality rate per 100,000 person years)*	Women *(mean mortality rate per 100,000 person years)*
Lowest mortality	Health professionals (225) Business and public service professionals (228) Functional managers (233) Financial institution and office managers (234) Corporate managers and directors (250) Teaching professionals (262)	Culture, media and sports occupations (133) Business and public service professionals (159) Teaching professionals (180) Science, research, engineering and technology professionals (180) Business and public service associate professionals (188) Science and technology associate professionals (203)
Highest mortality	Elementary cleaning occupations (592) Administrative occupations: communications (604) Elementary agricultural occupations (623) Elementary personal services occupations (650) Elementary process plant occupations (672) Elementary construction occupations (701)	Elementary administration occupations (383) Assemblers and routine operatives (386) Managers and proprietors in agriculture and services (397) Elementary process plant occupations (405) Textiles and garments trades (483) Plant and machine operatives (517)

Source: Adapted from Katikireddi *et al.* (2017, pp. e503–e505).

Inequalities in the quality of work

The Chartered Institute of Personnel and Development (CIPD) developed the Good Work Index as a way of measuring the quality of work (Norris-Green and Gifford, 2021). It comprises seven indicators:

- pay and benefits, e.g. wages, pensions and work-related benefits
- employment contracts, e.g. temporary, variable or flexible contracts and job security
- work-life balance, e.g. job intensity, flexible working and the ability to manage competing priorities
- job design and the nature of work, e.g. workload, autonomy, resources, a sense of purpose, complexity and opportunities to develop skills and careers
- relationships at work, e.g. positive or negative relationships with line managers, colleagues and customers
- employee voice, e.g. participation in management meetings, forums and trade unions
- health and wellbeing, e.g. experience of physical health problems, exhaustion, stress and depression

These indicators are used in the CIPD's annual survey of workers to examine to what extent people working within different occupational groups experience good work (Figure 14.1). The CIPD 2020 survey (Williams *et al.*, 2020) found that, overall,

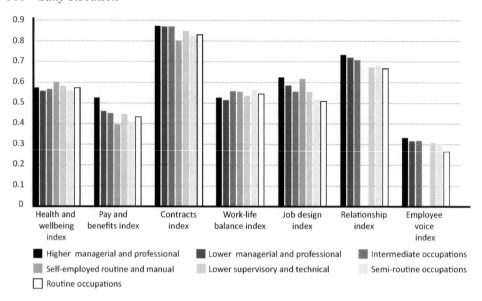

Figure 14.1 Quality of work by socio-economic classification, 2020

Source: Adapted from Williams *et al.*, 2020, p. 6

those in higher managerial and professional occupations experienced better work, and those in routine and manual occupations had the poorest experience of work. The latter were three times more likely to be low paid or to have insufficient paid work hours compared to the higher managerial and professional occupations. Pay is an important indicator of health. There is a large body of evidence showing people with higher income and/or wealth experience much better health outcomes, such as average longer life expectancy and better self-reported health, than those who receive low pay and those living in poverty (Marmot *et al.*, 2020; Tinson, 2020).

Aside from pay, the results of the remaining six indicators were more mixed. For example, perceptions of health and wellbeing did not vary much across all occupational groups, and work-life balance was best among those working in routine and manual occupations. People working in animal care, housekeeping and sports reported the best health and wellbeing, and they experienced good working relationships and a good work-life balance. Those working in legal services, health and conservation reported the poorest work-life balance.

The annual report from the Health and Safety Executive, for 2020/21, described workers' reports of stress, depression and anxiety in Great Britain as being highest among professional and associate professional occupations in public service (HSE, 2021b). These included nurses, therapists, teaching professionals, welfare professionals, care professionals, police officers and those working in customer services. In 2021, the Northern Ireland Statistics Research Agency examined workers' depression, anxiety and stress in Northern Ireland using self-reported emotional, psychological or mental health conditions from the Census and prescription data (IJpelaar *et al.*, 2021). In contrast with the Great Britain data, they found workers' self-reported emotional, psychological or mental health conditions were lowest among the professional occupations and highest among workers employed at an elementary level in sales and customer services. The latter were also receiving the greatest number of prescription medicines for mental health problems. The common finding is that jobs which involve high levels of communication with the public are associated with poorer mental health.

Together, these studies suggest that both poorer job quality and earlier death are more likely among some of the lowest paid, elementary, routine, manual jobs such as working in factories, cleaning or as a labourer on a farm or building site. While pay clearly favours those in managerial and professional jobs which benefits health, for many workers across all occupations there are aspects of their jobs that are not experienced positively. These differences vary across individual occupations and do not simply reflect their broader socio-economic classification.

Working during the COVID-19 coronavirus pandemic

Due to the COVID-19 coronavirus pandemic, during 2020 the UK periodically 'locked down' forcing some people into unemployment, some received government money through the furlough scheme while they could not work, some worked from home and key workers such as health and social care, education, childcare, transport, utilities and financial services continued to keep vital services running. The CIPD 2021 survey (Norris-Green and Gifford, 2021) found little notable difference compared to their 2020 survey, but key workers experienced a poor work-life balance, less flexible working, more exhaustion and higher workloads with lower resources compared to others. Those working from home gained more autonomy, better workplace relationships and flexible working patterns, but they experienced higher workloads, exhaustion and a blurring of their work and life.

> *In the UK, stress, depression and anxiety; musculoskeletal disorders, breathing and lung problems and injuries are the most common work-related health concerns. Elementary, routine and manual jobs are associated with earlier deaths, and managerial and professional jobs with higher pay, but work-related poor health does not reflect a simple gradient of socio-economic status.*

Work environments and health

The Health and Safety at Work Act 1974 is the primary legislation that covers work-related health and safety in Great Britain. It sets out the responsibilities of employers to protect the health and safety of their employees and the public, employers' responsibilities to themselves and other employers and the responsibilities of the self-employed (HSE, 2021d). There are many regulations that make up secondary legislation, called statutory instruments. Northern Ireland has similar laws. The laws are enforced by the Health and Safety Executive (GB and NI) and local authorities. An unhealthy work environment often comprises a combination of physical and psychosocial factors. Each industry and occupation will have its own work-related health risks. Table 14.2 presents some of the most common work-related causes of poor health across eight British industries.

Physical environment

The physical working environment can present a range of potential hazards to workers', and visitors'/customers', health if not designed or handled with care. For example, we need to consider the design of workstations, loud noise, vibration, poorly maintained

Table 14.2 Examples of causes of injuries, illness and death at work by British industries

Industry	Common causes of injuries, illness and death
Agriculture	Contact with electricity power lines, being struck by moving vehicles, trees or bales, falls from a height, drowning, contact with machinery, animal injuries, being trapped by something collapsing, slips/trips/falls
Catering and hospitality	Slips/trips, knives, manual handling/lifting, products causing skin irritation/dermatitis
Construction	Inhaling asbestos, silica and diesel engine fumes causing cancers; dusts, chemicals, fumes and paints causing breathing and skin problems; manual handling/lifting, noise, vibration
Cleaning	Slips/trips, products causing skin irritation/dermatitis, manual handling/lifting/awkward postures, falls from a height
Food and drink manufacturing	Slips/trips/falls, manual handling of containers/products; machinery, falling objects, tools/knives, workplace transport accidents, noise, disinfectants, inhaling dust from grain, flour or wood, excessive demands and lack of control leading to work-related stress
Health and social care	Touching/inhaling cytotoxic drugs, products causing skin problems/dermatitis; sharps, needles or blade injuries; inhaling diathermy emissions, manual handling/lifting/back injuries, legionella, unsafe equipment, slips/trips/falls, abuse/violence
Police	Assault, slips/trips, handling accidents, stress
Textiles	Fabrics, fibres or liquids causing fire, inhaling wool and cotton dust, corrosive or hot chemicals, handling dyed/chemically treated fabric, knives, high temperature machines, unsafe equipment, manual handling of bales

Source: HSE (2021e).

equipment/machinery, poor maintenance of floors or lighting, too high or low temperatures, waste and clutter, poor cleanliness, unsafe storage of materials, moving vehicles, inaccessible evacuation exits, ultra-violet sunlight if working outside, inadequate lifting equipment, micro-organisms and dangerous chemicals. Some of the methods used to prevent poor health in the workplace include

- carrying out regular risk assessments to identify potential hazards and the level of risk to people
- recording and monitoring accidents and sickness
- reducing the causes of potential harm, e.g. fixing loose carpets and poor lighting, or using different materials/equipment or changing ways of working
- protecting people who need to engage with potentially harmful objects, chemicals or organisms with ventilation, protective clothing, goggles, gloves and/or by avoiding lone working
- using equipment for heavy lifting
- health and safety training and information, e.g. posters

We help to prevent accidents and diseases by legally requiring workplaces to report work-related accidents, diseases and dangerous incidents to the Health and Safety

Executive (GB and NI). This is in line with the Reporting of Injuries, Diseases and Dangerous Occurrences Regulations (RIDDOR) (HSE, 2021d) (see Chapter 10). Employers, or the self-employed, must report accidents which cause an observable physical injury such as an open wound or death. They must report certain work-related occupational diseases, once medically diagnosed, which include

- carpel tunnel syndrome and hand-arm vibration syndrome, associated with vibrating power tools
- diseases associated with biological agents to which, for example, laboratory workers may be exposed
- occupational asthma caused by inhaling dust and fumes
- occupational cancers, e.g. mesothelioma or lung cancer due to exposure to asbestos
- occupational dermatitis caused by chemicals or biological irritants
- severe cramp of the hand or forearm, associated with repetitive movements
- tendonitis or tenosynovitis of the hand or forearm associated with demanding repetitive tasks

They must also report dangerous occurrences such as the collapse or failure of lifting equipment, instances when equipment touches overhead power lines and the release of a harmful substance into the air or water. Incidents concerning gas must be reported where someone is hospitalised or dies, and registered gas engineers must report any gas appliances that are thought to be dangerous. Control of Substances Hazardous to Health (COSHH) is a set of regulations that govern the control of hazardous substances in the workplace (Figure 14.2). It is a criminal offence for these to be breached.

Psychosocial environment

The psychosocial environment concerns how workers are treated and how they feel. It includes culture, interpersonal relationships and how jobs are designed. In turn, these are shaped by the wider societal, economic and political context. The environment affects workers in two ways. It directly affects their physiology, that is how

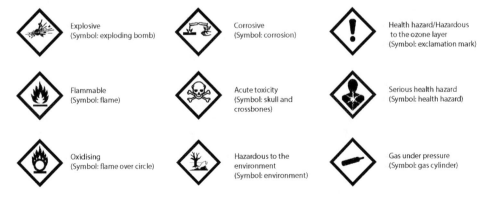

Figure 14.2 Nine hazard pictograms to indicate a hazardous chemical

Source: UN Economic Commission for Europe (2021). Reproduced with permission from the United Nations.

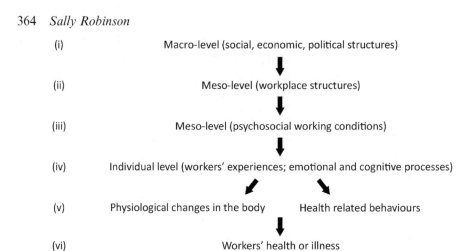

(i) Macro-level (social, economic, political structures)

(ii) Meso-level (workplace structures)

(iii) Meso-level (psychosocial working conditions)

(iv) Individual level (workers' experiences; emotional and cognitive processes)

(v) Physiological changes in the body   Health related behaviours

(vi) Workers' health or illness

Figure 14.3 How the psychosocial work environment influences workers' health

Source: Adapted from Rugulies (2019, p. 2).

their bodies function, and it influences their health-related behaviours. For example, chronic stress directly affects the endocrine, metabolic and immune systems of the body and is associated with eating fewer fruit and vegetables and engaging in less physical activity. Together, these are strongly associated with coronary heart disease (Chandola *et al.*, 2008).

Figure 14.3 shows the chain of influences on workers' health. At the macro-level (i), an example of UK law is the Working Time Regulations 1998 which limits working time to a maximum of 48 hours per week averaged over 17 weeks (Legislation.gov.uk, 1998a). Although the wealthiest and well-known workplaces can have significant political and social influence, most workplaces have opportunities to influence the local community and the health of their workers at the meso-level (ii and iii) and the individual level (iv). Recently recorded reasons for workers' stress, depression and anxiety were at the meso-level and these included tight deadlines and too much responsibility, violence, threats/bullying, a lack of support, uncertainty, a lack of clarity about the job and a lack of control over their work (HSE, 2021b). During 2021, these were made worse by the COVID-19 coronavirus pandemic. General Practitioners cited work-related mental health problems as being mostly precipitated by workload pressures, poor interpersonal relationships and changes at work (HSE, 2021b). In 2021, nearly four-fifths of UK workers had taken stress-related absence in the previous 12 months due to

- workload (59%)
- management style (32%)
- demands related to homeworking due to the COVID-19 coronavirus pandemic (31%)

(CIPD, 2021a)

Concepts that help workplaces to decide where to focus their health promoting efforts at the meso-level include the demand/control model, effort/reward model, organisational justice and workplace social capital.

Demand/control model

The demand/control model is based on a wealth of evidence that shows workers' health is influenced by the balance of the demands on a worker and the control they have over their work (Karasek, 1979; Karasek and Theorell, 1990).

- Demand means how demanding the job is, e.g. stressors such as interruptions, pressures, conflicts, levels of sustained concentration and workload
- Control means the amount of discretion a worker has, e.g. autonomy, scope to make decisions, authority and having influence over their own and others' work and conditions

There are four combinations (Figure 14.4):

- *low control/high demand* is a 'high strain/stress job' where there may be insufficient time to cope with the workload, workers are unable to influence the work or the environment, and there are few opportunities to develop new skills. High strain/stress jobs are associated with cardiovascular disease, depression and health-harming coping behaviours such as smoking
- *low control/low demand* is a 'passive job' where workers are under-stimulated and may develop 'learned helplessness'. Passive jobs are associated with depression
- *high control/high demand* is an 'active job' where workers can influence their work and the environment to meet the high demands. Active jobs are associated with high levels of job satisfaction because the job helps them to achieve their goals and become accomplished
- *high control/low demand* is a 'low strain/stress job' where workers may be able to influence the demands of their job if they feel under-stimulated. Low strain/stress jobs are associated with good physical and mental health

(Ahlin *et al.*, 2018; Karasek and Theorell, 1990; Pikhart and Pikhartova, 2015; Söderberg, 2014)

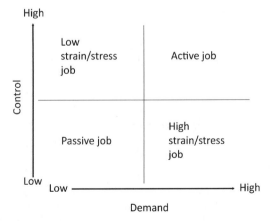

Figure 14.4 Demand/control model

Source: Adapted from Karasek (1979, p. 288).

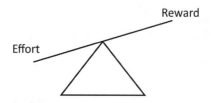

Figure 14.5 Effort/reward imbalance at work

Effort/reward model

Effort-reward is a sociological model that argues work is based on a contract of reciprocity, that is costs and gains (Siegrist, 2002). It recognises that work provides opportunities for rewards:

- pay
- self-efficacy, e.g. job satisfaction because of a belief that they are, and can be, successful in their job
- self-esteem, e.g. recognition, adequate pay and potential promotion
- self-integration, e.g. social identity and being part of a network
- security
- career opportunities

If rewards are experienced as less than the effort, there is an imbalance (Figure 14.5). Effort may include

- having no choice but to stay in a job due to high unemployment, the availability of only part-time or zero hours contracts when full time work is needed, or having no opportunities to re-skill or gain qualifications (macro level)
- being asked to carry out more duties or longer hours than anticipated when a work contract was signed (meso level)
- feeling demands are exceeding a worker's coping abilities or not receiving sufficient encouragement or praise (individual level)

If the effort is great at both the structural (macro and meso) and individual level, the impact of the imbalance will be greater. There is a body of research demonstrating that an imbalance of more effort and less reward is associated with exhaustion, stress, pain, poor self-rated health, cardiovascular disease, alcohol dependence and mental health problems such as depression; as well as workplace bullying (Dragano *et al.*, 2017; Ge *et al.*, 2021; Notelaers *et al.*, 2019; Rugulies *et al.*, 2017; Siegrist, 2002).

Organisational justice

Organisational justice refers to the extent to which decision-making includes input from those who will be affected by the decision and whether decisions are ethical, accurate and fairly applied without bias. Workers' feelings, behaviours and relationships can be affected by their experience of justice within their workplace. Experiencing injustice is associated with poor self-rated health, mental health problems and sickness absence from work (Elovainio *et al.*, 2002). This understanding takes 'reward for effort' further by showing that the procedures for *how* rewards are shared is also important to health.

Workplace social capital

Social capital is an umbrella concept which includes trust, social support, recognition and reciprocity. It includes social relationships at work, the leadership styles of managers, the social atmosphere at work, belonging to networks, sharing, and being accepted, respected and supported by fellow workers (Rydström *et al.*, 2017). A substantial review of the evidence concluded that social capital encourages better physical and mental health, and protects against early death (Ehsan *et al.*, 2019). For example, Ekbladh's (2010) research with workers on long term sick leave found the aspects of work that supported their work-related performance, sense of wellbeing and job satisfaction were the social interactions at work and the meaning of work. One respondent said,

> "It's an important job and she is proud about being regarded as competent by others."

(p. 128)

The most interfering, were the demands of work and unsatisfactory rewards.

Figure 14.6 shows some of the psychosocial experiences reported by workers in England in 2018. In summary, a workplace characterised by stress, excess demand, low control, an imbalance in effort and reward, interpersonal conflicts and low social support directly and indirectly encourages cardiovascular disease, mental health

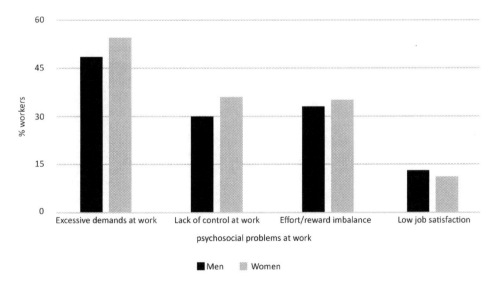

Figure 14.6 Work-related psychosocial experiences of workers in England aged 50 to 69 years, 2018

Source: Oldfield *et al.* (2018).

problems and contributes to wider health inequalities (Bell, 2017; Marmot and Bell, 2010; Pikhart and Pikhartova, 2015).

The physical and psychosocial workplace environment is a powerful influence on workers' health.

Individuals in the workplace

Workers are individuals with their own biology, psychology and social context. Each has multiple identities beyond their work identity which relates to their age, sex, gender, ability/disability, race, ethnicity, language, religion, sexual orientation, socio-economic status, education, family, friends, social groups and so forth. People experience health promoting and health negating experiences across their whole lives, what we call the life course approach (Kuh *et al.*, 2003). The workplace is one of the many social determinants of people's health alongside their living conditions, culture, education, their local community, public amenities, health and social services; and the wider cultural, political, economic and natural climate (Robinson, 2021). Workers do not enter a workplace with equal health, and the line between their working lives and the rest of their lives is permeable. Both within and outside of their work and workplace, they may have

- biological challenges, e.g. illness, a physical disability or pregnancy
- psychological challenges, e.g. anxiety, substance dependency, a cognitive impairment or a mental disorder
- social challenges, e.g. poverty, poor housing, caring responsibilities or discrimination

People's work-related experiences can either exacerbate the positive or the negative aspects of their health. A good work experience can improve their health; a poor one will worsen their health. This applies to anyone, but the UK seeks to protect potentially vulnerable workers in the workplace (and elsewhere) through legislation such as the Human Rights Act 1998 and the Equality Act 2010 (Legislation.gov.uk 1998b; 2010). The Health and Safety Executive (2021f) defines vulnerable workers as

- new and expectant mothers
- people with disabilities
- young people
- migrant workers
- gig economy, agency and temporary workers
- workers who are new to the job
- lone workers
- older workers

On a broader scale, as we have seen, different and unequal health outcomes emerge across different occupations, but it may be that certain occupations attract the healthier, better educated and wealthier people and others attract those whose circumstances limited their education, qualifications, wealth and therefore their health. Once in work, it makes sense for a workplace to promote the health of workers because healthier workers are associated with greater productivity, a prosperous business and a stronger economy which supports the health and wellbeing of the population (Burton, 2010) (Box 14.1).

Box 14.1 Supporting a migrant workforce

An occupational health nurse worked with a predominantly migrant workforce at a fresh food manufacturing site in England. She writes about their needs and how to support them.

Some migrant workers did not understand UK healthcare services and were unaware that they could register with a GP and access primary care for free. Both language and culture were barriers. Some would self-medicate with traditional remedies, illegal drugs, antibiotics and alcohol obtained via the internet, which resulted in various types of unnecessary or harmful self-medication including overdoses. Some would end up at Accident and Emergency units when their symptoms became unbearable.

Some workers with low-paid work or zero hours contracts held down more than one job, sometimes working one shift then going straight onto the next. Some skipped meals to ensure their families ate. They needed to travel to work because they had to live in places with affordable accommodation, but these were not always safe neighbourhoods. Three employees were robbed and assaulted, sustaining serious head injuries. Many more were fearful of crime, especially when crimes against migrants increased during the Brexit referendum.

Many migrants came from countries where their cultural norms included smoking, drinking strong caffeinated and/or energy drinks and eating high sugar foods. It is important to remember what many migrants may have lost. Some may feel they have lost their personal and cultural identity; they may have lost social status compared to the work and life they had before, some may feel frustrated because they are not using their full capabilities and some have left families behind. Feeling isolation is exacerbated by a new language and culture. Consuming alcohol, tobacco and sugar can be ways of coping.

Some strategies which can support the health of the migrant workforce are:

- *Listen* to their social histories; understand their thinking, feelings and behaviour; build rapport and trust
- *Communicate* with patience; learn a few words in their language; use translation services; make the business case for introducing courses for English for Speakers of Other Languages (ESOL); have key documents translated; consider the implications of the worker bringing a child or another adult to translate their health details
- *Assess health risks* after clear communication and understanding has been established. Refuse to undertake a formal assessment until these are in place. Use empathic, objective language; acknowledge workers' strengths such as resilience; explore potential health risks in their accommodation and workplace; consider occupational or other exposures to health risks before they came to the UK; be sensitive to their culture, faith and health beliefs
- *Refer* to sources of support such as social or faith networks, cultural cafés and healthcare services
- *Work with employers* to create a health promoting and pleasant workplace, e.g. utilise key services such as an Employment Assistance Programme which can provide confidential help for many health and wellbeing concerns; provide culturally appropriate meals in harmony with healthier eating advice;

be aware when workers are fasting; avoid assuming that workers from the same country will support one another; be inclusive and try to minimise or eradicate anything that can create feelings of difference or discrimination
- *Sources of information* designed to support migrant workers include

  - Migrant Help www.migranthelpuk.org
  - Unison www.unison.org.uk/get-help/knowledge/vulnerable-workers/migrant-workers
  - Health and Safety Executive www.hse.gov.uk/migrantworkers

(Source: Brownett, 2017)

Adverse and protective factors

Bell (2017) explains some individuals may be more vulnerable to an unhealthy workplace than others because they have more adverse factors in their lives, such as

- adversity in their early life
- difficult relationships
- adverse life events
- financial worries
- natural disasters
- serious illness

Together, these encourage poor emotional and mental health which increase unhealthy behaviours. These can be made worse by

- living in poor housing and a poor neighbourhood
- poor social capital
- social isolation

Others fair better because they have fewer adverse factors and more protective factors in their lives. These include having

- coping abilities
- self-efficacy
- resilience
- the ability to learn and develop social skills

Together, these encourage mental wellbeing, a sense of control over one's life and healthy behaviours. These can be further enhanced by

- social support at work
- family
- neighbourhoods

Enhancing protective factors can be achieved through education (empowerment model of health promotion) and improving the psychosocial work environment (social change model of health promotion). The aim is to encourage

- empowerment, e.g. having the resources for health and 'having a voice' which can contribute to decisions

---

Box 14.2 Building workers' resilience

Building workers' resilience means fostering

- their self-efficacy
- a positive affect/mood and optimism
- their sense of coherence, a belief that what happens is rational, has meaning and is manageable because resources are available
- their social support
- positive interpersonal relations with managers

Educational programmes to develop resilience should

- be based on experiential/active learning
- encourage self-awareness, reflection, relaxation, mindfulness and principles of cognitive-behavioural therapy
- include goal-setting, coaching and small group discussion
- be approximately eight to 10 sessions over a four to five-week period
- include the full support of senior management

(Source: Gifford and Young, 2021)

- control, e.g. having a sense of control and having real control over the design of the work and the work environment
- self-efficacy, e.g. believing that one can be successful and accomplish tasks
- resilience, e.g. feeling capable of dealing with setbacks, the ability to rebound from adversity (Box 14.2)
- social relationships, e.g. encourage social networks which help to buffer the harms associated with isolation and stress
- community belonging, e.g. creating a work community in which workers feel a sense of belonging

(Bell, 2017)

(See Chapters 6, 7 and 8)

Health-related behaviours

Workers' health-related behaviours are influenced by their workplace and their wider psychosocial environment. Recent studies examining the health-related behaviours across UK occupations found

- those in routine and manual occupations smoked more than twice as much as those working in managerial and professional occupations (ONS, 2020) (Table 14.3)
- the highest proportion of heavy alcohol drinkers were among the skilled trade occupations, especially males, and the lowest proportion was among those working in professional occupations (Thompson and Pirmohamed, 2021) (Table 14.4)

Table 14.3 Current UK smokers by occupation, 2019

Socio-economic classification	England	Wales	Scotland	Northern Ireland	Total, UK
Managerial and professional	9.3%	10.1%	8.7%	8.0%	9.3%
Intermediate	14.2%	13.9%	13.1%	14.2%	14.1%
Routine and manual	23.2%	25.2%	25.1%	23.0%	23.4%

Source: ONS (2020).

Table 14.4 Heavy alcohol consumption[a] among UK workers aged 40 to 46 years, by occupation, 2006 to 2010 ($n = 100,817$)

Rank	Occupations most associated with heavy drinking	Occupations least associated with heavy drinking
1 (highest)	Publicans and managers of license premises	Accounts and wages clerks, book-keepers and other financial clerks
2	Industrial cleaning process occupations	Nurses
3	Plasterers	Information and communication technology managers
4	Sports and leisure assistants	Chartered and certified accountants
5	Bar staff	Educational assistants
6	Refuse and salvage occupations	Secondary education teaching professionals
7	Weighers, graders, sorters	Teaching professionals (n.e.c.[b])
8	Auto electricians	IT strategy and planning professionals
9	Roofers, roof tilers and slaters	Mechanical engineers
10	Vehicle body builders and repairers	Software professionals

[a] Heavy alcohol consumption was defined as >50 units for men and >35 units for women, per week
[b] Not elsewhere classified, e.g. private music teachers or teaching English as a foreign language
Source: Thompson and Pirmohamed (2021).

- healthy eating recommendations were less likely to be followed by those working in skilled/partly skilled and unskilled manual occupations than those in professional, managerial or skilled non-manual occupations (Yau *et al.*, 2019)
- on working days, those working as managers, directors and senior officials spent significantly more time sitting than those who worked as associate professionals and in technical occupations, secretarial work, skilled trades, sales and customer services and elementary administration and service occupations (Kazi *et al.*, 2019) (Table 14.5)

The data suggest that unhealthy behaviours, except sitting, are more common among the skilled, unskilled, semi-routine and routine occupations. These are relatively lower paid jobs, and less healthy behaviours are strongly associated with living among poorer or disadvantaged groups and in areas of greater deprivation (Bell, 2017; ONS, 2017). Zhang and colleagues (2021) carried out a large study of UK and American adults and concluded that socio-economic status had a greater influence on preventing disability and early death from cardiovascular disease than health-related behaviours: smoking, alcohol, physical activity and diet. These findings point to the importance

Table 14.5 UK average sitting times by occupation, 2019 (*n* = 1,200 workers; 10 worksites)

Groups of occupations	Average sitting time per day (hours)		
	Sitting at work	Working day total	Non-working day total
Managers, directors and senior officials (*n* = 109)	7.1	10.8	6.9
Professions (*n* = 394)	6.8	10.9	7.9
Associate professionals and technical occupations (*n* = 115)	5.9	10.0	7.6
Secretarial and related occupations (*n* = 115)	5.9	10.3	6.8
Skilled trades (*n* = 12)	4.8	8.4	7.3
Sales and customer service (*n* = 249)	6.0	10.2	8.0
Process, plant and machine operatives (*n* = 4)	4.7	8.9	7.3
Elementary administration and service occupations (*n* = 21)	2.1	4.9	6.7

Source: Adapted from Kazi *et al.* (2019, p. 28).

of the setting (social change model of health promotion) when trying to encourage healthier behaviours, rather than relying on individual instruction (preventive model of health promotion) or education (educational model of health promotion) alone. As Bell (2017) explains,

"… smoking tobacco, misuse of alcohol, unhealthy diet and lack of physical exercise are well-known risks to health. But each of these behaviours has its own complex web of causation, incorporating individual, community and societal-level factors. These include psychosocial pathways … behaviours respond to the social environment mediated by individual motivations, capabilities and opportunities."

(p. 32)

Thinking point:

Consider an example of your health-related behaviour. Think about the social and psychological influences that shaped this behaviour. For example, consider friends, family, education, living environment, media, marketing, price, what you know about it, how you feel about it, the value you place on it and what benefits you gain from it. Then consider how the social context may have influenced your psychological perspectives, experiences and choice to engage with it.

The International Labour Organization argues that health-related behaviours associated with stress; the use of alcohol, drugs and tobacco; physical inactivity and violent behaviour are more effectively addressed when they are integrated with work-related health and safety policies and management practices that recognise the importance of the workplace setting and its wider social environment (Forastieri, 2012).

Workplaces can improve workers' health by fostering personal protective factors and a healthy psychosocial environment within and beyond the workplace.

Healthy workplaces

A safe and healthy workplace provides good quality work and supports the health of workers. Here we describe the evidence-based characteristics of good quality work and two evidence-based models of a healthy workplace.

Good quality work

Good quality work is described by the UK's Good Work Index (Norris-Green and Gifford, 2021) and the Scottish Fair Work Framework (Fair Work Convention, 2016). Both seek to address the most well-evidenced psychosocial factors that affect the quality of working life. Good and fair work

- is accessible to all who wish to work
- gives people job security, e.g. a fair and secure income, flexible working, sick pay and pensions
- provides opportunities for training, mentoring and development, and for career progression
- provides a sense of fulfilment, e.g. having control over the work and opportunities to problem solve and develop confidence
- gives workers a voice, e.g. views are sought as part of constructive dialogues within a transparent work environment
- provides a supportive environment with social support, dignity and respect for workers' family and personal lives including a work-life balance
- is mentally and physically healthy

Healthy workplaces

Across the UK, workplaces are being encouraged to become healthy workplaces through awards:

- Northern Ireland Workplace Wellbeing Awards
- Healthy Working Wales Workplace Awards
- Scotland Healthy Working Lives Awards
- England Healthy Workplace Awards

Each has its own criteria and workplaces can be helped by initiatives such as Work Ready (Box 14.3) and occupational health services. Health professionals who provide occupational health services include occupational health nurses, doctors who specialise in occupational medicine, occupational physiotherapists, occupational psychologists, occupational hygienists, ergonomists and occupational health technicians (CIPD, 2021b). They work within small and large organisations across the private, public or voluntary sector, or they can be self-employed. Examples of their work include

- primary health promotion, e.g. undertaking 'stress audits', advising employers how to improve the psychosocial environment, advising on workplace design, risk assessments and risk management, workforce health need assessments, health education and wider programmes to support health and wellbeing and the health surveillance required by law such as when workers are exposed to hazards

---

Box 14.3 Work Ready

Work Ready aims to help workforces to become healthier, happier and more productive. It is designed and led by registered dietitians who visit the workplace to carry out a holistic workplace nutritional needs assessment. This includes

- understanding the workplace's objectives for health and wellbeing
- understanding the characteristics of the workers and the work environment
- reviewing existing health promotion in the workplace
- working with the occupational health team, workers and anyone who is leading health and wellbeing in the workplace
- speaking to staff champions, if available
- examining the facilities for food and drink in the workplace
- assessing policies which relate to health and wellbeing

Dietitians can advise about which types of nutrition-related initiatives would provide most value to the workforce, provide practical food demonstrations appropriate to the workers' needs, give advice about the food and drink provision in the workplace, and provide training on team building including 'workplace champion' teams to encourage future development.

One worker said, "I found it very helpful to have all the advice drawn together as one normally picks bits up in dribs and drabs. The full picture is very persuasive and makes me want to do something about it."

(Source: British Dietetic Association, 2021)

- secondary health promotion, e.g. providing information about health screening and offering counselling
- tertiary health promotion, e.g. communication to support recovery from sickness and enable someone to return to work
- healthcare, e.g. assessing whether work has negatively affected someone's health using communication and examination, carrying out screening tests, providing minor treatment, making referrals for treatment or care and carrying out assessments to determine whether someone is fit for work

(CIPD, 2021b; RCN, 2021)

CIPD Wellbeing model

The UK's Chartered Institute of Personnel and Development (CIPD) believes a healthy workplace is about,

"Creating an environment to promote a state of contentment which allows an employee to flourish and achieve their full potential for the benefit of themselves and their organisation."

(Suff and Miller, 2016, p. 21)

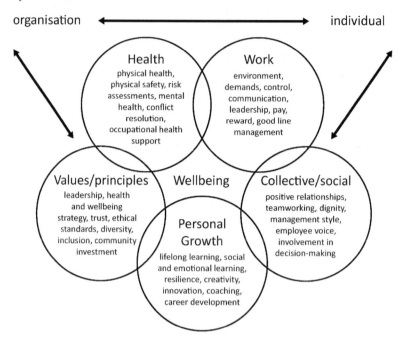

Figure 14.7 CIPD wellbeing model

The CIPD encourages those who work in Human Resources to take an active role in workplace health and wellbeing, because they know the workers and can influence management practices, and they work alongside occupational health services. The CIPD's Wellbeing model comprises five overlapping domains designed to help organisations think about how to create a healthy workplace (Figure 14.7). Each domain includes elements to be addressed at the individual and organisational levels because one affects the other. A healthy workplace depends on constructive interactions between all workers, including managers. Senior managers need to ensure health and wellbeing is a strategic priority, both for its own sake and for a productive business, and be role models who actively participate in healthier change.

WHO Healthy workplace model

The World Health Organization (WHO) includes a healthy workplace as one of its healthy settings, as discussed in Chapter 8. A healthy workplace is where managers and workers collaborate in a process of continual improvement aimed at protecting and promoting the health, safety and wellbeing of all workers as well as the sustainability of the workplace (Burton, 2010). It differs from the CIPD Wellbeing model by giving stronger emphasis to the workplace as part of a wider community where each can support one another (Figure 14.8). At its heart are three principles:

- ethics, doing what is moral, legal and 'right'
- leadership engagement, meaning gaining commitment from the leaders and influential stakeholders
- worker involvement

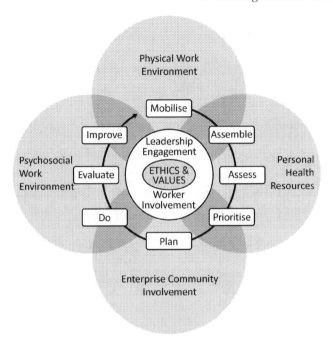

Figure 14.8 WHO Healthy workplace model

There are four areas where employers can collaborate with employees to influence the health of all workers most effectively, as well as building the productivity, efficiency and competitiveness of the organisation. These are

- the physical work environment
- the psychosocial work environment
- personal health resources in the workplace, e.g. health-related behaviours, information, resources and opportunities to support mental and physical health
- enterprise community involvement, e.g. activities, expertise and resources the workplace can offer to the local community and vice versa, such as assistance with transport, dealing with work-related pollution, offering opportunities to develop knowledge and skills, and augmenting local health services

A healthy workplace is created through a process of continual improvement which is based on engaging workers. This is an example of planning health promotion, as discussed in Chapter 8.

- *Mobilise* active and enthusiastic commitment from influential key people for a healthy workplace
- *Assemble* people and resources, perhaps set up a representative/diverse healthy workplace team
- *Assess* the current situation, needs and assets, perhaps using the 'stages of change' model (see Chapter 5), and articulate the desired future
- *Prioritise* the actions which need to be addressed first

- *Plan* some long-term goals
- *Do* it
- *Evaluate* how successful the action was, whether it met the objectives
- *Improve* the healthy workplace by making any necessary adjustments based on the evaluation, and go back to 'mobilise'

(Burton, 2010)

Summary

This chapter has

- described the most common work-related health concerns in the UK
- discussed the inequalities in health and health-related behaviours across different occupations
- examined how the physical and psychosocial work environment can harm and support workers' health
- identified workers as individuals who enter the workplace with their own vulnerabilities and protective factors
- described examples of protecting and promoting the health of workers
- described the features of good quality work and a healthy workplace

Further reading

Clarke, S., Probst, T.M., Guldenmund, F. and Passmore, J. (eds) (2020) *The Wiley Blackwell handbook of the psychology of occupational safety and workplace health.* Chichester: John Wiley & Sons

Useful websites

Chartered Institute of Personnel and Development. Available at: www.cipd.co.uk
Health and Safety Executive. Available at: www.hse.gov.uk
Health and Safety Executive Northern Ireland. Available at: www.hseni.gov.uk
NHS at Work Network. Available at: www.nhshealthatwork.co.uk

References

Ahlin, J.K., Westerlund, H., Griep, Y. and Hanson, L.L.M. (2018) 'Trajectories of job demands and control: risk for subsequent symptoms of major depression in the nationally representative Swedish Longitudinal Occupational Survey of Health (SLOSH)', *International Archives of Occupational and Environmental Health*, 91(2), pp. 263–272

Bell, R. (2017) *Psychosocial pathways and health outcomes: informing action on health inequalities.* UCL Institute of Health Equity/Public Health England. Available at: https://www.institute-ofhealthequity.org/resources-reports/psychosocial-pathways-and-health-outcomes-informing-action-on-health-inequalities/psychosocial-pathways-and-health-outcomes.pdf (Accessed 10th June 2022)

British Dietetic Association (2021) *Workplace health. Work ready.* Available at: www.bdaworkready.co.uk (Accessed 11th June 2022)

Brownett, T. (2017) 'Recollections of managing the health of migrants in a blue-collar workplace', *Occupational Health and Wellbeing*, 69(1), pp. 27–29

Burton, J. (2010) *WHO healthy workplace framework and model: background and supporting literature and practice*. Geneva: World Health Organization

Chandola, T., Britton, A., Brunner, E. *et al.* (2008) 'Work stress and coronary heart disease: what are the mechanisms', *European Heart Journal*, 29(5), pp. 640–648

Chartered Institute of Personnel and Development (2021a) *Health and wellbeing at work 2021*. Available at: https://www.cipd.co.uk/Images/health-wellbeing-work-report-2021_tcm18-93541.pdf (Accessed 11th June 2022)

Chartered Institute of Personnel and Development (2021b) *Occupational health*. Available at: https://www.cipd.co.uk/knowledge/culture/well-being/occupational-health-factsheet (Accessed 11th June 2022)

Dragano, N., Seigrist, J. Nyberg, S.T. *et al.* (2017) 'Effort-reward imbalance at work and incident coronary heart disease', *Epidemiology*, 28(4), pp. 619–626

Ehsan, A., Klass, H.S., Bastianen, A. and Spini, D. (2019) 'Social capital and health: a systematic review of systematic reviews', *SSM Population Health*, 8 doi:10.1016/j.ssmph.2-19.100425

Ekbladh, E. (2010) 'Perceptions of the work environment among people with experience of long term sick leave', *Work*, 35(2), pp. 125–136

Elovainio, M., Kivimäki, M. and Vahtera, J. (2002) 'Organizational justice: evidence of a new psychosocial predictor of health', *American Journal of Public Health*, 92(1), pp. 105–108

Fair Work Convention (2016) *Fair work framework 2016*. Available at: https://www.fairwork-convention.scot/wp-content/uploads/2018/12/Fair-Work-Convention-Framework-PDF-Full-Version.pdf (Accessed 11th June 2022)

Forastieri, V. (2012) *Trainer's guide. SOLVE: integrating health promotion into workplace OSH policies*. Geneva: International Labour Office. Available at: https://www.ilo.org/wcmsp5/groups/public/—ed_protect/—protrav/—safework/documents/instructionalmaterial/wcms_178397.pdf (Accessed 12th June 2022)

Ge, J., He, J., Liu, Y., Zhang, J., Pan, J., Zhang, X. and Liu, D. (2021) 'Effects of effort-reward imbalance, job satisfaction and work engagement on self-rated health among healthcare workers', *BMC Public Health*, 21(195) doi:10.1186/s12889-021-10233-w

Gifford, J. and Young, J. (2021) *Employee resilience: an evidence review*. Summary report. Chartered Institute of Personnel and Development. Available at: https://www.cipd.co.uk/Images/employee-resilience-discussion-report_tcm18-91717.pdf (Accessed 12th June 2022)

Health and Safety Executive (2021a) *Health and safety at work. Summary statistics for Great Britain 2021*. Available at: https://www.hse.gov.uk/statistics/overall/hssh2021.pdf (Accessed 12th June 2022)

Health and Safety Executive (2021b) *Work-related stress, anxiety or depression statistics in Great Britain, 2021*. Available at: https://www.hse.gov.uk/statistics/causdis/stress.pdf (Accessed 12th June 2022)

Health and Safety Executive (2021c) *Occupational lung disease statistics in Great Britain, 2021*. Available at: https://www.hse.gov.uk/statistics/causdis/respiratory-diseases.pdf (Accessed 13th June 2022)

Health and Safety Executive (2021d) *Information and services*. Available at: https://www.hse.gov.uk (Accessed 12th June 2022)

Health and Safety Executive (2021e) *A-Z of guidance by industry*. Available at: www.hse.gov.uk/guidance/industries.htm (Accessed 13th June 2022)

Health and Safety Executive (2021f) *Vulnerable workers*. Available at: https://www.hse.gov.uk/vulnerable-workers (Accessed 13th June 2022)

IJpelaar, J., Barry, R., Hughes, J., McAuley, R. and Lyness, D. (2021) *Mental health status of Northern Ireland population in employment: occupations and industries*. Available at: https://www.nisra.gov.uk/sites/nisra.gov.uk/files/publications/Mental%20health%20status%20of%20population%20in%20employment.pdf (Accessed 12th June 2022)

Karasek, R.A. (1979) 'Job demands, job decision latitude, and mental strain: implications for job redesign', *Administrative Science Quarterly*, 24(2), pp. 285–308

Karasek, R.A. and Theorell, T. (1990) *Healthy work: stress, productivity, and the reconstruction of the working life.* New York: Basic Books

Katikireddi, S.V., Leyland, A.H., McKee, M., Ralston, K. and Stuckler, D. (2017) 'Patterns of mortality by occupation in the UK, 1991–2011: a comparative analysis of linked census and mortality records', *Lancet Public Health*, 2(11) doi:10.1016/S2468-2667(17)30193-7

Kazi, A., Haslam, C., Duncan, M., Clemes, S. and Twumasi, R. (2019) 'Sedentary behaviour and health at work: an investigation of industrial sector, job role, gender and geographical differences', *Ergonomics*, 62(1), pp. 21–30

Kuh, D., Ben-Shlomo, Y., Lynch, J., Hallqvist, J. and Power, C. (2003) 'Life course epidemiology', *Journal of Epidemiology and Community Health*, 57(10), pp. 778–783

Legislation.gov.uk (1998a) *The working time regulations 1998.* Available at: https://www.legislation.gov.uk/uksi/1998/1833/contents/made (Accessed 13th June 2022)

Legislation.gov.uk (1998b) *Human Rights Act 1998.* Available at: https://www.legislation.gov.uk/ukpga/1998/42/contents (Accessed 13th June 2022)

Legislation.gov.uk (2010) *Equality Act 2010.* Available at: https://www.legislation.gov.uk/ukpga/2010/15/contents (Accessed 13th June 2022)

Marmot, M., Allen, J., Boyce, T., Goldblatt, P. and Morrison, J. (2020) *Health equity in England: the Marmot review 10 years on.* London: Institute of Health Equity

Marmot, M. and Bell, R. (2010) 'Challenging health inequalities – implications for the workplace', *Occupational Medicine*, 60(3), pp. 162–164

Norris-Green, M. and Gifford, J. (2021) *CIPD good work index 2021.* London: Chartered Institute of Personnel and Development. Available at: https://www.cipd.co.uk/Images/good-work-index-research-report-2021-1_tcm18-96100.pdf (Accessed 12th June 2022)

Notelaers, G., Törnroos, M. and Salin, D. (2019) 'Effort-reward imbalance: a risk factor for exposure to workplace bullying', *Frontiers in Psychology*, 10 doi:10.3389/fpsyg.2019.00386

Office for National Statistics (2010) *Standard occupational classification 2010. Volume 3. The national statistics socio-economic classification (rebased on the SOC2010) user manual.* London: Palgrave Macmillan

Office for National Statistics (2017) *An overview of lifestyles and wider characteristics linked to healthy life expectancy in England: June 2017.* Available at: https://www.ons.gov.uk/peoplepopulationandcommunity/healthandsocialcare/healthinequalities/articles/healthrelatedlifestylesandwidercharacteristicsofpeoplelivinginareaswiththehighestorlowesthealthylife/june2017 (Accessed 12th June 2022)

Office for National Statistics (2020) *Smoking habits in the UK and its constituent countries.* Available at: https://www.ons.gov.uk/peoplepopulationandcommunity/healthandsocialcare/healthandlifeexpectancies/datasets/smokinghabitsintheukanditsconstituentcountries (Accessed 13th June 2022)

Oldfield, A., Rogers, N., Phelps, A. *et al.* (2018) *Data collection 2002–2016 English Longitudinal Study of Ageing: Wave 8.* Available at: https://ukdataservice.ac.uk/search/?q=english+longitudinal+study+of+ageing (Accessed 13th June 2022)

Pikhart, H. and Pikhartova, J. (2015) *The relationship between psychosocial risk factors and health outcomes of chronic diseases. A review of the evidence for cancer and cardiovascular diseases. A Health Evidence Network (HEN) synthesis report.* Copenhagen: World Health Organization (Europe)

Public Health England (2018) *Definitions, references and indicator sources for work, worklessness and health: local infographic tool.* Available at: https://assets.publishing.service.gov.uk/government/uploads/system/uploads/attachment_data/file/714730/Work_worklessness_and_health_local_infographic_data_sources_and_references_June_2018.pdf (Accessed 13th June 2022)

Robinson, S. (2021) 'Social context of health and illness', in Robinson, S. (ed) *Priorities for health promotion and public health.* London: Routledge, pp. 3–33

Royal College of Nursing (2021) *Occupational health.* Available at: https://www.rcn.org.uk/clinical-topics/public-health/occupational-health (Accessed 13th June 2022)

Rugulies, R. (2019) 'What is a psychosocial work environment?', *Scandinavian Journal of Work, Environment and Health*, 45(1), pp. 1–6

Rugulies, R., Aust, B. and Madsen, I.E. (2017) 'Effort-reward imbalance at work and risk of depressive disorders. A systematic review and meta-analysis of prospective cohort studies', *Scandinavian Journal of Work, Environment and Health*, 43(4) doi:10.5271/sjweh.3632

Rydström, I., Dalheim, L., Dellve, L. and Ahlstrom, L. (2017) 'Importance of social capital at the workplace for return to work among women with a history of long-term sick leave: a cohort study', *BMC Nursing*, 16(38) doi:10.1186/s12912-017-0234-2

Siegrist, J. (2002) 'Effort-reward imbalance at work and health', in Perrewé, P.L. and Ganster, D.C. (eds) *Historical and current perspectives on stress and health.* Bingley: Emerald, pp. 261–291

Söderberg, M. (2014) *Psychosocial work conditions – cardiovascular disease, perceptions and reactive behaviour.* Gothenburg: University of Gothenburg

Suff, R. and Miller, J. (2016) *Growing the health and well-being agenda: from first steps to full potential.* Chartered Institute of Personnel and Development. Available at: https://www.backinactionuk.com/wp-content/uploads/cipd-health-wellbeing-agenda.pdf (Accessed 13th June 2022)

Thompson, A. and Pirmohamed, M. (2021) 'Associations between occupation and heavy alcohol consumption in UK adults aged 40–69: a cross-sectional study using the UK Biobank', *BMC Public Health*, 21(190) doi:10.1186/s12889-021-10208-x

Tinson, A. (2020) *Living in poverty was bad for your health before COVID-19.* The Health Foundation. Available at: https://www.health.org.uk/sites/default/files/2020-07/Living%20in%20poverty%20was%20bad%20for%20your%20health%20before%20COVID-19.pdf (Accessed 13th June 2022)

United Nations Economic Commission for Europe (2021) *GHS pictograms. Globally harmonised system of classification and labelling of chemicals.* Available at: https://unece.org/transportdangerous-goods/ghs-pictograms (Accessed 13th June 2022)

Waddell, G. and Burton, A.K. (2006) *Is work good for your health and well-being?* London: The Stationery Office

Williams, M., Zhou, Y. and Zou, M. (2020) *CIPD good work index 2020. UK working lives survey.* Chartered Institute of Personnel and Development. Available at: https://www.cipd.co.uk/Images/good-work-index-full-report-2020-2_tcm18-79210.pdf (Accessed 13th June 2022)

World Health Organization/International Labour Organization (2021) *WHO/ILO joint estimates of the work-related burden of disease and injury, 2000–2016.* Geneva: World Health Organization/International Labour Organization

Yau, A., Adams, J. and Monsivais, P. (2019) 'Time trends in adherence to UK dietary recommendations and associated sociodemographic inequalities, 1986–2012: a repeated cross-sectional analysis', *European Journal of Clinical Nutrition*, 73(7), pp. 997–1005

Zhang, Y., Chen, C., Xiong-Fei, P., Guo, J., Li, Y., Fanco, O.H., Liu, G. and Pan, A. (2021) 'Associations of healthy lifestyle and socioeconomic status with mortality and incident cardiovascular disease: two prospective cohort studies', *BMJ*, 372(604) doi:10.1136/bmj.n604

15 Promoting health in the National Health Service

Sally Robinson

Key points

- Introduction
- The health system
- A healthy National Health Service
- Preventing disease and promoting health within healthcare
- Health promoting healthcare practitioners
- Summary

Introduction

This chapter describes how the UK National Health Service (NHS) was originally set up as a disease-centred care service. This led to 'health' being understood by many as being synonymous with care. Today the NHS is working to become a 'health' service and positioning itself as one part of a wider UK intersectoral health system. We discuss what a healthy NHS looks like and how it includes both pathogenic and salutogenic approaches to supporting people's health and quality of life. The chapter concludes by explaining how healthcare practitioners can become more health promoting.

The health system

A health system,

> "... consists of all organizations, people and actions whose *primary intent* is to promote, restore or maintain health. This includes efforts to influence determinants of health as well as more direct health-improving activities. A health system is therefore more than the pyramid of publicly owned facilities that deliver personal health services. It includes, for example, a mother caring for a sick child at home; private providers; behaviour change programmes; vector-control campaigns; health insurance organizations; occupational health and safety legislation. It includes inter-sectoral action by health staff, for example encouraging the ministry of education to promote female education, a well known determinant of better health."
>
> (WHO, 2007, p. 2. Reproduced with permission from the World Health Organization)

DOI: 10.4324/9780367823696-19

The World Health Organization (2007) suggests the concept of an organised health system began about a 100 years ago. These are political and social institutions. The aim of a health system is to improve health and health equity, and it includes health promotion (including health education), health protection, drawing attention to the social and environmental determinants of health and influencing them, healthcare public health (planning healthcare services), social protection and healthcare services.

The creation of the National Health Service and consequences for care and health

In the UK, the National Health Service (NHS) began in 1948. It was revolutionary because it

- was available to the whole population free of charge at the point of service
- brought hospitals under the control of central government
- was paid for by central government through a national insurance scheme

The NHS was created at a time when the medical model of health and illness was unquestioningly revered (Robinson, 2021a). People, including politicians, supported the scientific approach which comprised the objective study of the body like a machine; diagnosing the fault; fixing the body with surgery, medicines or physical manipulation; and providing personal care and rehabilitation to return the body back to having an 'absence of disease or infirmity'. Although supported by a wide range of professions allied to medicine and associated scientists, doctors were the most visible, influential and powerful. In the same way that the medical model adopts a reductionist approach, that is developing expertise in specific systems of the body, organs, cells and genes; so medicine and the NHS around which is was designed, developed specialities such as gastro-intestinal or oncology consultants and departments. There were many positive and negative consequences to the way in which the NHS was set up, but they include

- it reinforced medicine and the medical model as the dominant model of health and illness in the UK
- it reinforced the idea that health means an 'absence of disease'; if a doctor could not identify/diagnose a germ or bodily malfunction, the person was deemed to be healthy
- the National Health Service was misnamed; it was primarily a national care service which provided diagnostics, treatment, rehabilitation and personal care
- it emphasised hospitals as being at the centre of the system, giving them high status around which was the lower status 'community'
- health became synonymous with illness; an inquiry into someone's health elicited a response about their illness status
- health became synonymous with healthcare and medical care
- health seemed to be a matter for healthcare professionals, the NHS and no one else
- the whole health system was perceived as being the NHS
- it detracted from attending to the underlying social, economic and environmental determinants of health, not least by politicians

(Robinson, 2021a)

To understand the full implications of these consequences, we need to be clear about the meanings of 'care' and 'health'.

Care

Illness is a subjective experience. It is about feeling unwell. Disease is diagnosed by a doctor with reference to the symptoms described by the patient and the signs that the doctor observes. Healthcare practitioners aim to help people through care, that is through diagnosis, treatments and a wide range of related physical, emotional and social support. They often use touch in their work. Core to this work is an understanding of anatomy, microbiology, pathology, biochemistry, neuroscience, illness-related behaviour; and the psychology and sociology of illness, medicine, rehabilitation and care.

Carers undertake all or some of the following: they

- work face to face with individuals, families or occasionally groups, based on an initial assessment or diagnosis which has identified a need for care
- work with people who are physically, mentally, emotionally or socially vulnerable
- provide personal care, e.g. helping with washing, dressing and eating
- provide treatment, e.g. the clinical skills of prescribing and administering medicines, injections, surgery, wound dressings, sonography, specialised arts or psychological therapies/counselling, prescribed physical exercises or occupational activities

Carers are expected to demonstrate the skills for care which are to

- be caring and provide the right care for people across the life course
- be compassionate, empathic and respect people's dignity
- be competent in providing care; have the correct knowledge and skills
- communicate well, be good listeners and respect person-centredness: 'no decision about me without me'
- have courage to 'do what is right', be an advocate for people and embrace new ways of working
- be committed to improving care for all

(CBCNO and DHCNA, 2012)

Care includes health education, usually secondary and tertiary health education rather than primary (see Table 7.1 p.169). It is often in the form of patient education, meaning it focusses on explaining a procedure, treatment, an aspect of personal care or a rehabilitation plan. Patient education is sometimes called clinical health promotion within a patient pathway (Tønnesen, 2011).

Health

Health is a subjective experience. It means different things to different people. For example, it may be about feeling well, happy, fit, socially included, content or secure; being pain free, peaceful or warm; having a job, home and friends; and it may (or may not) include having no disease or bodily malfunction. Core to understanding and promoting people's health is an understanding of, and listening to, people; the psychology of health and health-related behaviours; the social, political, economic and environmental context in which people live; how social, environmental, biological and psychological factors influence people's health positively or negatively; the ability to

---

Box 15.1 The creation of the NHS as separate from public health (the public's health)

"The creation of the NHS was in many respects a major public health achievement ... It was also believed that a single national service would give greater scope for preventing illness and for integrating different services to meet health needs. However, the principal focus of the NHS was on diagnosis and treatment ... Consequently, there was a lack of leadership and coordination of public health at a national level, especially after 1951 when the Ministry of Health's responsibilities for environmental health, housing, water and other public health-related services were transferred to other departments.

"To make matters worse, divisions between different parts of the health service were institutionalized. The three main parts of the NHS – hospital; services, family practitioners (GPs, dentists, pharmacists and opticians), and community and public health services – had separate administrative structures, and collaboration between them was poor. At this time, local authorities were responsible for managing community services, including district nursing, health visiting, ambulance services, maternity and child welfare clinics, the school health service and health education. During the 1960s, attempts were made to bring local authority community health professionals into closer contact with GPs. However, collaboration remained problematic, and for the most part hospitals, primary care and community/public health occupied different worlds."

(Source: Baggott, 2013, pp. 3, 4)

---

detect who is healthy and who is at most risk of becoming unhealthy through social disadvantage or exposure to risks. It does not include touch. Communication is core to promoting and protecting health and, at times, this can be complemented by care.

The study and practice of care is not the same as the study and practice of health. Both are interdisciplinary subjects which were once much closer, but they became separated due to the rise of the medical model in the 19th century. Apart from a few professionals such as Specialist Community Public Health Nurses, those who study 'health' often have little expertise in 'care'; those who study 'care' often have little expertise in 'health' (Box 15.1). The NHS needs healthcare practitioners to learn more about health and they need to work in partnership with those who specialise in health.

A modern health system

Watching the development of health systems across the world during the 20th century, was the World Health Organization. Since its inception in 1946, it had argued that health was holistic and not, "... merely the absence of disease or infirmity" (WHO, 1946, p. 1). It was a positive concept which included a person's physical, mental and social wellbeing. The World Health Organization was concerned about the medicalisation of health systems, an extremely expensive approach which emphasised cure and hospitals rather than prevention, and relied on relatively few highly educated medical experts in disease and infirmity (Table 15.1). It would not achieve its mission to achieve 'health for all' people across the world, as discussed in Chapter 1. From the 1978

Table 15.1 Comparison of the NHS in the 1950s to a modern health system

NHS 1950s	Modern health system
'Care for all'	'Health for all'
Aim: treat disease and malfunctions	Aim: promote good health and wellbeing, prevent disease and malfunctions through early intervention; treat disease and malfunctions
Medical model of health and illness	Medical and social models of health and illness
Disease-centred	Health-centred
Medical professional-centred	Person-centred
Top-down, expert-led, hierarchical system	Participation of people in planning their system
Universal care	Universal health
Free for all, at the point of needing care	Equal chances of health for all
NHS as an island with hospitals placed at the centre, each surrounded by their local community healthcare service	Integration of the healthcare sector into the wider health system embedded among the population
Sectors beyond healthcare not recognised as relevant	Intersectoral and interagency; all parts of the health system are recognised as contributing to population health
Tertiary care, acute and hospital-based care, was prioritised with the aim to cure people because it was believed this would produce a fall in the demand for healthcare	Within healthcare, primary care is prioritised because it has most potential to prevent disease and promote health through early intervention, and it is at the interface between all elements of the health system and secondary and tertiary healthcare

Declaration of Alma-Ata to today, the World Health Organization has been consistent about the optimum characteristics of any health system.

- *Health* is a human right. It is a holistic and positive concept, which can be supported by treatment, care, rehabilitation, disease prevention, health protection, health education, and social and environmental change. It is 'everybody's business'
- *Participation* means that people have the right and the duty to be actively involved in the planning and implementation of their health system
- *Person-centred* means the individual, person or community should be at the centre of decisions that affect them, as opposed to a system which is profession-centred or centred on the needs of an organisation
- *Life course* – a health system should support people across their life course and provide extra support at critical times of life
- *Universality* means 'health for all'. Countries need to ensure health is accessible and affordable to all people
- *Universal health coverage* means ensuring that people can access affordable healthcare. Essential healthcare services include maternal, newborn and child health
- *Equity* refers to addressing unfair inequalities in health, often relating to social inequities such as those associated with gender discrimination or socio-economic status, which are fuelled by culture, politics and power. Vulnerable groups need to be identified and supported

- *Integration* and *intersectoral* are phrases used to emphasise how the health system comprises a range of different agencies and sectors which need to work together in partnership to achieve improved health for all. It is also called a 'whole-of-society' approach and includes education, trade, agriculture, social care, housing and so forth
- *Healthcare is one part of a wider health system* and it should reflect the characteristics above. Primary care, delivered in people's local communities, is recognised as being the most cost efficient and effective type of care for achieving better health outcomes for the most people and reducing health inequalities. Primary care needs to be supported by integrated healthcare services, and then the integrated healthcare services need to work in partnership with the wider health system

(Nolte *et al.*, 2020; WHO, 1978; 2007; 2019a; 2019b)

Today, the UK health system includes public health; much of the work of local government including social care, community safety, clean water, sanitation, housing, environment and education; and many charities, private businesses, health-related independent regulatory authorities/'watchdogs', health-related advisory and research organisations, community groups and healthcare providers. Most of the health system protects and promotes people's health through communication, education and a wide range of activities from policymaking to community action which bring about healthier social and environmental changes. Most contributors do not carry out care.

Those who work in public health are expected to be aware of the whole health system and to encourage its components to work together for optimum population health. This includes identifying population groups that may require healthcare and alerting healthcare providers. For example, the public health workforce such as epidemiologists and health protection professionals will have anticipated the COVID-19 coronavirus pandemic, alerted vaccine developers/producers, prepared for a public information campaign (primary health education) and ensured healthcare providers were preparing to undertake a mass vaccination programme. The healthcare workforce provided the vaccine-related care.

Integrating healthcare into the health system

In the UK, healthcare is provided by private businesses and the publicly funded NHS. The NHS has undergone many reorganisations during its lifetime, partly due to political preferences, mostly because demand has always outstripped supply and due to constant tensions between hospitals and primary care; prevention and treatment; public and private; and the vested interests of professional groups such as doctors (Baggott, 2004). In 1999, responsibility for the NHS was devolved to Scotland, England and Wales. The Northern Ireland NHS was always independent. As the NHS has its roots and traditions in care, not in health, and in the medical model of health and illness, we have seen governments gradually transforming the NHS to become part of a modern health promoting health system.

Some examples include

- 1992 *Health of the Nation* (England), a public health White Paper which called for cross-government working and for 'healthy alliances' across health authorities, local authorities, other local public services, the voluntary sector, employers and media. Using the World Health Organization's 'settings approach', alliances could work towards achieving healthy schools, workplaces, prisons and so forth. An evaluation, in 1998, showed the NHS/health authorities and others were not effectively working together

- 2003 *NHS Scotland* was launched. It integrated healthcare with existing public health and health education organisations
- 2009 *Public Health Wales* became part of NHS Wales
- 2009 *Health and Social Care (Reform) Act (Northern Ireland)* established the Northern Ireland Public Health Agency, and the Health and Social Care Board became responsible for healthcare and social care
- 2012 *Health and Social Care Act* (England) moved forward the integration of healthcare, social care and public health under the heading 'health and care'. It created local health and wellbeing boards, comprising representatives of healthcare (NHS), public health, adult social care and children's services. The Act emphasised the role of primary care by funding and enabling local healthcare/ general practice services to work together to buy the services its local community needed. These services might be provided by hospitals, local authorities, NHS mental health providers, the private sector, charities, NHS community services and so forth. The Act formally supported the participation of the public in health and social care matters and made clear that public health departments in local authorities would lead on the monitoring, evaluating and planning of healthcare services along with their strong remit to reduce health inequalities across the life course
- 2013 the 2020 *Vision for Health and Social Care* (Scotland) aimed to integrate healthcare and social care, provide person-centred services, support self-management and community care, reduce health inequalities and encourage disease prevention. Today, NHS Scotland includes Public Health Scotland
- 2014 *NHS Five Year Forward View* (England) called for greater disease prevention, peer/patient support, increased person-centred care; and new models of care based on integrating care services and rethinking where and how to deliver care in ways that better meet the people's care needs, e.g. providing more specialist healthcare outside of hospitals and integrating healthcare, social care and rehabilitation services in care homes. More widely, it encouraged partnerships between the local NHS, local authorities, charities and others to develop ideas about how they could work together to improve people's holistic health in their geographical area
- 2019 *NHS Long Term Plan* (England) set out aims to enhance prevention, reduce health inequalities, remove the divide between primary care and other community health-related services, provide more person-centred care and move to integrated care systems which aim to meet health and care needs in an area
- 2021 *A Healthier Wales* aimed for a wellness system across the life course which included preventing illness, early intervention, equitable and seamless healthcare and social care services, more home-based care and greater self-management
- 2021 *Build Back Better* discussed UK funding to deal with the post-COVID-19 coronavirus pandemic and backlogs for healthcare, an integrated care system and plans for a *National Prevention Service* focussed on health checks and changing behaviour. Separately, the *Office for Health Improvement and Disparities* (England) and the *UK Health Security Agency* were launched in the same year.

(Baggot, 2013; H.M. Government 2021; Legislation.gov.uk 2012; NHS 2014; 2019; Scottish Government, 2013; Welsh Government, 2021)

It is worth noting that the media, politicians, governments and those who influence governments contribute to an array of confusing terminology. For example, we see and hear the healthcare service described as the health service, the NHS or healthcare described as the health system and the health system described as health and

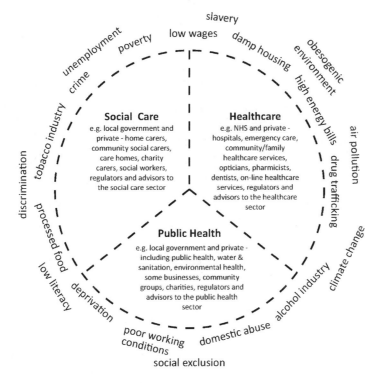

Figure 15.1 The health system should draw attention to the social and environmental determinants of health

social care (healthcare and social care). What was named the Health and Care System for England in 2013 (Gov.UK, 2013), comprising public health, healthcare and social care, broadly reflects the World Health Organization's definition of a health system. Figure 15.1 is a version of this.

> *The NHS was set up as a disease-centred care service. Current UK policy aims to integrate the NHS into the wider health system.*

A healthy National Health Service

A healthy NHS is integrated into the wider health system. It shares the load of promoting the health of the population and preventing disease equally with other sectors and agencies. It recognises that its unique contribution to population health is to provide healthcare, but this is not more important than the contributions made by other sectors and agencies. Healthcare practitioners are as valuable to the population's health as sanitation workers, health and safety inspectors, community arts practitioners, teachers, cooks, environmental health officers, social workers and gardeners. It recognises that while healthcare is their business, health is everybody's business.

Becoming a healthy NHS also means enhancing the 'health' within the healthcare organisation. The concept of a health promoting hospital emerged from the World Health Organization's *Ottawa Charter for Health Promotion* and the launch of its 'settings approach', as discussed in Chapter 8. A healthy setting is one where each element, the people (staff, visitors, patients) and the physical and social environment are health promoting. It is characterised by partnerships, community participation, equity and empowerment. The first international conference culminated in the *Budapest Declaration on Health Promoting Hospitals* in 1991. The health promoting hospitals movement later became the International Network for Health Promoting Hospitals and Health Services. They explain,

> "Health promoting hospitals and health services (HPH) orient their governance models, structures, processes and culture to optimize health gains of patients, staff and populations served and to support sustainable societies."
>
> (INHPHHS, 2020, p. 4)

The Network set the standards to which health services should aspire:

Standard 1. Demonstrating organisational commitment for HPH, e.g. optimising health gains for patients, staff and populations by ensuring their models of governance, policies, structures, processes and culture optimise health.

Standard 2. Ensuring access to the service, e.g. ensuring services are available, accessible and acceptable to all.

Standard 3. Enhancing people-centred healthcare and user involvement, e.g. striving for patient-centred care and patient health. Enabling service users to participate and contribute to the service.

Standard 4. Creating a healthy workplace and healthy setting, e.g. developing a setting which improves the health of patients, relatives, staff, support workers and volunteers (Figures 15.2–15.5 illustrate hospital art).

Standard 5. Promoting health in the wider society, e.g. contributing to promoting the health of the local population.

(INHPHHS, 2020)

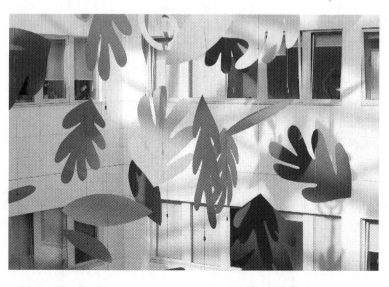

Figure 15.2 'Falling Leaves' by Sian Tucker at Chelsea and Westminster Hospital, London

Source: Sian Tucker, 'Falling Leaves', suspended in the academic atrium at Chelsea and Westminster Hospital. Reproduced with permission from CW+, the charity for Chelsea and Westminster Hospital NHS Foundation Trust

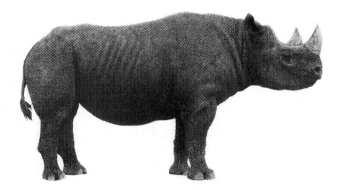

Figure 15.3 'Jos' by Jonathan Delafield Cook at Chelsea and Westminster Hospital, London

Source: Jonathan Delafield Cook, 'Jos', in the ground floor atrium at Chelsea and Westminster Hospital. Reproduced with permission from CW+, the charity for Chelsea and Westminster Hospital NHS Foundation Trust

Health promoting hospitals

Yaghoubi and colleagues (2019) carried out a review of 23 international studies published between 2000 and 2016 to collate the evidence about what enables hospitals to become health promoting hospitals (HPHs), some of the challenges they face and their reported outcomes. Their review focussed on hospitals, not wider healthcare services.

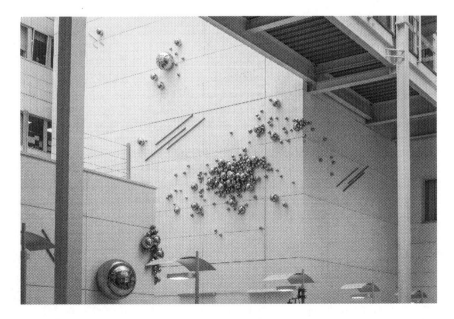

Figure 15.4 'Assembly450' by Joy Gerrard at Chelsea and Westminster Hospital, London

Source: Joy Gerrard, 'Assembly/450', in the first and second floor atrium at Chelsea and Westminster Hospital. Reproduced with permission from CW+, the charity for Chelsea and Westminster Hospital NHS Foundation Trust

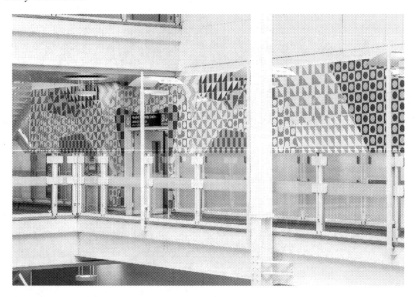

Figure 15.5 'Radiance' by Adam Nathaniel Furman at Chelsea and Westminster Hospital, London

Source: Adam Nathaniel Furman, 'Radiance', in the Reuben's Maternity Centre at Chelsea and Westminster Hospital. Photography by Gareth Gardner. Reproduced with permission from CW+, the charity for Chelsea and Westminster Hospital NHS Foundation Trust

Leadership

The support of hospital leaders is essential. They have the most opportunities to implement the Network's HPH standards, but managers largely ignore the concept. Those hospitals that have been more successful had the leadership and support to drive the required hospital development. Managers are sometimes resistant because health is not immediately profitable for them.

Policy and strategy

Hospitals need to integrate health into their goals, values and mission statements. From this, the appropriate resources, both financial and non-financial, from the local community can support their health promoting strategies. For example, they could set up health promotion committees. It helps to have government policies which support the drive towards HPHs.

People

Staff involvement in developing the HPH is vital. Staff with specialist knowledge and skills are needed to implement changes and evaluate them. Excellent communication and education skills are required. Engaging the hospital workforce in health promoting interventions increases their motivation and job satisfaction, and a lack of motivation is one reason why HPHs can stall. Staff education, enablement and empowerment are established as important factors for success, as is empowering patients and people in the local community. Fundamental are accurate assessments of the needs of patients, giving clear information to patients and providing good follow-up care post-discharge.

Partnerships and resources

Having sufficient people, time and skills are important, as are partnerships with other health-related providers and between the clinical staff and administrative staff. It is important to encourage people in the local community and social organisations to work with their local hospital and help towards creating a HPH. A challenge is persuading hospitals to allocate budgets to 'hard to measure' future health and disease prevention rather than immediate and 'easy to measure' treatments which attract positive attention.

Processes

A HPH improves health by improving its structure, culture and processes. Evaluation, for example patients' evaluation of care, is a key activity (Box 15.2).

Box 15.2   #Hello my name is

Dr Kate Granger was a doctor, specialising in elderly medicine, who was diagnosed with terminal cancer at the age of 29 in 2011. After one of many operations, she became aware of how many members of the hospital staff did not introduce themselves to her before providing care. She said, "It made me feel like I didn't really matter, that these people weren't bothered who I was and I ended up, at times, feeling like I was just a diseased body in a hospital bed." In August 2013, she and her husband started the '#Hello my name is' campaign on social media, asking for people to pledge their support. It aimed to change the NHS culture, and staff's behaviour, towards being more compassionate and person-centred.

Brian, a porter in the Emergency Department, was the first to introduce himself to Kate when she arrived in pain. He fetched her an extra pillow and blanket and ensured she was comfortable before he left. She said, "When somebody did introduce themselves it made such a difference to how I was feeling about myself. It made me feel more human again." Research shows that people who have better working relationships with their healthcare professionals have better outcomes, and compassionate care costs no money and can provide job satisfaction.

The core values of the campaign are:

- timely and effective communication, bespoke to the patient, starting with a simple introduction
- the little things matter, such as sitting at someone's level
- the most important person is the patient, and everything should be done with them in mind
- see the patient as a person, a human being, an individual with friends and family

Kate died in 2016, but her husband continues the '#Hello my name is' campaign, which is now embedded into many healthcare organisations across the world.

(Source: youtube.com/hashtag/hellomynameis; www.hellomynameis.org.uk)

Outcomes

Some of the activities reported by hospitals that are working towards becoming HPHs include

- creating a patient-centric culture
- promoting the general concept of a HPH
- creating an organisational structure in line with the HPH aims
- providing educational and counselling services for patients
- creating a healthy physical and psychosocial environment for staff and patients
- providing skills training to enhance patient and staff relations
- introducing environmental health and nutritional standards for the hospital
- including the hospital quality improvement team in the HPH project
- attending to patients' cultural and social backgrounds
- providing transparent and appropriate information to patients
- providing follow-up and convalescent care after discharge
- enabling people to manage their chronic illnesses and improve their health-related behaviours
- providing health promotion guidelines for specific disease groups
- evaluating patients' satisfaction
- considering the local community's culture and values
- introducing a system for staff recommendations
- enabling staff to improve their own health-related behaviour
- providing services in various settings beyond the hospital
- collaborating with local community organisations
- holding workshops with other hospitals
- continuous evaluation of the HPH process, impact and outcomes
- focussing on quality indicators instead of productivity
- using the media to disseminate disease prevention information

(Yaghoubi *et al.*, 2019)

The International Network of Health Promoting Hospitals and Health Services supports health services that want to become more health promoting.

Preventing disease and promoting health within healthcare

Irving Zola introduced the concept of the river to explain how healthcare practitioners were so focussed on heroically rescuing people from the river who had become ill, travelled 'downstream' and were now drowning, that they failed to notice what was causing people to fall into the river, 'upstream', in the first place (McKinlay, 1975) (Figure 15.6). Initially the NHS, influenced by the medical model, was focussed on treating and preventing biological causes of disease. Over the last four decades we have seen the NHS give more attention to disease prevention, which has meant focussing on risk factors and risk behaviours. In summary, the message suggests if people could avoid behaviours such as smoking, alcohol, unhealthy eating and sedentary behaviour, they would suffer less and the costs of healthcare would reduce, or at least the rate of increase would slow down. It is supported by a sound body of evidence (NHS, 2019). At the same time, we have also witnessed growing evidence that the social determinants

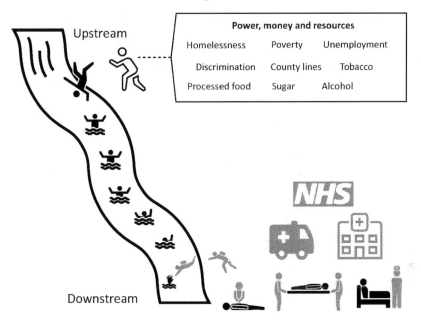

Figure 15.6 Zola's river

of health are upstream, at the source of the river. People's social position, which reflects their power, money and/or resources, determines how they live and work and then the type of accommodation, neighbourhood, employment and education they experience (Marmot *et al.*, 2020). Along with the industries that promote tobacco, processed food, alcohol and so forth, these factors encourage some people to the water's edge; they are more vulnerable to developing poorer health than others and then falling into the river. In summary, these two positions reflect the medical model and the social model of health and illness (Robinson, 2021a). The UK health system, and its better integration of services, is trying to bring the medical and social models together to prevent disease and promote better health for all. These two models, and the river analogy, tend to dominate how we approach public health in the UK today.

All Our Health

All Our Health is a collection of online resources (Gov.UK, 2022). It is described as comprising evidence-based training and guidance for UK healthcare professionals to prevent illness, protect health and promote wellbeing. It advises:

- think prevention first
- be aware of the health needs within the local community including those who may be vulnerable or feel socially excluded, e.g. by reading the local health profiles
- know what activities can help to protect and promote health, e.g. screening, reducing alcohol consumption or avoiding the causes of disease such as air pollution
- know the local resources and services; work with and work within the local community, e.g. make referrals, share resources, and jointly plan and deliver non-clinical interventions with charities, community groups and individuals

Examples from the online collection include

- *Healthy beginnings* explains how children living in more deprived areas are more likely to be exposed to more avoidable risks and have poorer health outcomes by the time they go to school. Healthcare practitioners can reduce health inequalities by providing support during preconception, pregnancy and the first 1,001 days of life. For example, support needs to include parental and children's emotional and social wellbeing and children's early communication skills as these influence their whole life course
- *Healthcare public health* includes encouraging healthcare professionals to access training to become more confident in preventing and managing cardiovascular disease including discussing the risk factors such as smoking, obesity and alcohol; encouraging health checks for high blood pressure or raised blood cholesterol; knowing where to refer patients; identifying who is at greater risk of developing cardiovascular disease in the local community and working with partners in the local community such as community weight services or leisure centres
- *Supporting health, wellbeing and independence* includes encouraging professionals to explain how we reduce the risks of developing dementia through physical activity, healthy eating, no smoking, minimal alcohol, health checks for diabetes and high blood pressure, and being socially active. It includes knowing local services and sources of help, supporting carers and creating dementia-friendly environments
- *Health protection* includes understanding the health impacts of air pollution, knowing what advice to give during a high pollution episode, registering for air pollution alerts and supporting Clean Air Day and other initiatives to reduce air pollution. Health protection also includes how to prevent infections and reduce antimicrobial resistance
- *Health improvement* includes encouraging professionals to understand and educate about the benefits of screening; good oral, sexual and reproductive health; physical activity; and avoiding tobacco, obesity, excess alcohol and the misuse of illicit drugs
- *Improving the wider determinants of health* includes the importance of health for all, ensuring practitioners use their skills of empathy and kindness to enable those who may feel socially excluded to access the health system. Healthcare practitioners need to assess people holistically, beyond their immediate complaint, and provide bespoke interventions. Practitioners need the knowledge and skills to best support people with learning disabilities and mental health needs. This theme also includes understanding community concerns such as homelessness, county lines and health in local workplaces
- *Place-based services of care* means healthcare practitioners offering services in the community rather than offering them within traditional NHS settings. This means working in partnership with local people to listen, plan, design, deliver and evaluate initiatives aimed at improving health. Initiatives may be 'non-clinical' such as social prescribing (see Chapter 2 and Box 15.3), and they may be led by members of the community such as peer support networks. Place-based services are person-centred/community-centred and strengths-based, and often start with building trust and relationships

Aaron Antonovsky (1996) argued that Zola's river analogy is pathogenic. It is concerned with those who are drowning, those who are upstream and could be prevented from travelling further, and those on the water's edge about to fall in. Risk factors, which could be biological, behavioural, psychological or social in nature, will cause people to move downstream towards disease, with the eventual outcome of death. Pathogenesis means the focus is on preventing risk factors for a disease. It is disease-centred.

Box 15.3 Social prescribing

In 2021, the former Chief Pharmaceutical Officer for England, Dr Keith Ridge, found that 10 per cent of prescriptions for medicines, in primary care settings, were either inappropriate or the ailment could be better addressed with a non-medical intervention. The over-medicalisation of health has been a concern since Ivan Illich wrote about iatrogenesis in 1976 – 'medicine causes harm'. More recently, concerns about the dangers of over-prescribing, including anti-microbial resistance where antibiotics no longer work; concerns about spiralling healthcare costs; the rise of long-term conditions including chronic pain and emotional distress for which treatment is limited; as well as demands for improved social care have encouraged practitioners to look to non-medical solutions including the arts and health (see Chapter 11). Social prescribing, which was endorsed by the NHS in 2019, enables practitioners to refer individuals to social prescribing link workers, sometimes called care navigators, who are often attached to General Practitioner surgeries. They make an assessment and then match individuals to services and opportunities in their local community.

Referrals to link workers can be made by the individual themselves, local authorities, pharmacies, general practice/primary care services, hospital discharge teams, the police and fire services, social services, housing associations and social enterprise organisations. Social prescribing can include baking, singing, gardening, art, reading groups, physical activity, dancing, social/support groups, debt advice, confidence-building courses, walking groups, befriending schemes and groups focussed on particular interests such as metalwork or even laughter yoga.

Helena, a social prescribing link worker in Newcastle Upon Tyne, is based in a GP surgery. She describes her work as focussing on what really matters to a person and identifying the barriers that are preventing them from achieving it. She explains her work as a process of building a one-to-one relationship and working with the individual throughout their journey. Helena's background was working as a public health specialist, where she had acquired an in-depth knowledge of the local community and the available social opportunities. Over a six-month period, she helped 120 individuals.

Jim's house was full of boxes, rubbish and piles of paper. His drains were blocked, and he wasn't paying his rent. It transpired that Jim had lost the landlord's telephone number so he couldn't report the blocked drain and was unable to discuss the rent. A care navigator helped Jim to clean and sort out his house, found the telephone number, and the rent and drain were sorted. She also introduced him to a local community café which he started to attend regularly. He began to engage with local people and his siblings, and his emotional and physical health markedly improved.

Dr Marie-Anne Essam, a general practitioner, describes social prescribing as, "… the most effective, wide reaching and life changing initiatives to date … Social prescribing changes people and places for the better … we can … 'demedicalise' aspects of our NHS, and see resilience grow …"

One of the challenges of social prescribing is raising awareness among healthcare practitioners to refer people to the service. Another is a reluctance to engage with social prescribing because practitioners are waiting for better evidence that it works, holding it to the same rigorous standards of medical effectiveness. Others argue it is a holistic approach, and there is already sufficient evidence that it helps many people, and the NHS cannot afford *not* to engage with social prescribing.

(Source: DHSC, 2021; Illich, 1976; NHS, 2022)

For example, disease prevention is concerned with preventing cardiovascular disease in those who are well and preventing those with cardiovascular disease from developing further unpleasant symptoms. The disease is the focus, regardless of other aspects of a person's health and their life, or whether the person will die from a traffic accident.

Thinking point:

To what extent is All Our Health pathogenic?

Salutogenesis

Antonovsky (1996) described how salutogenesis was central to health promotion. The origins of the word 'salutogenesis' lie in the Latin word 'salus' which means health and in the Greek word 'genesis' which means origin. In contrast to Zola's river analogy, Antonovsky argued we are all in a river; it is 'the river of life' as we travel from conception to death, and possibly beyond. Disrupters, such as illness, disease, bad news, a bereavement, being made homeless, experiencing discrimination or undertaking an unhealthy behaviour which causes back ache, will disrupt a person's life causing them dis-ease while their life continues. If they are fortunate, they will recover, return to 'ease' and continue onwards with their life (Figure 15.7). Rather than focussing on specific disrupters, such as how to prevent a single disease, a cause of unhappiness or backache, which is the pathogenic approach, Antonovsky was concerned with what resources support 'ease', a good life. He argued we need to (i) understand the causes of dis-ease, the disrupters, and (ii) we need to ensure that all people have the best tools to navigate their lives, to swim in the river of life with ease. If we can do this, we may achieve a good quality of life for all. The perception of having good health is central to people's perceptions of having a good quality of life. As we go through life and we experience disruptions, such as an illness, we learn how to cope with it, how to avoid it in future and what makes us feel better. We learn and we continue to learn. So, for Antonovsky, the work of achieving health is a personal and unique process of life-long learning which contributes to achieving a sense of 'ease' and a good quality of life. Now we have moved away from a disease-centred model to one that is truly person-centred.

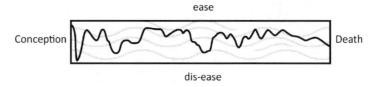

Figure 15.7 Navigating Antonovsky's river of life between ease and dis-ease

To carry out salutogenic, person-centred health promotion is to acknowledge the complexity of humans. Healthcare practitioners cannot claim to be promoting the health of a person with advanced cancer if they ignore aspects of the person beyond the disease. They must engage with all aspects of the person. As discussed in Chapter 1, health is person-centred, time dependent, positive and holistic. However, this presents challenges to those who are often working within a healthcare organisation that is pathogenic and disease-centred in orientation. Antonovsky writes,

> "The provider of care must indeed be highly empathic and sensitive to withstand the pressure to forget the human being who has the disease. The health promoter, irrespective of her personal bent, is pressured to be concerned with the person."
> (Antonovsky, 1996, p. 14)

For example, a midwife working with a feminist model of healthcare wants to empower a pregnant woman to be at the centre of her care and make her own choices. However, her choices might create a professional risk for the midwife who is governed by the clinical protocols and policies of the NHS.

Salutogenesis means focussing on those assets, resources and strengths which will help a person, or a community, move towards better health. Today, salutogenesis can be thought of as an umbrella term for a broad range of concepts, theories and elements with the same purpose (Figure 15.8).

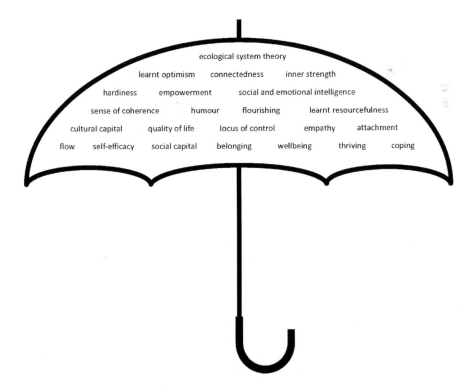

Figure 15.8 The salutogenic umbrella

Source: Adapted from Eriksson and Mittelmark, 2017, p. 103

Sense of coherence

One salutogenic concept is the sense of coherence. Antonovsky's (1996) research sought to find out what human characteristics support a good quality of life. This led him to a collection of characteristics which he called having a sense of coherence. For people with a strong sense of coherence, their world makes sense at a cognitive (thinking), emotional (feeling) and instrumental (practical) level. The world is perceived as being meaningful, comprehensible and manageable. They will

- make sense of it and be motivated to cope with it (meaningfulness)
- understand it (comprehensible)
- believe they have the resources to handle it (manageable)

Sense of coherence is explained as,

> "One has a pervasive, enduring though dynamic feeling of confidence that the stimuli from one's internal and external environments ... are structured, predictable, and explicable; the resources are available ... to meet the demands; and these demands are ... worthy of investment and engagement ..."
>
> (Mana *et al.*, 2021, p. 2)

In the context of healthcare, the more a person can comprehend a disease, a situation, a health-related intervention, a treatment or other aspect of care; manage it and make sense of it, the greater their chances of being better able to cope with it (Box 15.4).

A person's sense of coherence comes from their life experiences, their prior learning about what gives their life meaning, what type of resources are helpful for them to have a good quality of life, how much information they think they need and so forth. They recall these at times of 'dis-ease', seek them out, use them, and then evaluate and learn again. A sense of coherence is shaped and reshaped. It helps people towards their vision of a good quality of life, including good health. Research has shown that people are likely to develop a strong sense of coherence when they have good connections with the place they live. This means there is a synergy between themselves and

---

Box 15.4 Hospice ward manager

"By focussing on the individual, involving them in their care planning, supporting their relationships and building on their strengths, it is possible to promote their health and wellbeing. We try to empower patients to take some control over their situation. It's important that we provide information and education about health, dying and death, not only for our patients but for their families and the wider community. Patients can express fear of hospices, believing them to be miserable foreboding places where people just go to die. Although this perception usually changes quite quickly on admission, much unnecessary anxiety has already been experienced by the patient. Such misconceptions apply not only to hospices, but to death, dying and bereavement in general. Ideally, education about these matters needs to be a component of promoting health, and it needs to take place before a person is dying or requires admission to a hospice."

(Reproduced with permission)

their groups, their socio-economic and cultural surroundings, and the psychological and emotional context of their lives (Lindstrom, 2011). People's sense of coherence increases across their life course, and those with the highest sense of coherence are among older people. A strong sense of coherence is central to having a healthy orientation to life. The evidence shows it is associated with

- living longer
- choosing healthier behaviours such as less alcohol and tobacco, healthier eating and more physical activity
- managing stress and life events better
- improving resilience
- better management of an acute or chronic disease such as diabetes, cardiovascular disease, cancer and mental disorders
- perceptions of having a good quality of life
- perceptions of good health
- being better able to cope with the regular stressors of life
- being less emotionally distressed during the COVID-19 coronavirus pandemic
                    (Eriksson and Lindström, 2006; Lindstrom, 2011; Mana *et al.*, 2021)

Those personal or community characteristics which support a strong sense of coherence are called generalised resistance resources. These include

- material resources, e.g. money
- ego identity, having an integrated but flexible sense of self
- knowledge, intelligence and skills
- coping strategies
- social support
- cultural stability
- a commitment to, and cohesion with, one's cultural roots
- ritualistic activities, e.g. habits and routines
- religion and philosophy, e.g. having some answers to the complex nature of life
- an orientation towards good health and preventing disease
- a person's general constitution and genetics

                                                                          (Idan *et al.*, 2017)

How to strengthen someone's sense of coherence is a topic of current research. For example, in Norway researchers took two groups of patients receiving outpatient care for mental health problems (Langeland *et al.*, 2006). One group received standard care ($n = 47$) and the other received standard care plus participation in salutogenic talking-therapy groups ($n = 59$). The aim of the groups was to increase the individuals' awareness of their potential, their external and internal general resistance resources and their ability to put these resources into action. The results showed that coping with everyday living improved significantly among those who had participated in the intervention. There is some evidence to suggest that a sense of coherence may be increased by

- working in ways that enhance people's sense of security and belonging, perhaps within a group or building connections with a community
- creating opportunities to discuss feelings

- encouraging self-reflection, e.g. considering what helped last time they were in pain
- experiential/active learning by doing and participating
- working with an empowerment model of health promotion to enable individuals to put their prior learning into action

> (Idan *et al.*, 2017; Super *et al.*, 2016; Thompson *et al.*, 2021)

Thinking point:

To what extent is All Our Health salutogenic?

Promoting health combines preventing disease, preventing a deterioration in people's quality of life and supporting people's assets to enable them to meet their goals for health and a good quality of life.

Health promoting healthcare practitioners

Promoting health is not only about communicating to achieve biological/medical/ behavioural outcomes; it is a communication process that includes psychological and social dimensions. Healthcare practitioners need to

- work with what people know, believe and feel as well as what motivates them
- understand how people's social situations may have led them to needing health-care. This includes knowing what the local health profiles show (see Chapter 9), understanding how the social determinants of health are a powerful influence on people's health-related choices and behaviours, and lending their support to actions for a healthier society
- recognise promoting health is a process as well as an outcome. It is about 'how' practitioners communicate, not just 'what' they communicate

Here, we consider some examples of how healthcare practitioners may work with individuals in a healthcare context.

Changing health-related behaviours

It is often unrealistic to expect people to change their health-related behaviour in one conversation. There are many steps to people deciding to change a health-related behaviour and then putting it into practice. These are shown in Table 7.4 (p.180) and in the models and theories of health-related behaviour change, discussed in Chapter 5. Sometimes, the aim of one conversation is simply to open a door, to raise awareness. The next conversation opens the door wider. Bit by bit, an individual becomes more aware of an issue, and

- after the next conversation, they build their knowledge
- after the next, they may begin to change how they feel about the prospect of changing behaviour
- after the next, they clarify what they want to do and why they are motivated to do it
- after the next, they make a decision
- after the next, they are ready to act and start to develop a new skill or behaviour

This process may occur quickly, in the space of an hour, or it may take years. Each conversation, no matter who it is with, adds up.

In the UK, Making Every Contact Count (MECC) (PHE *et al.*, 2016) is about having short conversations about health-related behaviours such as stopping smoking, healthy eating or improving mental health, which are appropriately timed and sensitively judged. A priority for healthcare practitioners is to build a trusting relationship with individuals. This must not be jeopardised by insensitive and poorly timed conversations and nor, says MECC, must it be about telling someone how to live their life. 'Light-touch' health-related conversations need to become normalised within healthcare. MECC advises practitioners to

- sit or stand at the individual's level
- try to be friendly and, if appropriate, smile
- ask open questions to understand the individual, explore their personal situation and learn what matters to them.
- treat the person as an equal in this conversation
- avoid interrupting
- be aware that the tone and pace of your voice is appropriate; avoid speaking too fast, so the individual has time to take information in and to think
- take care not to judge the individual
- check if there is something else the individual wants to talk about
- check that you have each understood one another
- either provide information, direct them to a service or enable them to consider ways towards finding their own solutions

The types of questions which might be helpful include,

"What are your goals? What is the number one priority for you?"

"I'm noticing that you are struggling with your breathing. What do you think might be causing this?"

"I think you might find breathing easier if you were carrying a little less weight. How do you feel about trying to lose some weight?"

"You mentioned earlier that you have been struggling since your wife died. Would you like to tell me a little more about this?"

"So, to sum up, you are feeling lonely and struggling with managing meals. Have I understood correctly?"

"I understand your reasons for not taking the medicine for your high blood cholesterol. Would you be open to considering some alternative non-medical ways forward?"

"It's really good that you have mentioned this. Now, if you like, we can work on this together and try to improve the situation."

"We have a leaflet about increasing physical activity as part of everyday life. Would you be interested in it?"

Practitioners need to find out and keep in mind each person's own goals for their own health. They need to find out about the person's generalised resistance resources; foster their sense of belonging, capabilities and inner strengths; and support their self-confidence and self-esteem. They need to help individuals to understand their situation and make any proposed change meaningful and manageable for them, for example encouraging them to identify what positives or rewards would be meaningful to them if they made a change. For example,

> "You say that you successfully stopped smoking five years ago. That's brilliant. What or who helped you to give up smoking?"

> "What *can* you do comfortably?"

> "What would it mean to you if you could achieve this?"

> "Would you like some information about the support group that meets on Wednesdays?"

> "I think you are doing really well. Have you thought of a reward for yourself when you meet your goal?"

It is understandable that some healthcare practitioners feel under-prepared to discuss health issues; health is often only a small part of their healthcare education. It was partly to meet this need that the companion book to this one, *Priorities for Health Promotion and Public Health* (Robinson, 2021b), was written and opportunities for short continuing development courses are more numerous than they used to be (e.g. HEE, 2022).

The process of promoting health as an intrinsic part of care

Healthcare practitioners often cite a lack of time and resources as barriers to promoting health. It is true that some health promotion may take the form of a longer conversation; it may be an 'add on' such as an additional clinic, service, event, a special day, or a week such as Mental Health Awareness week, Movember or Dry January; but once we understand health promotion as a process – of learning and empowering – as well as outcomes, we see that many healthcare practitioners are already using many of the core communication skills needed to promote health within their care. Those who

- listen to people
- talk with people
- are 'with' people
- are advocates for people
- smile
- introduce themselves
- make human connections
- demonstrate good two-way, equal communication
- demonstrate kindness and empathy
- demonstrate and share their problem-solving skills
- have resilience

- ask for help from others
- apologise when they get something wrong
- demonstrate curiosity about people and their worlds
- are motivated to help individuals and groups to attain what health means to them

are promoting health.

To what degree healthcare practitioners should be role models for good health, 'practising what they preach' is hotly debated. For example, nurses in one study (Wills *et al.*, 2019) said,

> "We should act what we say."
>
> (p. 428)

> "… being told to lose weight by a thin person is not very motivating – patients think you don't understand."
>
> (p. 428)

> "It's how I talk to patients that matters."
>
> (p. 428)

> "I give enough to this place, so what I eat and look like is my business."
>
> (p. 428)

Some argue that the priority is for nurses to be 'human' not perfect, empathic and someone who understands the challenges involved in changing people's health-related behaviour (Kelly *et al.*, 2016). Others are asking whether it is fair to expect a healthcare practitioner to be a role model for health if their employers do not provide a health promoting setting in which to become one. There are countless ways in which the NHS can become more health promoting for staff, visitors and patients, as discussed above. For staff, this includes a healthy working environment and culture including having adequate staffing; stability; opportunities to learn about, develop and experience healthy attitudes and behaviours in the workplace; and invitations to contribute new ideas for improving health in the NHS.

With the support of a health promoting setting, healthcare practitioners can learn more about health, build on their existing skills and encourage the NHS to live up to its name as a National Health Service within the wider UK health system.

Summary

This chapter has

- described some of the consequences of creating the NHS as a disease-centred care service rather than one focussed on health
- defined a health system and illustrated how current UK policy aims to integrate the NHS into a wider health system
- outlined the characteristics of a healthy NHS

- discussed the difference between pathogenesis and salutogenesis and their importance to promoting health within healthcare
- provided examples of how healthcare practitioners can prevent disease and promote health
- suggested there is a need for healthcare practitioners to learn more about health and acknowledged that many use health promoting skills in their care

Further reading

Allied Health Professions Federation (2019) *UK allied health professions public health strategic framework 2019–2024*. Available at: https://www.health-ni.gov.uk/sites/default/files/publications/health/uk-ahp-public-health.pdf

Bowden, J. and Manning, V. (eds) (2016) *Health promotion in midwifery. Principles and practice*. 3rd edn. London: Routledge

Evans, D., Coutsaftiki, D. and Fathers C.P. (2017) *Health promotion and public health for nursing students*. 3rd edn. London: Sage

Useful websites

International Network of Health Promoting Hospitals and Health Services. Available at: www.hphnet.org

Making Every Contact Count. Available at: https://www.makingeverycontactcount.co.uk

National Academy for Social Prescribing. Available at: https://socialprescribingacademy.org.uk

The Kings Fund: public health. Available at: https://www.kingsfund.org.uk/topics/public-health

References

Antonovsky, A. (1996) 'The salutogenic model as a theory to guide health promotion', *Health Promotion International*, 11(1), pp. 11–18

Baggott, R. (2004) *Health and health care in Britain*. 3rd edn. Basingstoke: Palgrave

Baggott, R. (2013) *Partnerships for public health and well-being*. Basingstoke: Palgrave/Macmillan

Commissioning Board Chief Nursing Officer and Department of Health Chief Nursing Adviser (2012) *Compassion in practice*. London: Department of Health/National Health Service

Department of Health and Social Care (2021) *Good for you, good for us, good for everybody*. Available at: https://assets.publishing.service.gov.uk/government/uploads/system/uploads/attachment_data/file/1019475/good-for-you-good-for-us-good-for-everybody.pdf (Accessed 14th June 2022)

Eriksson, M. and Lindström, B. (2006) 'Antonovsky's sense of coherence scale and the relation with health: a systematic review', *Journal of Epidemiology and Community Health*, 60(5), pp. 376–381

Eriksson, M. and Mittelmark, M.B. (2017) 'The sense of coherence and its measurement', in Mittelmark, M.B., Sagy, S., Eriksson, M., Bauer, G.F., Pelikan, J.M., Lindström, B. and Espenes, G.A. (eds) *The handbook of salutogenesis*. Springer, pp. 97–106. Available at: https://link.springer.com/chapter/10.1007%2F978-3-319-04600-6_12 (Accessed 10th June 2022)

Gov.UK (2013) *The health and care system explained*. Available at: https://www.gov.uk/government/publications/the-health-and-care-system-explained/the-health-and-care-system-explained (Accessed 12th June 2022)

Gov.UK (2022) *Collection. All our health: personalised care and population health*. Available at: https://www.gov.uk/government/collections/all-our-health-personalised-care-and-population-health#about-all-our-health (Accessed 13th June 2022)

Health Education England (2022) *Making every contact count*. Available at: https://www.e-lfh.org.uk/programmes/making-every-contact-count (Accessed 13th June 2022)

H.M. Government (2021) *Build back better. Our plan for health and social care.* Available at: https://www.gov.uk/government/publications/build-back-better-our-plan-for-health-and-social-care (Accessed 10th June 2022)

Idan, O., Eriksson, M. and Al-Yagon, M. (2017) 'The salutogenic model: the role of generalized resistance resources', in Mittelmark, M.B., Sagy, S., Eriksson, M., Bauer, G.F., Pelikan, J.M., Lindström, B. and Espenes, G.A. (eds) *The handbook of salutogenesis.* Springer, pp. 57–70. Available at: https://www.ncbi.nlm.nih.gov/books/NBK435841 (Accessed 13th June 2022)

Illich, I. (1976) *Limits to medicine: medical nemesis: the expropriation of health.* London: Marion Boyars

International Network of Health Promoting Hospitals and Health Services (2020) *2020 standards for health promoting hospitals and health services.* Available at: www.hphnet.org/wp-content/uploads/2020/12/2020-HPH-Standards.pdf (Accessed 10th June 2022)

Kelly, M., Wills, J., Jester, R. and Speller, V. (2016) 'Should nurses be role models for healthy lifestyles? Results from a modified Delphi study', *Journal of Advanced Nursing*, 73(3), pp. 665–678

Langeland, E., Riise, T., Hanestad, B.R., Bortvedt, M.W., Kristoffersen, K. and Wahl, A.K. (2006) 'The effect of salutogenic treatment principles on coping with mental health problems. A randomised controlled trial', *Patient Education and Counseling*, 62(2), pp. 212–219

Legislation.gov.uk (2012) *Health and social care act 2012.* Available at: https://www.legislation.gov.uk/ukpga/2012/7/contents/enacted (Accessed 13th June 2022)

Lindstrom, B. (2011) 'Salutogenesis and NCDs', Introductory paper presented at *Project Planning Meeting for NCD Flagship Projects* (23rd March). St Petersburg, Russia. Available at: http://www.ndphs.org/?mtgs,ncd_project_planning_1 (Accessed 11th June 2022)

Mana, A., Bauer, G.F., Magistretti, C.M. *et al.* (2021) 'Order out of chaos: sense of coherence and the mediating role of coping resources in explaining mental health during COVID-19 in 7 countries', *SSM-Mental Health*, 1 doi:10.1016/j.ssmmh.2021.100001

Marmot, M., Allen, J., Boyce, T., Goldblatt, P. and Morrison, J. (2020) *Health equity in England: the Marmot review 10 years on.* London: Institute of Health Equity

McKinlay, J.B. (1975) 'A case for refocussing upstream: the political economy of sickness', in Enelow, J.D. and Henderson, J.B. (ed) *Applying behavioral science to cardiovascular risk.* New York: American Heart Association, pp. 9–25

National Health Service (2014) *Five year forward view.* Available at: https://www.england.nhs.uk/wp-content/uploads/2014/10/5yfv-web.pdf (Accessed 10th June 2022)

National Health Service (2019) *The long term plan.* Available at: https://www.longtermplan.nhs.uk (Accessed 13th June 2022)

National Health Service (2022) *Case studies.* Available at: https://www.england.nhs.uk/personalisedcare/upc/comprehensive-model/case-studies (Accessed 14th June 2022)

Nolte, E., Merkur, S. and Anell, A. (eds) (2020) *Achieving person-centred health systems.* Cambridge: Cambridge University Press/World Health Organization (Eur)

Public Health England, NHS England and Health Education England (2016) *Making every contact count (MECC): consensus statement.* Available at: https://www.england.nhs.uk/wp-content/uploads/2016/04/making-every-contact-count.pdf (Accessed 14th June 2022)

Robinson, S. (2021a) 'Social context of health and illness', in Robinson, S. (ed) *Priorities for health promotion and public health. Explaining the evidence for disease prevention and health promotion.* London: Routledge, pp. 3–33

Robinson, S. (ed) (2021b) *Priorities for health promotion and public health. Explaining the evidence for disease prevention and health promotion.* London: Routledge

Scottish Government (2013) *A route map to the 2020 vision for health and social care.* Available at: http://www.sspc.ac.uk/media/Media_473395_smxx.pdf (Accessed 14th June 2022)

Super, S., Wagemakers, M.A.E., Picavet, H.S.J., Verkooijen, K.T. and Koelen, M.A. (2016) 'Strengthening sense of coherence: opportunities for theory building in health promotion', *Health Promotion International*, 31(4), pp. 869–878

Thompson, K., Herens, M., van Ophem, J. and Wagemakers, A. (2021) 'Strengthening sense of coherence: evidence from a physical activity intervention targeting vulnerable adults', *Preventive Medicine Reports*, 24 doi:10.1016/j.pmedr.2021.101554

Tønnesen, H. (2011) 'Clinical health promotion – what does it mean?', *Clinical Health Promotion*, 1(2), pp. 39–40

Welsh Government (2021) *A healthier Wales: our plan for health and social care.* Available at: https://gov.wales/sites/default/files/publications/2021-09/a-healthier-wales-our-plan-for-health-and-social-care.pdf (Accessed 10th June 2022)

Wills, J., Kelly, M. and Frings, D. (2019) 'Nurses as role models in health promotion: piloting the acceptability of a social marketing campaign', *Journal of Advanced Nursing*, 75(2), pp. 423–431

World Health Organization (1946) *Constitution.* Geneva: World Health Organization

World Health Organization (1978) *Declaration of Alma-Ata. International conference on primary health care. Alma-Ata, USSR, 6–12 September 1978.* Available at: https://www.who.int/docs/default-source/documents/almaata-declaration-en.pdf (Accessed 13th June 2022)

World Health Organization (2007) *Everybody's business. Strengthening health systems to improve health outcomes.* Geneva: World Health Organization

World Health Organization (2019a) *Stronger collaboration, better health. Global action plan for healthy lives and well-being for all.* Geneva: World Health Organization

World Health Organization (2019b) *Promote health. Keep the world safe. Serve the vulnerable. Thirteenth general programme of work 2019–2023.* Geneva: World Health Organization

Yaghoubi, M., Karamali, M. and Bahadori, M. (2019) 'Effective factors in implementation and development of health promoting hospitals: a systematic review', *Health Promotion International*, 34(4), pp. 811–823

Index

Note: Locators in *italics* represent figures and **bold** indicate tables in the text

2-Day Diet 342–343
2030 Agenda for Sustainable Development 20,
    21, 21, **200**, 201, 213, 304–306

abnormality 270
absorption 324
academia, research and teaching 114
academic public health 30
acceptance 184
Acheson, Donald 230, 232
active engagement 276
Adams, J. 122
advocacy 29, 188–189, 199, 219–221, 305
affective: communication 134; learning 134,
    179
age-specific mortality rate 72
aggression 4–5
airborne transmission of infectious agent 67
Ajzen, I. 118, 120
alcohol: control 305–306; Global Alcohol
    Action Plan 305; health warnings 311–313
Alcoholics Anonymous (AA) 316–317
All Our Health 395–398
Alzheimer's disease 72
American Psychological Association 113–114
anabolism 325
analytical studies 80–82
AND/OR Boolean operators 94
anger 124
An-Nafi, Ign 69
annual public health reports 225, 232
antibodies 256–257, *257*
antigen 256–257, 268
antimicrobial resistance (AMR) 261–262
Anti-social Behaviour Crime and Policing
    Act 2014 302–303
Antonovsky, A. 169, 396, 398–400
Antonovsky's river of life between ease and
    dis-ease *398*
anxiety 124, 209, 356–357
appraisal tool **96**

Aristotle 113, 177, 280
arts and health 275–278; art forms with
    examples 275, *276*; contribution 280–282;
    engagement across prevention 276–277,
    281; future of 290; history 278–280; in
    hospital 280; interventions 277; online,
    digital and electronic arts 286–287;
    performing arts 282–285; radio and
    community health promotion 286–287;
    visual arts, design and craft 288–290;
    works in **280**
art therapy 277
association 75
Astbury, N.M. 339
attitude 119

Bacon, Francis 89
Bacteroides bacteria 344
basal metabolic rate (BMR) 325–326
Baumeister, R.F. 5, 7
BBC Music Day, 2019 283–284
Becker, M.H. 116
behaviour 119
Behavioural Insights Team (The Nudge
    Unit) 127
behavioural intention 119
behaviour change: behaviour approach 173;
    health-related behaviours 12, 113, 115, 152,
    402–404; *see also* models and theories of
    behaviour change
Belfast Healthy City 214
Bell, R. 370
benevolence **5**
Bhopal disaster, 1984 262
bill of mortality 69–70, *70*
bioecological model of human
    development *6*
biological body 8
biological factors 15
biopsychosocial model 11, 14–15, 114, 280
biopsychosocial model *14*

Black Death 254
body fat: excess **346**; visceral fat 324, 328
body mass index (BMI) 323
Boer War (1899–1902) 227
bonding 208
bovine spongiform encephalopathy (BSE) 232, 259
Bowling, A. 106
Boyce, N. 69
Bradshaw's taxonomy of needs 207
Braille 137
brain 3–5
Brandes, K. 125
breast cancer 116–118, 270
breast screening 270
breathing or lung problem 357
Brexit referendum 369
bridging 208
British Psychological Society 114
British Sign Language (BSL) 139
Bronfenbrenner, U. 5
Brug, J. 122
bubonic plague of 1352 254
Build Back Better, 2021 388
Buncefield oil storage depot 264
Burton, A.K. 355–356
Bushman, B.J. 5, 7

calorie(s): consumption 346; expenditure 329, 346–347; overconsumption of 242, 323, 345
campylobacter bacteria 259
campylobacter food poisoning 253
cannabinoid type 1 receptors 331, 346
carbohydrates 324, 330, 342
cardiovascular disease 15, 74, 76, 124, 174, 196, 209, 286, 288, 324, 329, 340, 343, 356, 365–367, 372, 396, 398, 401
care 14, 50, 145, 148, 153, 167, 189, 205, 216, 231–232, 240, 278, 290, 360–361, 375, 382, 384, 393, 396, 399, 404–405
career routes 56, **57–58**
Carpenter, C.J. 118
case-control studies 82, *82*
case-finding 268
case study 102
catabolism 325
causation 75
cause: component 75; and effect 63, 72, 75–77; necessary 75; sufficient 75
census 78, 80, 231, 358, 360
Central Council for Health Education 166, 227
cervical screening 270
Chadwick, Edwin 225–226, *226*
Chartered Institute of Personnel and Development (CIPD) 375, *376*; CIPD

Wellbeing model 375–376, *376*; Good Work Index 359, 374
chemical, biological, radiological and nuclear (CBRN) hazards 262; common exposures in the UK 264–265; emergency planning and response 262–265
Chernobyl disaster, 1984 263
cholera 225
chronic obstructive pulmonary disease (COPD) 284–285
clinical trials 84
clostridium 259
Cocaine Anonymous (CA) 316
Cochi, S.L. 257
cognitive: communication 133; learning 179; skills 6, 188
cognitive learning 134, 179
cohort studies 81
common diseases from food 259–260
common-sense model 113, *123*, 123–126
communicable diseases 66, 74, 114, 225, 249–251; agencies 252; control measures 254; managing pandemics 254–255; outbreak management 252–253; pathogens 250–251; point source outbreak 253–254; surveillance and management 251–254; transmission 250–251
communication/health communication 133–136, 148; aim 134; clear content 134–135; communication models and theories 150–151; communication process 135–136; continuum *148*; digital communication 145–146; elaboration likelihood model 150; group work 141–142; health belief model 149; heuristic-systematic model 150–151; interpersonal communication 137, 144, 147; intrapersonal communication 137; mass communication 142–145; non-verbal communication 139; one-to-one communication 139–141; one-way communication 136–137; with people 139–142; purpose 134–137; self-efficacy 151; social marketing 146–147; theories of behaviour change 149–150; theory of planned behaviour 149; transtheoretical model 149–150; two-way communication 136–137; types of 137–139; verbal communication 137–138; World Health Organization' Strategic Communications Framework 147–148
community action 209
community-based 209, 210, 227
community consultation 209
community development 29, 50, 54, 199, 219–211, 221
community development worker **36**
community disempowerment 211
community empowerment 186–189

Community Empowerment Act, 2015 212
community infections 229
community trials 84
comparative need 207
competencies 28
competencies for working in health promotion and public health 42; International Union for Health Promotion and Education (IUHPE) 49; Public Health Skills and Knowledge Framework (PHSKF) 42–43; UK Public Health Register (UKPHR) Practitioner Standards for Registration 49; WHO-ASPHER competency framework 45–49
CompHP Competencies and Professional Standards 53
comprehensive or detailed HIAs 243
conative learning 134, 179
conformity **5**
confounders 81
confounding 81
congruence 184
consciousness raising 120
consent form 110
contemplation 121, 149
Conti, Leonard 23
continuing professional development (CPD) 50, 52, 56, 59
continuous dieting/continuous energy restriction 335–340
control group 83
Control of Substances Hazardous to Health (COSHH) 264, 363
convenience sampling 108
Convention against Illicit Traffic in Narcotic Drugs and Psychotropic Substances 1988 306
Convention on Psychotropic Substances 1971 306
Copernicus 89
coping: approach 124; avoidance 124
core conditions: acceptance 184; congruence 184; empathy 184
counselling 114
counterconditioning 120
covert observation 106
COVID-19 coronavirus pandemic 29, 65, 118, 208–209, 228, 254–255, 361, 364; epidemiology 66; mass communication 143; media campaign 144; outbreak 66
Creative Arts Pilot Project 288–289
Crime and Disorder Act 1998 241
critical appraisal **91**
critical pedagogy 188
cross contamination 260–261
crude mortality rate 73
crude rates 72
cryptosporidium 259

cultural rules 5
cultural symbolism 9
culture 5, 9, 17, 127, 188–189, 265, 363, 390
Cylospora 259

Damghanian, M. 116
data 90
data analysis **91**
databases 92–95
death rates by occupation **359**
Declaration of Alma-Ata 386–387
deductive process **91**
demand/control model 364, *365*
dementia 72
demographic transitions 74
demography 63–64
Denis-Lalonde, D. 315
dental public health consultant **41**
depression 124, 356–357
de Quintana Medina, J. 128
Descartes, René 3, 89
descriptive studies 77–79
design of epidemiological studies 77; analytical studies 80–82; case-control studies 82–83; case reports and case series 79; clinical trials 84; cohort studies 81–82; community trial 84; cross-sectional studies 79–80; descriptive studies 78–79; ecological studies 80; experimental studies 83–84; observational studies 77–84; *see also* epidemiology
desk-based HIAs 243
determinants of health: environmental determinants 204, 216, 227, 383, 389; social determinants 31, **48**, 65, 190, 197, 211, 220, 232, 301, 368, 394, 402
Di Clemente, C.C. 120–121
dietary fibre **330**, 335, 342–343, **346**, 347
dieters 338
diet-induced thermogenesis (DIT) 325
dieting 323, 335, 338
dieting health warning 335
digestion 324
digital: arts 281, 286–287; communication 145–146; media 142; nudging 127
direct causal association 76
director of public health **41**
direct transmission of infectious agent 67
disability/ies/disabling, disability rights campaigners 368, 372, 396
disease, outbreak: agent 67; environment 67; host 67
disease-centred care service 382
disease-centred medical model 13
disease prevention 280; health education *versus* **169**; primary 115, **169**, 280, 308; secondary 115, **169**, 280; tertiary 115, **169**, 80

disease triangle *250*, 253
documentary analysis 106
double blind trial 84
Dowdle, W.R. 257
drinking guidelines/weekly drinking
    guidelines 314
drug-resistant pathogens 261
drugs 67, 122, 258, 297–318, 373; set and
    setting model 300; *see also* substance use
dual registration 54
dynamic social system 5

eating: compulsive 334; emotional 333;
    healthy 127, 146, 215, 281, 287, 372, 396,
    403; mindful 169, 202, 322, 332; mindless
    332
eating to lose weight 335; continuous dieting/
    continuous energy restriction 336–339;
    dieting health warning 336; fasting
    340–341; healthy weight loss diet 342;
    mediterranean diet 335–336; nutrients,
    hunger and satiety 341–342
Eatwell Guide 335–336
E. coli 0157 259–260
ecological fallacy 80
education 176
educational model 181–183
education for health 179
effort/reward model 366, *366*
Ejlerskov, K.T. 126
Ekbladh, E. 367
elaboration likelihood model 150
emergency planning and response 29,
    262–264
emotional health 177
empathy 184
empirical process **91**
empirical research 90
employment 355
empowerment 183–186; community
    disempowerment *211*; community
    empowerment 186–188; enablement 183;
    facilitation 183; self-empowerment 183
enablement 18, 158, 168, 183, 194, 199, 392
endemic of disease 66
energy balance 324–327, *324*
energy imbalance 327–328; calorie density
    of nutrients 331; consuming calories
    331–334; emotional eating 333–334; energy
    expenditure 331; expending calories
    329–330; fat cells 328; food and activity
    330–331; genes 328; mindless and mindful
    eating 332–334; portion sizes 331
energy restriction 340
Engel, George 13–14, 114
Engelen, B. 127
environmental health officers (EHOs) **37**, 259
environmental re-evaluation 120

epidemic of disease 66, 254
epidemiological transition 74
epidemiology 63; cause and effect 75–77;
    defined 63–68; disease outbreaks,
    epidemics and pandemics 66–67;
    experimental studies 83–84; history
    68–72; measures of disease frequency
    and deaths 72–74; outcome 75; purpose
    67–68; screening 84–86; social 65; study
    designs 77–83; uses 68; *see also* design of
    epidemiological studies
Epp, Jake 198
Equality Act 2010 241, 368
ethnography 101
Eugenics 164
European Healthy Cities Network *214*
evaluation **91**
evidence-based practices 92
evidence-based public health 92
Ewert, B. 127
exosystem 6
experimental studies *83*
expressed need 207

Facebook group 105
face-to-face communication 145, 189
Faculty of Public Health 231–232; speciality
    training programme 50
fad diets 339
Falcaro, M. 270
Fall, E. 125
false information 143
fasting 340–341
fat, dietary 174, 323, 342
fatal injuries *266*
fat cells 328, 331
fear 124
felt need 207
female deaths, causes of **74**
Fishbein, M. 118
Five Ways to Wellbeing 181
Flesch reading ease score 135
flexitarian planetary health diet 335
focus groups 105
food: common diseases from 259–260; food
    portion sizes 287, 331–332; Food Standards
    Agency 25, 259; Food Standards Scotland
    259; poisoning 76, 252–253, 259–260; safety
    46, 259–262; standards 259, 335
food poisoning 258, **260**
food safety and micro-biological hazards
    259; antimicrobial resistance (AMR)
    261–262; campylobacter bacteria 259;
    common diseases from food 259–260;
    cross contamination 260–261; *E. coli* 0157
    260; salmonella bacteria 259; vulnerable
    hosts 261
Fox, N.J. 8

Freire, Paulo 188
Freud, Sigmund 114
functional mapping *43*
functions 44

gastrointestinal symptoms 66, 259
gastrointestinal tract *325*
General Board of Health 159–160,
    160, 226
General Data Protection Regulation
    (GDPR) 110
General Dental Council (GDC) 50
generalisability **91**
General Medical Council (GMC) 50
germ theory 227
Ghaffari, M. 117
*Global Strategy for Health for All by the Year
    2000* 197
Global Strategy to Reduce the Harmful Use
    of Alcohol 305
Goffman, Erving 8
good listener 182
good quality work 374
Good Work Index 359, 374
Google Scholar 94
Graunt, John 69, *71*
Gray, D.E. 98
grey literature 93
grounded theory 102
groups: buzz 142; problem-solving 142
group work 141–142
Guilford, K. 117

Halpern, D. 127
Hanlon, P. 228
Hanlon method 238
harm minimization/reduction 122, 299–300,
    304, 308, 315–316
Harvie, Michelle 342
hazardous chemical *363*, 363
hazard(s): biological 262; chemical 262;
    food safety, hazard analysis for 266–267;
    Hazard Analysis and Critical Control
    Point (HACCP) 266; microbiological 249;
    nuclear 249, 262–265, 271; physical 267;
    radiological 262
health 11; concept 21; defined 12, 17;
    disciplines, fields of study, sectors and
    agencies **25**; holistic 24–25; as human right
    19; negative definition 23, 65; person-
    centred 21–22; positive 23–24; positive
    definition 23–24; time 22
Health and Care Professions Council
    (HCPC) 50
Health and care system for England 389
Health and Safety Executive 265
health and self-help *178*
Health and Social Care Act, 2012 240, 388

health belief model (HBM) 113, 115–118, *117*,
    149; limitations 118
healthcare 387–389; public health 29, *230*;
    services 216
health champion **34**
health continuum 280
health education 157–158, 167–171, 184;
    behaviour change approach 173; coercion
    to vaccinate 164–165; disease prevention
    versus **169**; early health education 166–167;
    educational model 176–183; empowerment
    model 183–189; Health Education Council
    190, 227; health promotion 190–191,
    194; indoctrination and instruction for
    mothers 161–164; mass health education,
    1848 to 1930 158–167; medical approach
    171–173; preventive model 171–175; process
    of learning 170–171; propaganda for
    population 159–161; social change model
    189–191
health exposure 75
health for all 18, 184, 198, **200**, 201, 232, 385–
    386, **386**, 395–396; *see also* Global Strategy
    for Health for All by the Year 2000
Healthier Wales, A, 2021 388
health impact assessments (HIA) 205,
    243; appraisal 244; monitoring 244–245;
    reporting 244; scoping 244; screening 244;
    stages *243*
health improvement 29, *230*; practitioner **39**
health-improving activities 382
Health in All Policies 204–205
health indicators **233**, 234
health literacy 151–153; accessible
    information standard 153; defined 152;
    mental capacity 154
Health Literacy Toolkit 153
health needs assessment (HNA) 234–241;
    steps of 236–240
Health of the Nation, 1992 387
health promoting healthcare service 216
health promoting hospitals 391–392;
    leadership 392; outcomes 394; partnerships
    and resources 393; people 392–393; policy
    and strategy 392; processes 393
health promotion 190–191, 194–195;
    characteristics 201–202; clinical health
    promotion 384; community consultation
    209; competencies for working
    42–50; defined 201; educational *195*;
    empowerment *195*; ethical practices
    204; ethics 202–203; global conferences
    200; healthy public policy 203–205; for
    individuals, groups or communities
    217–220; models *195*, 195–197, **196**; Ottawa
    Charter for Health Promotion 197–200;
    partnership working 205–206; place-
    based approaches 215–216; planning

217–220; political ideologies **202**; politics 202, 203; preventive *195*; primary health promotion 374; and public health 220–222, **221–222**; reorienting healthcare services 216; secondary health promotion 375; social change *195*, 317–318; strengthening community action 206–209; supportive environments 213–215; tertiary health promotion 375

health protection 29, *230*, 249, 255, 267; chemical, biological, radiological and nuclear (CBRN) hazards 262–265; communicable diseases 249–255; food safety and micro-biological hazards 259–262; risk assessment in workplace 265–267; screening 267–271; vaccination 256–259

health protection practitioner **37**

health-related awareness 194

health-related behaviours 12, 113, 115, 152, 402–404

health-related campaign 145

health-related learning 142, 194, 309

health system 14, 30, 216, 290, 382–389

health visitor **38**

health warnings 309–310; alcohol 311–313; on cigarettes 310–311, *312*; on e-cigarettes 311; tobacco 310–311

healthy arts framework 280, **282**

healthy eating 146

healthy living centres 211

Healthy New Town 215–216

healthy people in healthy society and healthy planet *22*

healthy settings: health promoting hospitals and health services 213; health promoting prisons 213; health promoting schools 213; health promoting universities 213; healthy cities 213–215; healthy homes 213; healthy islands 213; healthy markets 213; healthy municipalities and communities 213; healthy villages 213; healthy workplaces 213; movement 213, 215; social work setting 20

healthy society 11; bio-psychosocial model 13–16; medical model 12–13; World Health Organization 17–21

healthy weight loss diet 342

healthy workplaces 374–378

hedonism **5**

#Hello my name is 393

helping relationships 120

hepatitis A 259

Herman, C.P. 338

heuristic processing 150

heuristic-systematic model 150–151

high control/high demand jobs 365

high control/low demand jobs 365

Hill, Austin Bradford 76

Hippocrates 68

HIV *see* human immunodeficiency virus

Hobbes, Thomas 89

hospice 141, 400

host(s)/vulnerable hosts 261

Howell, Tony 342

Huang, J. 119

human development, bioecological model of *6*

human immunodeficiency virus (HIV) 252, 257, 286

human papillomavirus (HPV) 270

human rights 15, 18–19, 177, 306, 315

Human Rights Act 1998 368

human values **5**

hunger 5, 196, 332–334, 337, 341–342

hypothesis 90

ice breakers 142

ideal self 7, *8*

Illich, Ivan 184

illness 383

immunisation *see* vaccination

immunity (active, passive, herd) 256–259

immunoglobulin 256

incidence 66, 73, 74, 78, 80–83, 252

incidence studies 81

inclusion and exclusion criteria 94

indirect causal association 76

indirect transmission of infectious agent 67; airborne 67; vector borne 67; vehicle borne 67

inductive process **91**

inequalities: in communities 212; in health/ health inequalities 28, 32, 42; in quality of work 359–361; in society 203, 301; unfair/ inequity 197, 386

inequalities in work-related deaths 358–361

infant mortality rates 72–74

infectious agent: direct transmission of 67; indirect transmission of 67

infectious diseases *see* communicable diseases

influenza virus 254

informed consent 109–110

inspectors of nuisances 226, 231

intermittent energy restriction 340–341

International Labour Organization (ILO) 373

International Network for Health Promoting Hospitals and Health Services 390

International Standards on Drug Use Prevention 306

International Union for Health Promotion and Education (IUHPE) 49, 53, 55; *see also* CompHP Competencies and Professional Standards

interpretivism **91**, 97–98, **98**

interviews 104–105
inward gaze 211

James, William 114
joint strategic needs assessment 54, 240–241
Jones, C.J. 118
Jungner, G. 268

Karunamuni, N. 15
Koch, Robert 227

Latner, Janet 341
Laverack, G. 315
leader: authoritarian 141; participative 141; permissive 141
learning 179; active 142, 170, **309**, 371, 402; affective 179, **180**; cognitive 179, **180**; conative 179; domain of 179, **180**; health-related 134, 142, 168, 179, 194, 203, 309; as holistic process 179, 201; participatory 142, **170**, 189; process, facilitation 184; psychomotor/behavioural 179
leavism 357
lecturer in public health **39**
Leventhal, Howard 123–125
life course approach 301, 308, 368
life expectancy 64, *64*, 69
Lind, James 72
linking 208
listeria monocytogenes 259
literature, searching and reviewing 92; how to assess 95; how to search 94–95; literature review 97; where to search 92–94
literature review: narrative 91, 95; systematic 92, 95
Local Government Act 1929 227
local resilience forums (LRFs) 263
low control/high demand jobs 365
low control/low demand jobs 365
lung diseases 357

Maastricht Treaty and *Amsterdam Treaties* 241
macrosystem 6
maintenance 122
Making Every Contact Count (MECC) 403
malaria 66, 251; transmission cycle *250*
Marmot, Michael 65, 210
Maslow, A. 9–10
Maslow's hierarchy of needs *10*, 18, 207
mass communication 142–147
mass media 142
mass screening 268–269, **269**
material body 9
Mattson, M.P. 340
meal replacements 339
measles, mumps and rubella (MMR) vaccine 257

measles or mumps 250, 252, 256
measles vaccination 253
media: broadcast 142; digital 142; mass media campaigns 313; outdoor 142; print 142
mediation 199
medical officers 163, 166–167, 172, 226–227, 231
medical oncology 342
mediterranean diet 323, 335, 339, 343
memories 4
mental health 32–33, 146, 177
mesosystem 6
metabolism 325
method of agreement 76
method of concomitant variation 76
method of difference 76
microbiome 343, *344*
microorganisms 343–344
microsystem 6
Middle Eastern Respiratory Syndrome (MERS) 66, 254–255
migrant workforce 369–370
Mill, John Stuart 76
Ministry of Health Act 1919 227
misleading information 143
Misuse of Drugs Act 1971 298
mixed methods research 98, 107
models and theories of behaviour change 115; common-sense model 123–126; health belief model 115–118; nudge theory 126–128; theory of planned behaviour 118–120; theory of reasoned action 118–120; theory to colorectal cancer screening 119–120; transtheoretical model 120–123
models of health and illness: medical 12, 13, 65, 172, 383, 387; social 13, 395; traditional 13
models of health promotion: educational 170–171, 176–183; empowerment **170–171**, 183–189; preventive 170–175; social change 127, 136, 146, 189–191
models of substance use: medical 299–301; moral 298–299; social 301–304
Modern Slavery Act 2015 302
morbidity 72
Morris, Jeremy 68
mortality 69, 72
motivational interviewing 140
MPOWER 305
Mullan, B. 125
multi-voting technique 237
muscle 151, 277, 285, 326–327, 329, 337
musculoskeletal disorders 356–357, 361
music 282–286; listening, effect of 283
mutual aid 316

Narcotics Anonymous (NA) 316
narrative literature review **91**

narrative research 102
National Health Service (NHS) 115, 145, 227, 382; creation 383, 385; health promoting healthcare practitioners 402–405; health system 382–389; healthy 389–394; modern health system, comparison with **386**; preventing disease and promoting health 394–402
National Healthy Cities Networks 215
National Institute for Health and Care Excellence 125
National Institute for Health Research (NIHR) Centre for Engagement and Dissemination 109
National Statistics Socio-economic Classification (NS-SEC) 358
Nazi Germany 23
needle exchange *300*, 304, 315
needs: comparative need 207; expressed need 207; felt need 207; normative need 207; prioritization 238
negative predictive value 86
neurons *4*
NHS Five Year Forward View, 2014 388
NHS Long Term Plan, 2019 388
NHS Scotland, 2003 388
nicotine 16, 94, 190, 300, 302, 305, 314
Nightingale, Florence 280
nominal group technique 237
non-dieters 338
non-fatal injuries 267
non-verbal communication 105, 139, **140**
normative need 207
norovirus 259
Northern Ireland Public Health Agency 229, 388
Novichok poisoning, 2018 263–264
nuclear hazards 262–265
nudge theory 113, 126–128
nudging 146
Nursing and Midwifery Council (NMC) 50
nutrients: carbohydrates 324, 330, 342; fats 324, 331, 342; protein 324–325, 331, 333, 337, 341, 342
NVivo 105

obesity epidemic 324
obesogenic environment 127, 323, 344–345, 347
objectives 44, 90, 100, 146, **180**, 209, 217–219, 236
objectivity **91**
observation 106
observational studies 77, *77*
observation of reality 106
occupational health nurse **38**
occupational health services 374–376
occupational medicine 374

occupational therapy 15
occupations: and inequalities in health 358; managerial 360–361, 371; professional 360–361, 371; routine 358, 360, 371–372
odds ratio (OR) 83
Office for Health Improvement and Disparities 55, 221, 229, 233
Omran, A.R. 74
one-to-one communication 139–141
one-way communication 136–137
online databases 92, **93**
online forums 106
oral health promoter **36**
organisational justice 366–367
Ottawa Charter for Health Promotion 197–201, *198*, 241
outbreak of disease 66
outward gaze 211
overweight in individuals 323; eating to lose weight 334–343; energy balance 324–327; energy imbalance 327–334; excess body fat and health 323–324; fasting 340–341; healthy weight loss diet 342; microbiome 343–344; obesogenic environment 344–345; self-monitoring 343; tackling 345–347

pandemics 254–255; communication 255; contact tracing 255; of disease 66; isolating cases and contacts 255; non-pharmaceutical/societal interventions 255; quarantine 255; testing 255
participant information sheet 110
partnership 205–206; interagency 205, 386; interdisciplinary/multi-disciplinary 205; interprofessional/multi-professional 205; multi-agency 24, 205, 254, 262, 308, 315; partnership-working 28, 46, 199, 205–206, 308; team 205
Pasteur, Louis 227
pathogenic/pathogenesis 168, 382, 398–399, 406
pathogens 67, 249, 256, 259, 261
patient education 181
peer review 93
perceived behavioural control 120
performing arts 275, 281
period prevalence 79
person: bioecological model 5–7; defined 3–5, 9; health 10–11; ideal self 7, *8*; metaphysical aspects 3; self 7–10; self-concept 7–8, *8*; self-esteem 7, *8*; self-image 7, *8*; social-ecological model 5–6
person-centred: approach to health 22; aspiration 18; biopsychosocial model 15; care 153, 388; communication 139; counselling 9, 184; education 184; health promoting health care services 213; human rights 19
phenomenology 102

PHSKF *see* UK Public Health Skills and Knowledge Framework (PHSKF)
physical activity 78, 115, 117, 122–123, 125, 144, 152, 281, 325–331, 339, 343, 396
physical activity level (PAL) 325–326
physical health 177
pilot study **91**
place-based approaches 215
plague 69
Plato 113
point prevalence 79
Policing and Crime Act 2009 302
policy: healthy public policy 199, 203–205, 220, 241; policymakers 13, 47, 127, 190, 195, 204, 234, 278, 299; policymaking 203, 219, 387
Policy and Justice Act 2006 241
politics 174, 202, 301, 306
Polivy, J. 338
poll 99
Poor Law 227
Popay, Jennie 211–213
population-based screening test 84
population pyramid *65*
positionality **91**, 103
positive predictive value 86
positivism **91**, 97–98, **98**
poverty 14, 20, 32, 127, 160, 190, 231, 240, 305, 360
power **5**, 11, 19, 22, 118, 133, 141, 157–158, 183, **202**, 209, 212, 301, 317, 363
pragmatism **98**
pre-contemplation 121, 149
pregnancy and lactation 327
preparation 122
presenteeism 357
prevalence 73
prevalence surveys 79–80
primary research 90
probability or random sample 108
processes 7
Prochaska, J.O. 120–121, 123
Professional Standards Authority 51
Promesas y Traiciones 286–287
prospective cohort study 81
prostate cancer 268–269
protein 3, 331, 337, 341, 346
PSA-based screening programme 269
Psychoactive Substances Act 2016 298
psychological factors 15, 384
psychology 113–114; behavioural 402; clinical 114; of continuous dieting 338–339; defined 113; developmental 5; educational 114; forensic 114; functionalist approach 113; health 114–115; humanistic 9; neuropsychology 114; occupational 114; social 4–5, 114–115, 263; sport and exercise 114; structuralist approach 113–114

psychomotor/behavioural learning 134, 179
psychosocial environment 363, 371, 373
psychosocial work environment and workers' health *364*
Public Bodies (Joint Working) Scotland Act 2014 240
public health 225; analyst **38**; annual reports 232; challenges 258–259; consultant **40**; defined 229–231; domains and functions *29*, 29 ; functions *29*, 30, *43*; health impact assessment 241–245; health needs assessment 234–241; history 225–229; intelligence 30; joint strategic needs assessments 240–241; medicine 232; national public health profiles 233; practice 231; practitioners 30–31; principal **40**; reports 231–232; specialists 30; waves of **228**; workforce *31*
Public Health Act, 1848 226
Public Health Act, 1875 227
public health competency frameworks 49; CompHP core competencies for health promotion *49*; *UKPHR* Practitioner Standards for Registration 51; UK Public Health Skills and Knowledge Framework (PHSKF) 42–45; WHO-ASPHER Competency Framework 45–49
Public Health Outcomes Framework 234
Public Health Scotland 79, 229
Public Health Wales 150
Public Health Wales, 2009 388
public health workforce (UK) 28–29; career routes 56, **57–58**; domains 29; functions 30; job roles 32–41, **34–41**; workforce categories 30–32; workforce development 30
Public Involvement (PI) 109

qualitative methodology 98, 101, 103–106; case study 102; documentary analysis 106; ethnography 101; focus groups 105; grounded theory 102; interviews 104–105; narrative research 102; observation 106; phenomenology 102
qualitative research **91**
quality of life 17; environment 17–18; level of independence 17; physical 17; psychological 17; social relations 17; spiritual beliefs 17
quality of literature 95
quality of work by socio-economic classification 360–361
quantitative methodology 98–101
quantitative research **91**
questionnaire 89, 99, **99**

radiological hazards 262
Ramadan 340

randomisation 84
rapid or intermediate HIAs 243
rates of disease or death 72
readability 135
receptive engagement 276
recovery worker **35**
recreational arts engagement 277
recruitment 109
reflexivity **91**
registered public health specialist 51
registration of health promotion and public
   health professionals 50; continuing
   professional development (CPD) 56;
   dual registration 54; health promotion
   practitioner registration 53–54; UK Public
   Health Register (UKPHR) 51–53
reinforcement management 120
relapse 122
relative risk (RR) 82
reliability 85, **91**, 107
replicate **91**
Reporting of Injuries, Diseases and
   Dangerous Occurrences Regulations
   (RIDDOR) 363
research **91**
research article/paper **91**
research-based practices 89–92
research design **91**
research ethics 109; General Data Protection
   Regulation (GDPR) 110; informed consent
   109–110
research methodology and methods
   98–106
research philosophies 97; interpretivism
   97–98; positivism 97
research questions/question types 94–96, 99,
   107, 110
research sampling: convenience 108; mixed
   methods 107; probability or random
   sample 108; qualitative methodology 101–
   106; quantitative 98–101; recruitment 109;
   sampling 107–109; snowball 108; strategic
   108; validity and reliability 107
research terms **91–92**
reservoir 67, **228**
resilience 168; workers 371
retrospective approach 83
retrospective cohort study 81
revalidation 56
risk assessment in workplace 265; hazard
   analysis for food safety 266–267;
   workplace injuries, recording 266
risk factors 75
risk ratio 82
Rogers, Carl 9–10, 140, 184
role models 301, 376, 405
role play 142, 219

Rosenstock, Irwin 115–116
rough sleepers 121–122, 141, 186
Rousseau, Jean-Jacques 176
Rychetnik, L. 92

salmonella bacteria 259
salutogenesis 280, 398–402
salutogenic umbrella *399*
sanitary: associations 161–162; conditions
   226, 231; inspectors 159, 161, 226
satiety 341
Schmidt, A.T. 127
Schools for Mothers 164
Schwartz, Marlene 341
scientific method 90
Scottish Health Education Group 190, 227
Scottish Public Health Observatory 233
screening 84–86, **85**, 267–268; breast
   screening 268, 270; cervical screening
   270; mass screening programmes (UK)
   268–269; prostate cancer 268–269; tests
   85, 268; types 268; UK National Screening
   Committee criteria 268–269
Scriven, A. 136
secondary research 90
security **5**
sedentary/sedentary behaviour 12, 80, 144,
   227, 323, 327, 329–334, 394
selective screening 268
self 7
self-actualization 10, 18
self-awareness 103, 134, 194
self-concept 7–8, *8*
self-direction **5**
self-discipline 5
self-efficacy 116–118, 149
self-empowered person 186
self-empowerment 187
self-esteem 7, *8*
self-help 141, 146, 189, 316
self-image 7, *8*
self-liberation 120
self-management 125
self-monitoring of blood glucose 125
self-re-evaluation 120
self-regulation 124
self-regulatory model 123–126
sense of coherence 400
sensitivity 85
settings *see* healthy settings
Severe Acute Respiratory Syndrome (SARS)
   66, 254–255
Simple Measure of Gobbledygook (SMOG)
   Index 135
singing 283
singing for breathing 284–285
single blind trial 84

Single Convention on Narcotic Drugs 1961
    306
skills: life 169, 171, 183, 185, 188, 206, 286;
    personal 151, 188, 199, 220
Slim Me 339
smallpox 225, 252, 254
SMART Recovery 316
smokers by occupation **372**
smoking: cessation advisor **34**; cessation
    services 315; *see also* tobacco
smoking behaviour 120
Sniehotta, F.F. 120
Snow, John 72, 226
snowball sampling 108
social body 8–9
social capital 208, 367
social cynicism 118
social epidemiology 65
social factors 15, 65, 240
social health 177
social identity 9
social liberation 120
social marketing 146–147
social prescriber **35**
Social Services and Well-being (Wales) Act
    2014 240
societal health 177
society 5
socio-economic status 355
Socrates 113
Solihull online resources 52
Spanish flu 254
Specialist Community Public Health Nurses
    385
specificity 85
specific rate 72
spiritual health 177
stable behaviour 120
standardised mortality ratio (SMR)
    73–74
standardised rates 72
Standard Occupational Classification (SOC)
    358
standards, health services 390–391
starvation and preservation 336–337
Statistical Package for the Social Sciences
    (SPSS) 101
Stead, M. 144
stimulation **5**
stimulus control 120
Stopes, Marie 164, 166
Stoptober 2021 *313*
strategic sample 108
stress 356–357
Stronger Collaboration, Better Health 19
structuralism 113
subjective norms 120

subjectivity **91**
substance-related education 314–315
substance use 297; alcohol control 305–306;
    data collection and monitoring 308–309;
    drug control 306–307; early intervention
    308; harm minimisation 122, 300, 304, 308;
    harm reduction 315–316; health promotion
    interventions 309–318; international
    guidance 304–307; law enforcement,
    treatment and prevention 308; life course
    approach 308; mass media campaigns
    313; medical model 299–301; models of
    297–304; moral model 298–299; mutual
    aid 316–317; opportunistic interventions
    313–314; partnerships, multi-sectoral and
    multi-agency approaches 308; protection
    from commercial interests 308; reducing
    harmful outcomes 308; social change
    317–318; social model 301–304; Substance-
    related education 14–315; tobacco control
    305; UK principles for tackling tobacco,
    alcohol and drugs 307–309; universal and
    targeted approaches 306–308
surveillance, communicable disease 252
Sutton, G. 72
swine flu 254
synergistic interconnections 6
systematic processing 150
systematic review **92**, 94

teenage pregnancies *79*
thematic analysis 105
theoretical research 90, **92**
theory of planned behaviour (TPB) 113,
    118–120, 149
theory of psychoanalysis 114
theory of reasoned action (TRA) 113,
    118–120
Thorndike, A.N. 127
time/chronosystem 7
time variables 79
timing of meals 339
tobacco 76; control **47**, 302, 305; industry
    190, 305, 310; tackling tobacco 297–318;
    tobacco/cigarette health warnings 311–313,
    312, *312*; *see also* smoking
Tobacco and Related Products Regulations
    2016 302, 311
Tones, Keith 191
Tong, K.K. 118
total diet replacements 339
total energy expenditure (TEE) 325–326
training 176
transmission cycle of malaria *251*
transmission of infectious agent 67
transtheoretical model 113, 120–123, *121*,
    149–150

triangulation 107
trigger video 142
tuberculosis 74, 225, 252
two-way communication 136–137
type 2 diabetes 76
typhoid 225

UK Civil Contingencies Act 2004 262
UK General Data Protection Regulation
    (UK-GDPR) 110
UK Health Security Agency (UKHSA) 228,
    264
UK Mental Capacity Act, 2005 154
UK National Screening Committee
    (UKNSC) 85, 267; criteria 268–269
UK Public Health Register (UKPHR) 49
UK Public Health Skills and Knowledge
    Framework (PHSKF) 33, 42–43, 48
unemployment 355
universalism **5**

vaccination 256; Anti-Compulsory
    Vaccination League 165; anti-vaccine
    propaganda 165; coercion to vaccinate
    159, 164–165; herd immunity 257–258;
    how vaccination works 257; immunity
    256,*257*; public health challenges 258–259;
    Vaccination Act 1840 164–165
validity 85, **92**, 107
variables **92**
variant Creutzfeldt-Jakob disease (vCJD) 232
vector borne transmission of infectious agent
    67
vehicle borne transmission of infectious
    agent 67
Velema, E. 146
verbal communication 137–138, **140**
victim blaming 175
violence 54, 213, 356, 364
Vision for Health and Social Care, 2020 388
visual arts: design and craft 281; in mental
    health hospital setting 288–290
vomiting bug 259
vulnerable workers 368

Waddell, G. 355
Weal, R. 121
Weare, Katherine 176
wellbeing 17, 181
wellness 177
White, M. 122
wider public health workforce 30–32

Wilkinson, Kitty 161, 166, 181
Wilson, J.M.G. 268
Winslow, Charles-Edward A. 229
work: causes of injuries, illness and death
    362; good quality work 374, 378
work environments and health 361–368
workers: health 355–356, 364, 371, 378;
    health-related behaviours 371–373,
    402–404; stress 20, 364
workforce categories 30; public health
    practitioners 30–31; public health
    specialists 30; wider public health
    workforce 31–32
Working Time Regulations 1998 364
workload 20, 359, 361, 364–365
workplace injuries 357–358
workplaces, promoting health in 355;
    anxiety 356–357; depression 356–357;
    healthy workplace model 376–378, *377*;
    healthy workplaces 374–378; individuals
    in workplace 368–373; inequalities in
    work-related deaths 358–361; occupations
    and inequalities in health 358; physical
    environment 361–363; psychosocial
    environment 363–364; stress 356–357;
    work environments and health 361–368;
    workplace injuries 357–358; work-related
    poor health 355–361
Work Ready 374–375
work-related asthma 357
work-related deaths 356, 358
work-related poor health 355–361
work-related respiratory diseases 357
World Health Organization 11, 17–18, 313;
    constitution of 19; health as human right
    18; Health for all 18; healthy settings 20–
    21; healthy workplace model 376; Strategic
    Communications Framework 147–148
World Health Organization European
    Healthy Cities Network 214
World Health Organization Framework
    Convention on Tobacco Control 305
Worshipful Company of Parish Clerks 69
Wundht, Wilhelm 113

Yaghoubi, M. 391
yo-yo dieting 337

Zhang, Y. 372
Zika 252
Zola, Irving 394
Zola's river *395*, 396, 398

Printed in the United States
by Baker & Taylor Publisher Services